DATE DUE

JUL 10 1990		Due 6·12·93
		JUN 1 4 1994
JUL 24 1991		
		OCT 20 1994
SEP 23 1991		
		NOV 0 1 1995
NOV 17 1991		
DEC 06 1991		
JUN 0 4 1992		FEB 2 4 1997
		Due 5-30-97
SEP 0 4 1992		SEP 1 6 1998
DEC 06 1993		
NOV 29 1994		
		JUN 0 9 2002

DEMCO 38-297

INTERVENTIONAL ULTRASOUND

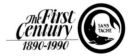

INTERVENTIONAL ULTRASOUND

Edited by

JOHN P. McGAHAN, MD

Professor
Division of Diagnostic Radiology
University of California
Davis Medical Center
Sacramento, California

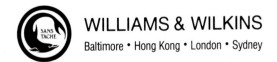

WILLIAMS & WILKINS
Baltimore • Hong Kong • London • Sydney

Editor: Timothy H. Grayson
Associate Editor: Carol Eckhart
Project Editor: Barbara Werner
Designer: JoAnne Janowick
Illustration Planner: Wayne Hubbel
Production Coordinator: Charles E. Zeller

Copyright © 1990
Williams & Wilkins
428 East Preston Street
Baltimore, Maryland 21202, USA

Accurate indications, adverse reactions, and dosage schedules for drugs are provided in this book, but it is possible that they may change. The reader is urged to review the package information data of the manufacturers of the medications mentioned.

Printed in the United States of America

Library of Congress Cataloging in Publication Data

Interventional ultrasound / edited by John P. McGahan.
p.   cm.
    Includes index.
    ISBN 0-683-05762-6
    1. Diagnosis, Ultrasonic. 2. Operative ultrasonography.
I. McGahan, John P.
    [DNLM: 1. Ultrasonic Diagnosis—methods.   WB 289 I617]
RC78.7.U4I586   1990
616.07′543--dc20
DNLM/DLC
for Library of Congress

89-14752
CIP

89 90 91 92 93
1   2   3   4   5   6   7   8   9 10

To Dad, Mom, Vicki, Johnny, Michele, Patrick, and Mollie

Preface

Ultrasound is widely recognized as one of the premier noninvasive imaging modalities used in modern medicine. Using this noninvasive imaging modality to guide interventional procedures may seem to be a contradiction. However, increased familiarity with sonography, combined with technical advances in ultrasound instrumentation, has led to increased use of ultrasound in guiding invasive procedures. "Interventional ultrasound" is used in many fields of medicine. For instance, ultrasound may be used by the radiologist to guide abdominal biopsy or drainage, by the surgeon to guide operative procedures, or by the obstetrician to direct needle placement into the uterus. This text is devoted to all practitioners using ultrasound in the guidance of invasive procedures.

The emphasis in this comprehensive text is methodology with a review of the techniques and materials needed to perform ultrasound guided invasive procedures. This text will provide a handy reference for anyone performing interventional ultrasound.

The first three chapters provide the foundation for interventional ultrasound: patient preparation, basic techniques, and the role of the sonographer and the cytopathologist in the success of aspiration/biopsy procedures.

After the foundation for any structure is complete, building can begin. Rather than starting from the bottom and building upwards, this text starts from the top and proceeds downward. The chapters are arranged in a cephalad to caudal direction of the body. Chapters 4 through 9 deal with interventional ultrasound applications in the brain, neck, thorax, and heart. Chapters 10 through 15 are presented by authors with proven experience and expertise in performing invasive procedures within the abdomen. Chapters 16 through 18 deal with newer applications of interventional ultrasound. These exciting chapters describe the use of endoluminal transducers to guide transrectal and transvaginal biopsy and deal with the interventional techniques in obstetrics. To complete this text from "head to toe," the final chapter presents the applications of interventional ultrasound in the extremities.

This text is designed as a reference for practitioners involved in applications of interventional ultrasound. Recent innovations and applications are well delineated by those who have had years of experience in performing interventional ultrasound. We hope that the readers will reap the benefits of the refinements presented here, and that the ultimate benefactors will be our patients.

Acknowledgments

My deepest appreciation is given to all the contributors who were so diligent in preparing timely, high quality chapters. Without their individual dedication to excellence, this text would not have been possible.

Thank you to the staff of Williams & Wilkins, especially Timothy Grayson, Carol Eckhart, and Charles E. Zeller for their guidance and editorial assistance in preparation of this book. I also thank all those with whom I perform interventional procedures in the Division of Diagnostic Radiology. These include present and former fellows, radiologists, obstetricians, urologists, surgeons, and neurosurgeons. I would also like to thank the members of our "team" of sonographers, both past and present, including: Sandy Maleski, Joen Traeger, Mike Cronan, Sylvia Crane, Elizabeth Taylor, and Mark Johnson.

Finally, I give my heartfelt thanks to the project codirector, my secretary, Karen Anderson. Karen diligently reminded me of deadlines and kept me on track with all the details. Without her assistance this text would still be "in preparation."

Contributors

Sergio Ajzen, M.D.
Assistant Professor, Escola Paulistia de Medicina, Sao Paulo, Brazil

James E. Boggan, M.D.
Associate Professor, Department of Neurological Surgery, University of California Davis Medical Center, Sacramento, California

William Bommer, M.D.
Associate Professor, Division of Cardiovascular Medicine, University of California Davis Medical Center, Sacramento, California

William E. Brant, M.D.
Assistant Professor, Division of Diagnostic Radiology, University of California Davis Medical Center, Sacramento, California

Robert L. Bree, M.D.
Chief, Radiology Service, VA Medical Center; Assistant Professor in Radiology, University of Michigan Medical School, Ann Arbor, Michigan

Patrice M. Bret, M.D.
Diagnostic Radiologist-in-Chief, Associate Professor of Radiology, Department of Diagnostic Radiology, Montreal General Hospital, McGill University, Montreal, Quebec, Canada

J. William Charboneau, M.D.
Associate Professor of Radiology, Department of Diagnostic Radiology, Mayo Clinic, Rochester, Minnesota

Ross Christensen, M.D.
Bay Radiology Medical Group, Chula Vista, California

Peter Cooperberg, M.D.
Professor of Radiology, Chief Department of Radiology, St. Paul's Hospital, Vancouver, BC Canada

Andou Coret, M.D.
Department of Radiology, Chiam Sheba Hospital, Tel Hashomer, Israel

Arthur C. Fleischer, M.D.
Professor of Radiology and Radiological Sciences, Chief, Ultrasound, Associate Professor Obstetrics and Gynecology, Vanderbilt University Medical Center, Nashville, Tennessee

Bruno D. Fornage, M.D.
Associate Professor, Chief, Section of Ultrasound, Department of Diagnostic Radiology, M.D. Anderson Cancer Center, Houston, Texas

Carl M. Herbert, M.D.
Assistant Professor Obstetrics and Gynecology, Center for Fertility and Reproductive Research, Vanderbilt University Medical Center, Nashville, Tennessee

Hans Jantsch, M.D.
Assistant Professor of Radiology, First Surgical Clinic, Department of Radiology, University of Vienna, Vienna, Austria

Philippe Jeanty, M.D., Ph.D.
Assistant Professor of Radiology and Radiological Sciences, Department of Radiology, Vanderbilt University Medical Center, Nashville, Tennessee

R. Brooke Jeffrey, Jr., M.D.
Professor of Radiology, Chief of Abdominal Imaging, Department of Diagnostic Radiology & Nuclear Medicine, Stanford University Medical Center, Stanford, California

Clifford S. Levi, M.D.
Associate Professor, University of Manitoba, Department of Radiology, Health Sciences Center, Winnipeg, Manitoba, Canada

Daniel J. Lindsay, M.D.
Assistant Professor, University of Manitoba, Department of Radiology Health Sciences Center, Winnipeg, Manitoba, Canada

Edward A. Lyons, M.D.
Professor, Department of Radiology, Health Sciences Center, University of Manitoba, Winnipeg, Manitoba, Canada

Junji Machi, M.D., Ph.D.
Research Assistant Professor, Department of Surgery, The Medical College of Pennsylvania, Philadelphia, Pennsylvania

Sandra E. Maleski, BS, RT, RDMS
Division of Diagnostic Radiology, Section of Ultrasound, University of California Davis Medical Center, Sacramento, California

John P. McGahan, M.D.
Professor and Chief of Abdominal Imaging and Ultrasound, Division of Diagnostic Radiology, University of California Davis Medical Center, Sacramento, California

Marilyn Morton, DO
Assistant Professor in Radiology, Department of Diagnostic Radiology, Mayo Clinic, Rochester, Minnesota

Berta M. Montalvo, M.D.
Associate Professor of Radiology, Chief, Body Ultrasonography Section, Division of Diagnostic Radiology, University of Miami School of Medicine, Miami, Florida

Robert M. Quencer, M.D.
Professor of Radiology, Neurological Surgery and Ophthanology, Department of Radiology, University of Miami School of Medicine, Miami, Florida

Carl C. Reading, M.D.
Assistant Professor, Department of Diagnostic Radiology, Mayo Clinic, Rochester, Minnesota

David Russell, RDMS
Pediatric Cardiology, University of Maryland Medical System, University of Maryland Hospital, Baltimore, M.D.

Bernard Sigel, M.D.
Professor and Chairman, Department of Surgery, Medical College of Pennsylvania, Philadelphia, Pennsylvania

Albert Siu, M.D.
Pathologist, Yolo Diagnostic Medical Group, Davis, California

Raymond L. Teplitz, M.D.
Professor, Department of Pathology, University of California Davis Medical Center, Sacramento, California

Eric vanSonnenberg, M.D.
Professor of Radiology and Medicine, Department of Diagnostic Radiology and Nuclear Medicine, University of California San Diego, San Diego, California

Gerhard R. Wittich, M.D.
Associate Professor of Radiology, Department of Diagnostic Radiology and Nuclear Medicine, Stanford University School of Medicine, Stanford, California

Witold M. Zaleski, M.D., FRCPC
Department of Radiology, Ottawa General Hospital, University of Ottawa, Ottawa, Ontario, Canada

Contents

Preface... vii

Contributors... xi

Chapter 1. **Principles, Instrumentation, and Guidance Systems** 1
John P. McGahan, MD
William E. Brant, MD

Chapter 2. **Fine Needle Aspiration/Cytology for Invasive Ultrasound Techniques** 21
Albert Siu, MD
Raymond L. Teplitz, MD

Chapter 3. **The Sonographer's Role in Invasive Procedures**... 35
Sandra E. Maleski, BS, RT, RDMS
John P. McGahan, MD

Chapter 4. **Intraoperative Cranial and Spinal Sonography** 43
John P. McGahan, MD
Berta M. Montalvo, MD
Robert M. Quencer, MD
James E. Boggan, MD

Chapter 5. **Neck and Parathyroid** 59
Marilyn J. Morton, DO
J. William Charboneau, MD
Carl C. Reading, MD

Chapter 6. **Interventional Ultrasound of the Breast** 71
Bruno D. Fornage, MD

Chapter 7. **Interventional Procedures in the Thorax**.......... 85
William E. Brant, MD

Chapter 8. **Interventional Echocardiography** 101
David S. Russell, MD
William Bommer, MD

Chapter 9. **Intraoperative Abdomen** 115
Junji Machi, MD, Ph.D.
Bernard Sigel, MD

Chapter 10. **Abdominal Abscesses: The Role of CT and Sonography** 129
R. Brooke Jeffrey, Jr., MD

Chapter 11. **Hepatobiliary Techniques** 145
Peter Cooperberg, MD
Andou Coret, MD
Sergio Ajzen, MD

Chapter 12. **Gallbladder** 159
John P. McGahan, MD

Chapter 13. **Pancreas** 171
Patrice M. Bret, MD

Chapter 14. **Percutaneous Gastrostomy** 193
Gerhard R. Wittich, MD
Eric vanSonnenberg, MD
Hans Janstch, MD

Chapter 15. **Urinary Tract** 199
Daniel J. Lindsay, MD
Edward A. Lyons, MD
Clifford S. Levi, MD

Chapter 16. **Guided Aspiration Biopsy with Transvaginal Sonography** 211
Arthur C. Fleischer, MD
Carl M. Herbert, MD
Robert L. Bree, MD

Chapter 17. **Prostate and Other Transrectally Guided Biopsies** 221
Robert L. Bree, MD

Chapter 18. **Obstetrics** 239
Witold M. Zaleski, MD
Philippe Jeanty, MD, PhD

Chapter 19. **Ultrasound-guided Intervention in the Extremities** 267
Ross A. Christensen, MD
Eric vanSonnenberg, MD

Index 275

1 Principles, Instrumentation, and Guidance Systems

JOHN P. McGAHAN
WILLIAM E. BRANT

Introduction

Fine-needle-aspiration biopsy has gained wide acceptance in clinical practice because of its simplicity, safety, and accuracy. While needle puncture and aspiration was first described in 1930, only more recently has the use of this technique increased with the development of newer guidance methods and refinements of aspiration and cytological techniques (1–4). Modalities such as ultrasound and computed tomography (CT) allow for precise needle placement in deep-seated lesions. In late 1972, both Holm (5) and Goldberg (6) independently devised transducers with a central hole through which a needle could be placed for aspiration or biopsy. The target lesion was visualized by a manual compound scanner and the transducer was angulated in the image plane indicating the direction of needle passage. The needle was inserted and the needle tip was displayed as a simultaneous A-mode moving deflection. Subsequent to these early reports the use of ultrasound guided aspiration and biopsy techniques has markedly increased (7, 8).

Recent advances in ultrasound instrumentation, including the use of high-resolution real-time equipment, have dramatically increased the applications of interventional ultrasound. Advanced electronics has led to the development of compact portable units that may be used to perform invasive ultrasound procedures throughout the hospital, including the intensive care unit and the operating room (9, 10). Newer biopsy attachments have allowed use of real-time monitoring of percutaneous needle placement in a number of anatomical locations. Specialized probes with biopsy attachments have been designed for applications such as transvaginal aspiration biopsy (11) and transrectal or transperineal biopsy of the prostate (12, 13). Simultaneously, new needles and catheters that are specifically designed for easy detection with ultrasound have been developed (8, 14).

ULTRASOUND ADVANTAGES AND DISADVANTAGES

One of the most important considerations when selecting the technique for guidance of aspiration, biopsy, or drainage procedures is the accuracy and safety provided by the guidance system. The inherent accuracy and safety of the procedure outweigh most other considerations such as expediency or cost of the imaging technology. Recent technological advances have included development of ultrasound guidance systems that allow for direct and precise sonographic visualization of a needle as it is passed into a target lesion (15–17). Direct needle visualization leads to precise needle placement in critical areas with avoidance of intervening structures and has increased the sonographic applications in interventional procedures. Some of the advantages and

1

disadvantages of use of ultrasound for guidance of invasive procedures are listed in Table 1.1.

Table 1.1.
ADVANTAGES AND DISADVANTAGES OF
ULTRASOUND GUIDANCE OF INVASIVE
PROCEDURES

Ultrasound advantages	Ultrasound disadvantages
• Accurate • Expeditious • Needle visualization • Real-time control • Portable • Inexpensive	• Limited by bone, air and bowel gas

An advantage of ultrasound is that procedures performed with sonographic guidance may be performed relatively expeditiously. A complete ultrasound guided aspiration or biopsy is often not much longer than a routine ultrasound examination. This is especially true for aspiration procedures in which ultrasound rapidly localizes fluid and guides needle aspiration. Biopsy or drainage procedures often take longer due to inherent technical complexity of the procedure, but are still facilitated by the ease of ultrasound guidance.

Recently, refinements in ultrasound instrumentation have allowed ultrasound scanners to become more compact and easily transportable throughout the hospital, and to intensive care units and the operating room (8–10). Neither CT, magnetic resonance imaging (MRI), or fluoroscopy are as yet portable and thus require patient transportation when they are used for guidance of invasive procedures. Nearly one-third of over 100 aspiration or drainage procedures performed under ultrasound guidance in our institution were performed at the patient's bedside (10). While it is inconvenient for the radiologist to leave the main radiology department of the hospital, the risk and inconvenience of transporting a critically ill patient to the radiology department must be considered. As more individuals become fa-

miliar with ultrasound, and units become more compact, it is likely that bedside ultrasound guidance of invasive procedures will increase.

Finally, ultrasound systems are relatively inexpensive as compared with other radiological equipment. In a busy radiology department, one ultrasound scanner may be dedicated to primary use in performance of aspiration, biopsy, or drainage procedures while other ultrasound scanners are used for diagnostic examinations.

The major disadvantage of ultrasound is the inability to view structures obscured by bone, air, or bowel gas. Consequently, the use of ultrasound to direct procedures may be limited in the chest, cranium, gaseous abdomen, or pelvis. For example, chest biopsies cannot be performed with ultrasound control unless the mass touches the peripheral pleura. In the midabdomen, a loop of bowel may obscure visualization with ultrasound. Therefore CT may be better for guidance of drainage procedures performed in these areas. Specific advantages and limitations of ultrasound in performance of difficult aspiration, biopsy, or drainage procedures will be discussed in subsequent chapters.

PATIENT PREPARATION

Proper patient consent must be obtained before aspiration, biopsy, or drainage. The procedure is explained in detail, including its risks, benefits, and alternatives. The fact that the patient understands the procedure is documented in the medical record. The patient should be asked about easy bruising, abnormal bleeding during tooth extraction or surgery, and any medication that may prolong bleeding time (18). Coagulation studies and a hematocrit are obtained when indicated, based on patient history and on the site and nature of the invasive procedure. For instance, the risk of hemorrhage from a diagnostic paracentesis is much less than the risk of hemorrhage from a large-bore catheter drainage. Each case must be individualized but, in general, prothrombin time (PT) should not be greater than 3 seconds of the control, the partial thromboplastin time (PTT) should be less than 45 seconds, and the platelets should be greater than 75,000/cc. Also, medications with antiplatelet activity should be checked closely as they may prevent normal platelet aggregation and prolong bleeding with a normal platelet count. Bleeding time is probably the single best test to check for any prolonged bleeding and if abnormal, a hematology consult should be obtained. Corrective measures for increased PT are to stop Coumadin, administer vitamin K, or fresh frozen plasma. Platelet transfusions may be used for a low platelet count (19).

Simple aspiration procedures such as thoracentesis and paracentesis usually require no preliminary patient preparation and only local anesthesia at the puncture site is needed. Although not mandatory, we ask patients to fast for 4 to 6 hours before abdominal biopsy. The use of analgesics and premedication for biopsy procedures is determined individually, depending upon the difficulty of the procedure and the wishes of the patient. Patients are often apprehensive and uncomfortable, and may experience some pain during the procedure. Intravenous catheters are placed prior to the procedure in patients who are elderly, have multiple medical problems, or in whom a difficult procedure is anticipated. An intravenous catheter for administration of intravenous analgesia is recommended for percutaneous drainage procedures. These are surgical procedures that may be associated with significant pain and discomfort.

Anesthesia

Choice of medication for patient comfort, relief of anxiety, and control of pain depends upon the procedure, the patient, and the attending physician. We find often that no medication is needed for those hospitalized patients undergoing a simple paracentesis or thoracentesis when the interventionalist has explained the procedure to the patient in detail. A simple aspiration with a 22-gauge needle performed under ultrasound control usually requires a single puncture and may cause no more pain or apprehension than an intramuscular injec-

tion or the starting of an intravenous line. Alternatively, in some patients undergoing a lengthy or complicated procedure, general anesthesia may be required. For instance, in performing a complicated drainage procedure on a child, we almost always have an anesthesiologist administer general anesthesia. Therefore, anesthesia for aspiration, biopsy, or drainage procedures must be individualized.

Medications to relieve anxiety or control pain may be given orally, intramuscularly, or intravenously. We strongly feel that the interventionalist should only administer medication with which he or she is thoroughly familiar. Closely reading package inserts for dosages and potential side effects is mandatory, and consultation with other health care professionals should be obtained before administering any unfamiliar medications.

Narcotics

Narcotics may be given as premedication by the intramuscular route or gradually titrated prior to the procedure using the intravenous route. Narcotics produce analgesia and sedation. The main side effect of narcotics is dose-dependent respiratory depression. For this reason, resuscitation equipment and naloxone (Narcan) must be immediately available.

Meperidine (Demerol) may be given via the intramuscular route in a dosage from 50 to 100 mg 1 hour before the procedure for an average size patient. The dosage for intramuscular premedication with morphine sulphate is 5 to 10 mg. Slightly larger doses may be given in some patients, and the dosage should be reduced for the elderly. Fentanyl is approximately 50 to 100 times more potent than morphine sulphate, with approximately 100 µg of fentanyl equivalent to 10 mg of morphine sulphate. In general, an intramuscular injection is safer than an intravenous injection, as it avoids the sudden rise in blood and brain levels of the medication. The intravenous dosage of fentanyl, morphine sulphate, or meperidine should be titrated slowly, based on the patient's initial response to the drug. For instance, 10 to

20 µg of fentanyl, 1 to 2 mg of morphine sulphate, or 10 to 20 mg of meperidine may be chosen as the initial dosage for intravenous injection.

The patient must always be closely monitored for respiratory depression. It is also important that the patient be monitored after completion of the procedure. Pain is a respiratory stimulus and the removal of the painful stimuli with termination of the procedure can potentiate respiratory depression. Respiratory depression secondary to narcotic administration is reversed with naloxone given as an initial dose of 0.4 to 2.0 mg and repeated in 2 to 3 minutes if adequate response is not obtained (20).

Tranquilizers

Procedure anxiety may be a principal reason for patient discomfort during an invasive procedure. This fear may be reduced by use of benzodiazepine tranquilizers. Diazepam (Valium) is a well-known member of this group that not only helps alleviate patient fear, but also may cause patient amnesia for the invasive procedure. Recently, a short-acting, more potent benzodiazepine derivative, midazolam HCI (Versed) has been produced. However, the package insert for Versed carries this strict warning:

Versed must never be used without individualization of dosage. Prior to intravenous administration of Versed in any dose, the immediate availability of oxygen, resuscitative equipment and skilled personnel for the maintenance of a patent airway and support of ventilation should be ensured. Patients should be continuously monitored for early signs of underventilation or apnea, which can lead to hypoxia/cardiac arrest unless effective countermeasures are taken immediately (21).

These medications may be given intramuscularly or intravenously and diazepam may be administered orally. Oral and intramuscular administration of diazepam rarely produces respiratory depression, although intramuscular injection of diazepam may be more painful than the invasive procedure itself. Therefore, intramuscular injection of diazepam is rarely used. The oral dosage of diazepam is 5 to 10 mg. Intravenous administration of these drugs should be closely monitored for respiratory depression, especially in the elderly. Careful use of diazepam will include gradual titration with patient response closely monitored. Intravenous dosage of diazepam may begin with as little as 1 mg in the elderly or 2 mg in the otherwise healthy adult. We have observed respiratory arrest in patients given as little as 2 mg of intravenous diazepam and yet we have seen other patients tolerate as much as 40 mg of diazepam administered intravenously. Clinical experience with midazolam has shown it to be from 3 to 10 times as potent per milligram as diazepam. Because of the serious and life-threatening cardiac and respiratory effects reported with midazolam, detection and correction of these reactions must be made for every patient, regardless of age or health status.

We have commonly used combinations of tranquilizers and narcotics for intravenous injection, but these combinations may produce profound respiratory arrest or circulatory collapse. If respiratory arrest occurs, the first response is to administer naloxone for any narcotics that have been administered. If this is not successful, physostigmine (Antilirium) is an effective, reversible anticholinesterase, and may be administered slowly intravenously. Unlike the narcotic reversant agent, naloxone, physostigmine has several side effects, including nausea, vomiting, and bradycardia. In any patients undergoing cardiorespiratory depression, general supportive measures, including patent airway, supportive ventilation, intravenous infusion of fluid therapy, patient repositioning, and judicious use of vasopressors appropriate to the clinical situation should be used.

A number of other medications or anesthetics may be used. Special circumstances include anesthesia in the pediatric age group and outpatient inhalation with nitrous oxide. Regional anesthesia, spinal epidural anesthesia, and general anesthesia may be needed in certain circumstances by interventionalists. Also, there are innumerable analgesic agents that are currently on the market with separate advantages and limitations. Before use of any of these medications, consultation with health care professionals familiar with these medications and reading appropriate literature for dosage and adverse effects is always necessary. The interventionalist needs to have a thorough knowledge of the drugs he or she chooses and must be prepared to manage their potential adverse effects.

GUIDANCE SYSTEMS

Ultrasound guided interventional procedures can be performed by a number of methods. These include indirect ultrasound guidance, freehand real-time needle placement, or use of sonographic needle guidance systems.

Indirect Ultrasound Guidance

During indirect ultrasound guidance, the ultrasound probe is used to select the site of the patient's skin for puncture. The ultrasound probe is removed and the site is marked with pressure from the hub of the needle (Fig. 1.1). The angle and the depth of the puncture are preselected from the ultrasound image. The biopsy site is prepped and draped. It is important that there be little delay so that the patient does not move from the time of removing the ultrasound probe to the time of needle insertion. To minimize the time interval, the ultrasound probe may be fitted with a sterile glove and Betadine or sterile gel used as an acoustic coupling agent. The ultrasound transducer may then be placed within the sterile field and removed immediately before needle insertion.

The patient must also suspend respiration in the exact position the ultrasound image was obtained. Attaining this exact position may be difficult but is necessary, especially when dealing with lesions close to the diaphragm where large movements may occur with respiratory excursions. The area is anesthetized with lidocaine and the aspiration or biopsy is performed. After aspiration/biopsy, the area is rescanned approximately 5 minutes after needle insertion to ascertain adequacy of drainage and check for any complications such as fluid leakage or hemorrhage (Fig. 1.2).

This indirect method of ultrasound guidance is the most common method used for performance of thoracentesis and paracentesis within our department. This method is useful for aspiration or drainage of large fluid collections or biopsy of large lesions. For instance, when performing diagnostic thoracentesis or paracentesis we have found that in most patients an adequate sample may be obtained using only a 22-gauge injection needle attached directly to a 12-cc syringe. Retraction of the syringe plunger is performed as the needle is introduced to supply negative suction at the needle tip and provide a sample immediately upon entry into the thoracic or abdominal fluid collection. If this method fails, either a larger diameter or longer needle is used. We have had a high retrieval rate with a low incidence of complication using this method for diagnostic paracentesis or thoracentesis (10). When per-

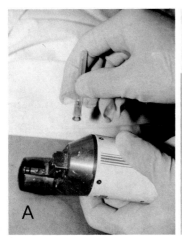 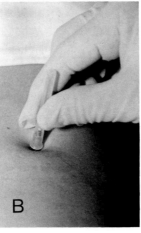

Figure 1.1. Indirect Ultrasound Guidance. **A**, The site of the patient's skin for puncture, the direction of the needle course, and the depth of needle placement are selected by real-time ultrasound examination. **B**, The ultrasound probe is removed and the site for puncture is marked by pressure using the needle hub. The site is then prepped and draped for needle insertion.

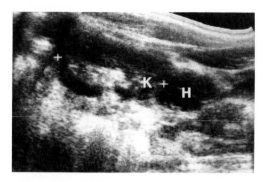

Figure 1.2. Post-biopsy Scan. Scan of the area of interest is always obtained after aspiration or biopsy. Here a delayed scan of the left kidney (*K*) demonstrates a hematoma (*H*) caudal to the inferior probe of the kidney. (Reproduced with permission from McGahan JP, Hanson FW: Ultrasonographic aspiration and biopsy techniques. In Dublin AB (ed): *Outpatient Invasive Radiologic Procedures: Diagnostic and Therapeutic.* Philadelphia, W. B. Saunders, 1989, p 99.)

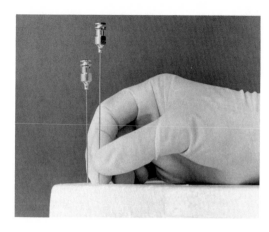

Figure 1.3. Tandem Needle Technique. A second needle is passed parallel with the first needle, which has already been placed into a suspected lesion.

forming biopsy of larger lesions using indirect ultrasound guidance, the tandem needle technique, fan needle technique or coaxial needle technique is occasionally used (Figs. 1.3, 1.4, and 1.5, 22, 23).

Freehand Puncture

Freehand puncture allows for direct visualization of the needle but requires specialized skills to assess the relationship between the needle and the image plane. Scanning is performed to optimize visualization of both the lesion and the needle. The needle may be positioned either adjacent to the transducer and parallel to the scan plane or remote from the transducer and perpendicular to the scan plane. Reading has found this technique to be highly accurate in aspiration biopsy of small lesions of the head and neck (24). This method has been used for needle placement in lesions as small as 1 cm in critical anatomical areas. This technique will be explained in further detail in Chapter 5.

Alternatively, the needle may be positioned perpendicular to the transducer scan plane. This is the method we often use in amniocentesis. As the needle is advanced, only the portion of the needle intersecting

the scan plane can be visualized as it is maneuvered toward the area of interest.

When the transducer and needle are both used within the sterile field, the transducer is placed within sterile coverings. The needle is advanced as the ultrasound probe is manipulated to keep the needle within the scan plane and directed at the lesion (Fig. 1.6). The transducer need not be placed in sterile coverage if it is kept remote from the sterile puncture site (24).

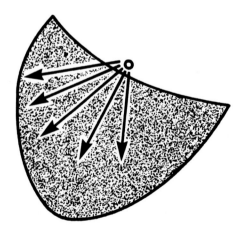

Figure 1.4. Fan Needle Technique. Multiple needles may be placed from one focus in a "fan" configuration in the detection of nondiscrete liver metastases.

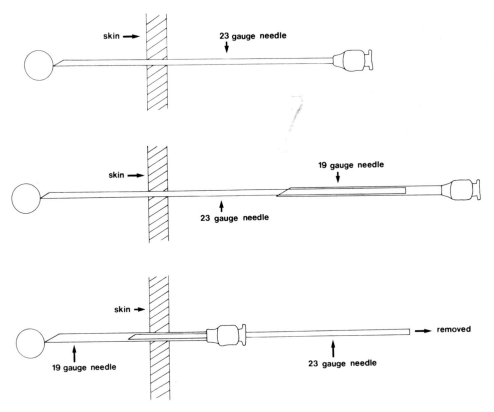

Figure 1.5. Modified Coaxial Technique. (*Top*) A small 22–23-gauge needle is passed percutane-ously into the middle of a suspected lesion. (*Middle*) After removal of inner stylet and the hub of the needle, an 18–19-gauge needle may be passed over the smaller needle to the edge of the sus-pected lesion. (*Bottom*) Once the large needle is properly positioned, multiple biopsy with a small needle may be performed or a small guidewire may be inserted for drainage procedures. (Repro-duced with permission from McGahan JP: Percutaneous biopsy and drainage procedures in the abdomen using a modified coaxial technique. *Radiology* 153:257–258, 1984.)

Needle Guidance System

Numerous needle guidance systems are currently available. These are of two major designs: a) dedicated biopsy transducers with holes or grooves built into the trans-ducer to hold the biopsy needle and b) at-tachable biopsy guides that may be easily fixed to the transducer. The dedicated bi-opsy transducers have several disadvan-tages, including the difficulty of sterilizing the transducer, the impossibility with many systems of visualizing the needle through-out its course, and the large patient contact area required for use of these linear array transducers (Fig. 1.7).

Attachable needle guides that fasten to transducers are in common use and widely available from all manufacturers. The nee-dle guides are designed with slots or grooves sized to needles of different sizes (Fig. 1.8). The guide holds the needle firmly and di-rects it along a predetermined course dis-played as a calibrated line on the video monitor of the ultrasound unit. The guide also serves to keep the needle within the scan plane of the ultrasound transducer. The angle, direction, and depth of the nee-dle can be continuously monitored in real time on the video output. The most superfi-cial 1 to 2 cm of the needle path may not be visualized because it is not usually included within the scan beam. This system can be used effectively to biopsy very small lesions (25). Attachable guides may be used with ei-

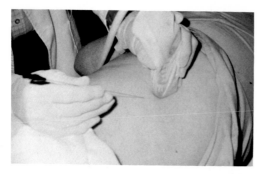

Figure 1.6. Free-hand Puncture. The needle is inserted to the side of the sterilely gloved transducer and advanced under ultrasound observation. When the needle can be inserted at a location remote from the transducer, the transducer need not have sterile coverings.

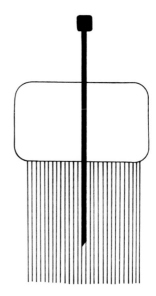

Figure 1.7. Dedicated Biopsy Transducer. This linear array dedicated biopsy transducer has a central hole to allow for passage of the needle. Since no crystals are present in the linear array where the needle is inserted, the needle itself cannot be visualized and its depth must be estimated.

ther linear array or sector transducers and specialized endoluminal probes.

The needle placement is similar to that used in other methods. The transducer need not be sterilized, but is covered by a sterile prefitted glove. Nonsterile gel is placed inside the glove to provide acoustic coupling between the transducer face and the glove. Sterile gel or povidone iodine solution is used as an acoustic coupling medium between the outside of the glove and the patient's skin. The sterile biopsy guide is attached to the transducer, and the area is rescanned to select the optimal puncture site. The skin is anesthetized with local anesthetic (1%–2% lidocaine). A small puncture is made in the skin with a scalpel blade to allow easy passage of the needle through the tough dermal tissues. The needle course is followed on the video monitor as it is placed into the target lesion.

Needle guidance attachments differ from manufacturer to manufacturer. A fixed attachment may contain several parallel slots that may be used for various gauged needles with a corresponding puncture line indicated on the ultrasound monitor. The appropriate needle (16-, 18-, 20-gauge) is placed through the appropriate slot for biopsy (Fig. 1.8). Alternatively, some guides have a single fixed-angle slot attachment that allows different size needles to be inserted (Fig.

1.9). Spring-loaded levers are adjustable for use with various size needles or catheters. Other manufacturers have not only slots to accommodate variable needle sizes but also adjustable guides that allow for needle insertion at variable angles of approach and to specific depths.

In general, all needle guidance attachments are designed so that the examiner can easily remove the guidance attachment and/or needle with one hand. The needle slot for the attachment must be large enough so the needle only has negligible resistance yet small enough to hold the needle in its desired path. The spring-loaded levers that hold the needle in place also must hold enough compression against the needle so it will not slip out of the guidance attachment during biopsy or aspiration.

Specially designed ultrasound needle guidance systems have been developed recently for use with endoluminal scanners. These may be used for either transperineal or transrectal biopsy of the prostate, or pelvic

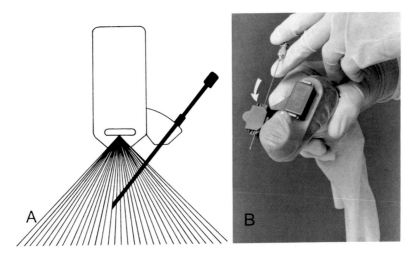

Figure 1.8. Sector Transducer Biopsy Attachment. **A,** Schematic drawing demonstrating a biopsy attachment for a sector transducer. **B,** A plastic "clip on" needle guidance attachment designed for ATL* ultrasound probe with three slots (curved arrow) designed for different sized needles. The first 1–2 cm of the needle is not visualized until it intersects the ultrasound beam. (See Figure 1.9). (Reproduced with permission from McGahan JP. Advantages of sonographic guidance. In McGahan JP (ed): *Controversies In Ultrasound.* New York, Churchill Livingstone, 1987, pp 249–267).

aspiration/biopsy with transvaginal transducers. If the needle is placed parallel to the long axis of the ultrasound probe and lies perpendicular to the ultrasound beam, nearly the entire shaft of the needle is well visualized because of increased acoustic reflection of the needle inserted perpendicular to the scan plane (Fig. 1.10). These transducers and biopsy guide attachments will be more completely described in Chapters 16 and 17.

Transducer Sterilization

Ultrasound-guided aspiration, biopsy, or drainage must be regarded as minor surgical procedures and sterile technique should be used. The ultrasound probes usually are not gas-sterilized. If the probe is placed within the sterile field, it should be thoroughly cleansed with absolute alcohol. Using the freehand method for real-time control, the biopsy is performed without use of sterile transducer coverings if the site of needle insertion is a significant distance away from the transducer face. Probe sterilization will require soaking the probes in chlorhexidine alcohol, Cidex, or Korsolin. Chlorhexidine alcohol usually is not effective against the hepatitis virus. While both Cidex and Korsolin are known to be effective against this virus, long periods of submersion are required.

Our standard procedure is to cleanse the transducer thoroughly with alcohol, place nonsterile acoustic gel on the scan head, and then enclose the entire transducer with a commercially available fitted sterile covering or a large sterile surgical glove. Sterile acoustic gel or liquid povidone iodine solution is used as acoustic coupling agent in the sterile field. Intraoperative ultrasound-guided procedures require similar techniques. Because of the larger sterile field and crowded conditions in the operating room, the entire transducer and its cable must be enclosed in sterile coverings. Ultrasound guidance of intraoperative procedures will be explained in more detail in Chapters 4 and 8.

*Advanced Technical Laboratories, Inc.; 22100 Bothell Highway S.E., P.O. Box 3003, Bothell, Washington 98041-3003

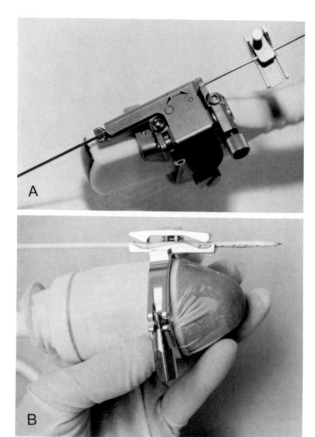

Figure 1.9. **A, B,** Two different fixed metal biopsy guidance attachments that allow for a variety of different needle sizes or catheters to be utilized for either aspiration/biopsy or drainage procedures.

NEEDLE VISUALIZATION— THEORETICAL AND PRACTICAL

Ultrasound visualization of a biopsy needle depends on complex interactions between the ultrasound beam, the biopsy needle, and fluid or soft tissues within the body. Reflection and scatter of the ultrasound beam from the needle play major roles in needle visualization. Reflection from a biopsy needle is determined by the acoustic impedance difference between body tissues and the metal of the needle, the angle of incidence between the needle and the ultrasound beam, and the size of the needle. Acoustic impedance is markedly different between metal and soft tissue, causing a large beam reflection (26, 27). When the needle is perpendicular to the ultrasound beam, nearly all of the reflected beam returns to the transducer, resulting in excellent needle visualization (Fig. 1.10). However, as the needle is rotated to intersect parallel to the ultrasound beam, a larger portion of the ultrasound beam will be reflected away from the transducer, and the needle is less easily seen. A needle placed exactly parallel to the ultrasound beam may not be seen at all (Fig. 1.7). Many biopsy guide attachments allow only narrow angles of incidence between the needle course and the ultrasound beam. The greater the angle of incidence, the greater the acoustic detection of the needle. Therefore, a freehand biopsy

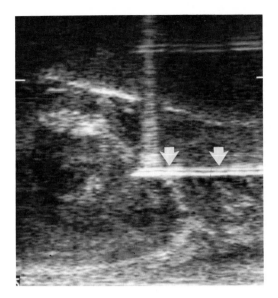

Figure 1.10. Image of the prostate obtained by a transrectal linear array transducer clearly demonstrates biopsy needle (*arrows*) placed transperineally entering the prostate. The needle is perpendicular to the linear array beam, increasing beam reflection and acoustic detectability of the needle.

may optimize needle visualization, as the needle may be placed in a position more perpendicular to the sound beam than the narrow angle of a biopsy guide attached to the transducer will allow.

Larger needles are easier to see. A large needle will intersect a greater portion of the width of the ultrasound beam, causing greater reflection. Needle visualization is best within the focal zone of the transducer where the ultrasound beam is thinnest. An advantage of electronically focused transducers is the ability to adjust the depth of the focal zone to match the location of the needle and improve needle detection.

The tip of most needles often produces an echo that is well visualized even when the shaft of the needle is not seen. This increased visibility is believed to be due to the multiple surfaces of the needle tip causing increased scattering of the ultrasound beam. With large, smooth metallic needles, reflection from the shaft is primarily responsible for needle visibility, while scatter is of mini-

mal importance. When the needle is passing through tissue at an angle nearly parallel to the ultrasound beam, most of the beam is reflected away from transducer and the needle is difficult to detect. Scattering will increase the portion of the reflected beam that will return to the transducer and be displayed in the image, thus increasing visibility of the needle. If the inner or outer surface of the needle or stylet is scratched or roughened, the surface inhomogeneities increase scattering and make the needle much easier to see sonographically (14). Spiral-shaped grooves within the needle may trap small gas bubbles that also scatter the beam and increase visibility (24). Practical applications of these theories have led to development of needles designed to increase their sonographic visibility (10, 14; Fig. 1.8). Some needles have tips roughened to increase acoustic detectability, while some designed by Cook Catheter (see Appendix to this chapter) have the entire shaft roughened and coated with Teflon, markedly increasing sonographic visibility and ease of use for ultrasound-guided procedures (14, 28; Fig. 1.11). The spiral windings of standard angiographic guidewires and the spiral grooves of the Rotex needle also result in excellent sonographic visualization (14, 24; Fig. 1.12).

Injection of air or water into the needle tip also improves needle visualization. When water is injected and the needle placed into a solid organ, such as the liver, there is a circumferential increase in echogenicity at the needle tip. Introduction of air into the needle may not be as helpful, as it causes an acoustic shadow which may prohibit sonographic visualization of the deeper structures. In practice, injection of air or water is rarely utilized.

Improvement of visualization of the needle may be obtained by gently jiggling the needle or moving the inner stylet up and down. If the biopsy needle has deflected out of the image plane, then rocking the transducer into the path of the needle may display it. Methods of improving needle visualization for aspiration or biopsy techniques are listed in Table 1.2.

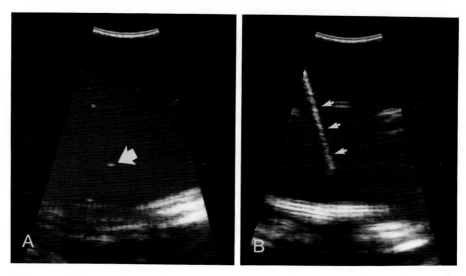

Figure 1.11. Needle Visualization. **A,** A standard 22-gauge Chiba type needle is placed into a water filled beaker with visualization of the echogenic tip (*arrow*). (The ultrasound gain settings are unaltered in Figures 1.11, 1.12, and 1.13). **B,** A 22-gauge roughened Chiba needle which has been coated with Teflon* demonstrates increased acoustic detectability of the shaft of the needle (*arrows*).

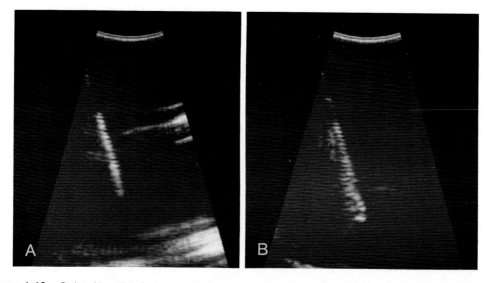

Figure 1.12. Rotex Needle. **A,** Inner stylet of a stainless stell Rotex** screw needle demonstrates excellent acoustic detectability when placed into a waterpath. **B,** Even after the inner stylet is placed into stainless stell cannula it still demonstrates excellent acoustic detectability when compared to standard thin-wall needles (see Figure 1.11).

*Cook Incorporated (See Appendix 1)
**Ursu Konsultab; Stockhom, Sweden A/C5606 10 007 03.

Table 1.2
Needle Visualization

Methods that may be used to improve needle visualization when using real-time ultrasound guidance

- Rock transducer
- Jiggle needle
- Move inner stylet
- Roughened needles
- Spiral stylet
- Insert guidewire (rare)
- Inject water or air (rare)

Experimental data have shown that certain catheter materials (Teflon) have better acoustic properties than others (nylon). Two examples of catheter material echogenicities are illustrated in Figure 1.13.

Needle Selection

A wide variety of needles is available for percutaneous aspiration, biopsy, and drainage procedures. These needles differ in length, inside and outside diameter, wall thickness, flexibility, needle tip and stylet design, sonographic visibility, and suitability for obtaining aspiration cytology or tissue cores for histology. Needle selection is determined in part by the type of lesion to be sampled and the type of specimen desired. Aspiration of a simple cyst can often be accomplished with a 22- or 23-gauge needle, while aspiration of an abscess with thick purulent debris will usually require a larger needle or catheter. Likewise, cytologic diagnosis of a liver metastasis is usally possible with a thin needle (22- or 23-gauge), but histologic diagnosis of hepatic cirrhosis will require a tissue core specimen obtained from a larger needle (14 to 18 gauge) to demonstrate tissue architecture. In general, thinner needles yield smaller specimens for diagnosis, but are associated with a lower incidence of complications. Large-bore needles provide larger specimens, but are associated with a higher rate of complications, especially hemorrhage (29, 30).

Bevelled-edge needles such as the Chiba, Menghini, or Turner needles have been shown by experimental data to yield more suitable specimens than nonbevelled needles with circumferential sharpened tips, like the Greene or Madayag needles (Fig. 1.14). However, a flexible needle with a bevelled edge, like the Chiba needle, often will bend as it courses through tissue following the direction of the bevel (31). This failure to run a straight course makes it difficult to trace with ultrasound. Some manufacturers make "stiff" needles to run a straighter

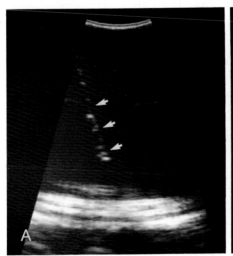 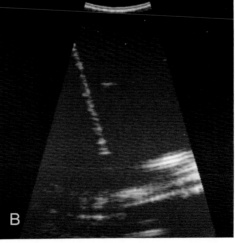

Figure 1.13. Catheter Echogenicity. A 5.0 Fr nylon catheter (**A**) is placed in a water beaker and demonstrates poor sonographic visibility (*arrows*) compared to a 5.0 Fr Teflon catheter (**B**).

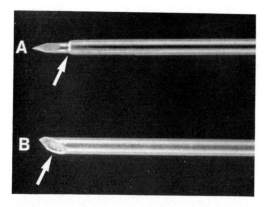

Figure 1.14. Needle Tips. The Greene needle (A) has a circumferential, non-bevelled tip (*arrow*) and an inner pointed stylet. The Chiba needle (B) has a sharp bevelled tip (*arrow*).

course through tissue. Others have designed sharply pointed stylets that are symmetrically bevelled on four sides to pass through tissue in a straight line. A variety of different tips has been designed to obtain cut biopsy tissue core samples for histology (Figs. 1.15–1.17). The Franseen needle (Figs. 1.15–1.17) has three cutting serrations at the tip. A sharp stylet fitted to the serrations of the needle tip is bevelled to track straight through tissue. The Tru-cut, Wescott, and Lee-Ray needles have a slotted tip (Fig. 1.15B) that side cuts the tissue to obtain histologic core samples.

Thin wall fine caliber needles constructed from advanced alloy metal yield larger tissue specimens than thicker walled needles. Cut biopsy needles such as the PercuCut needle (E-Z EM, Inc.; see Appendix 1) have slots with cutting edges in the needle tip designed to core out a tissue plug when the needle is rotated as it is advanced. The needles are relatively stiff and have trocar pointed stylets to tract straight through tissue. Needles as small as 20 gauge can obtain tissue samples from favorable tissue large enough for histologic diagnosis.

Needles with Teflon coating or surface roughening are especially well suited for ultrasound guided procedures because of their excellent sonographic visibility. The screw tip stylet of the Rotex needle (Figs. 1.12 and 1.16) has excellent sonographic visibility, but its use as a biopsy needle is confined to biopsy of solid lesions. Tissue specimens may prove to be difficult to remove or become macerated during removal from the screw stylet (29). This stylet may find its best use as an acoustic marker (24).

With many choices of needles from many manufacturers, it is prudent to become familiar with the use of a few needles that are easily obtainable locally. These can be effectively used with a minimum of experience for most aspiration, biopsy, and drainage procedures. Several U.S. needle and catheter manufacturers and distributors are listed in the Appendix to this chapter. Many of these manufacturers have distributors lo-

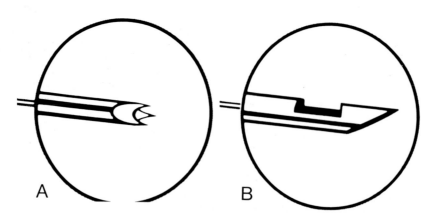

Figure 1.15. Needle Tips. Needle tips are designed to facilitate aspiration of tissue specimens. **A,** Franseen biopsy needle tip. **B,** Lee-Ray biopsy needle tip. (Reproduced with permission of Cook Catheter, Inc.; Bloomington, Indiana.)

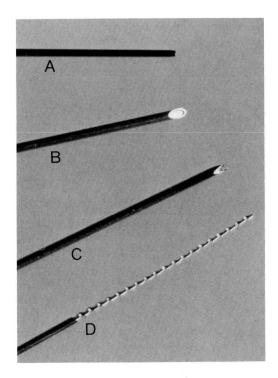

Figure 1.16. Needle tips. A variety of needles are available for percutaneous biopsy including: (A) the Greene needle with the stylet removed showing the nonbevelled tip, (B) the Chiba needle with a sharpened bevelled tip, (C) the Franseen needle with a cutting edge, and (D) the Rotex needle with the screw inner stylet

cated worldwide. The European and Asian addresses of these distributors are not included in the Appendix.

TECHNIQUE

Aspiration

The technique for aspiration of fluid depends upon the amount of fluid to be removed. Simple aspiration of a small amount of fluid can be performed by guiding the needle into the fluid collection, removing the inner stylet, attaching a syringe directly to the needle, and aspirating the fluid. If larger amounts of fluid are to be removed, attaching a three-way stopcock with tubing attached to a drainage bag will provide an effective closed system for repeated aspira-tion. Flexible plastic catheters that fit either outside or inside the needle can be left within the fluid collection during aspiration, allowing the needle to be withdrawn and thus decreasing the risk of tissue injury.

Biopsy

Biopsy is performed in a slightly different manner. When the needle is properly positioned, the inner stylet is removed and the syringe is attached to the needle, then 8 to 10 cc of negative suction is applied with a handheld syringe. Simultaneously, several 1-cm up-and-down movements within the lesion are made. A rotatory motion of the needle may be helpful when using a thin needle to obtain not only a cytological but a histological specimen (31, 32). This rotatory motion and use of larger needles may more reliably produce a histological specimen or core of tissue. Release of negative suction is needed as the needle is removed from the lesion so as not to aspirate more proximal contents. Some authors preload the syringe with 2 ml of saline to flush the specimen from the needle shaft into a test tube if no cytologist is available (23).

Biopsy with cutting needles is accomplished with a rotatory coring motion. For those needles with a biopsy notch on the inner obturator, biopsy is accomplished by advancing the obturator and then sliding the outer cannula over the obturator (33). Recently, automated biopsy guns have been manufactured that allow for an accurately cut biopsy specimen.

Specially designed needles such as the Surecut (Meadox Surgimed, Oakland, NJ, see Appendix 1) or the PercuCut self-aspirating needle (E-Z EM, Inc.; see Appendix 1) are designed for core tissue specimens. Use of these needles permits one-hand operation. The idea behind both needles is similar. In the Surecut system, the inner stylet of the needle is attached to the plunger of the syringe. In the PercuCut system, the inner stylet pierces a specially designed diaphragm in the hub of the needle. In either system retraction of the inner stylet of the needle produces negative suction at the needle tip, thus facilitating aspiration of the

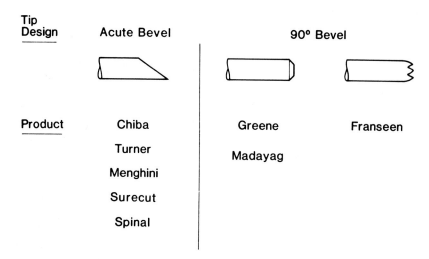

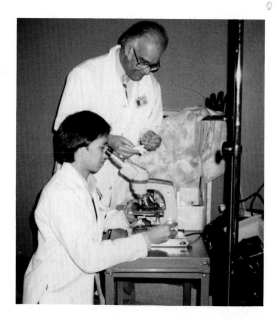

Figure 1.17. Artist's conception of the tips of various end cutting needle tips. (Reproduced with permission from Wittenberg J, Mueller PR, Simeone JF: Planning the biopsy. In Ferrucci JT Jr, Wittenberg J, Mueller PR, Simeone JF (eds): *Interventional Radiology of the Abdomen*, ed 2. Baltimore: Williams & Wilkins, © 1985, pp 36–49.)

specimen into the needle. These needles are unlike other aspiration biopsy systems in that suction is not released with removal of the needle from the body. The specimen is, therefore, contained in the needle tip, which may be removed with reinsertion of the inner stylet. Whichever system is utilized at our institution, the specimen is given to a cytologist who is present during the biopsy for immediate cytological staining (Fig. 1.18).

As the needle is placed, the distance of the lesion from the subcutaneous tissue is determined from the ultrasound image. The distance may be marked on the needle shaft or with steristrips or 1-cm markers (Fig. 1.19). Commercial needles now have rubber or plastic stops that may be used to ensure that the needle is not placed beyond the area of lesion to be biopsied.

An alternative to handheld suction with a syringe is use of a locking device that has been placed on the hub of the syringe to ensure constant and adequate suction. There are several commercially available systems (Fig. 1.20).

Biopty Gun

An automated biopsy gun has been used for successful ultrasound-guided prostate biopsies. The Bard/Radiplast Biopty Gun (Bard Urological Division, Covington, Georgia/Radiplast, Uppsala, Sweden) is used in conjunction with an 18-gauge biopsy-cut

Figure 1.18. A cytologist is usually present in the room to evaluate immediately adequacy of the tissue specimen obtained by ultrasound-guided biopsy.

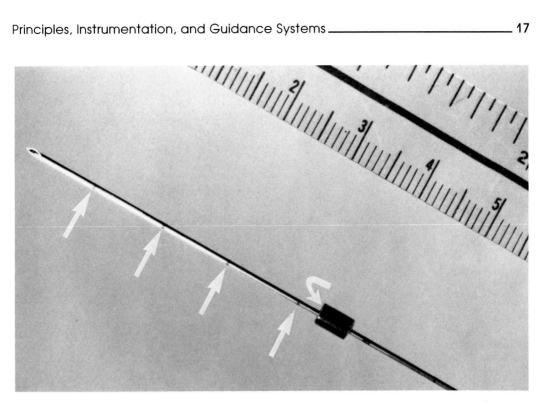

Figure 1.19. Needle with Biopsy Stop. The needle is designed with incremental markers (*arrows*) at 1 centimeter intervals along the shaft. These markers are helpful in determining the depth of needle placement. An attachable biopsy stop (*curved arrow*) is useful for avoiding inadvertent placement of the needle beyond the lesion.

needle. This is a miniaturized Tru-cut needle. (The needle and the gun are illustrated in Chapter 17.) These Biopty-cut needles consist of an inner trocar with a 1.7-cm sample notch. This inner trocar is placed into the outer cannula or sheath of the needle. The Biopty gun consists of a handheld device that automatically triggers a two-stage rapid firing of the Biopty-cut needle. The spring-loaded Biopty gun accepts the two separate hubs of the needle trocar and the cannula, which can be placed within the gun either before or after the mechanism is cocked. As the gun is fired, the inner trocar, with its sample notch, is thrust forward 2.3 cm. This is followed almost instantaneously by a simple forward thrust of the outer cannula, which shears off the tissue sample. Prostate biopsies (34) and percutaneous biopsy of other solid organs have recently proven successful with this automated gun system (35).

The Biopty-cut needle may be placed using ultrasound guidance. As the needle is not intended to be used separately from the gun, there is no locking mechanism between the inner trocar and the outer cannula of the needle. Therefore, interposition of a short section of a sterile plastic sheath that accompanies the needle between the trocar and the cannula portions has been advocated (35). The needle is placed in the desired location, which is confirmed under ultrasound guidance, with allowances made for the known 2.3-cm excursion, and the gun is attached and fired. Scoring of the needle tip with a scalpel may improve needle visualization for real-time ultrasound guidance. An 18-gauge needle is utilized and a core specimen obtained. This specimen is placed in formalin for pathological review. The disadvantage of this technique is utilization of a slightly larger needle—18-gauge as compared to the skinny biopsy needle. However, bleeding complications have not been a major problem in our experience. Advantages of this technique are elimination of the "crush" artifact and obscuration by blood that are common problems associated with

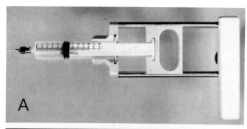

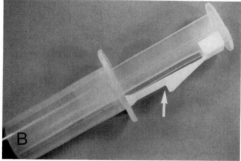

Figure 1.20. Suction Devices. Approaches used to facilitate the application of suction using one hand include: (A) Metal handle designed to hold syringe and apply suction by squeezing trigger (arrow) toward palm of hand, and (B) plastic clips on plunger of syringe designed to hold suction during aspiration/biopsy.

thin-needle biopsy techniques. Patient discomfort is thought to be decreased due to the rapid fire of the Biopty gun and the procedure time may be reduced.

Catheter Drainage

Catheter drainage may be performed using a variety of methods including either the Trocar or Seldinger technique. These will be specifically described in subsequent chapters.

ACKNOWLEDGEMENT

Special thanks to Karen Anderson for preparation of the chapter.

REFERENCES

1. Blady JV: Aspiration biopsy of tumors in obscure or difficult locations under roentgenoscopic guidance. AJR 42:515–524, 1939.
2. Letourneau JG, Elyaderani MK: General considerations of percutaneous biopsy and drainage. In Letourneau JG, Elyaderani MK, Castañeda-Zuñiga WR (eds): *Percutaneous Biopsy, Aspiration and Drainage*. Chicago, Yearbook, 1987, pp 1–29.
3. Martin HE, Ellis EB. Biopsy by needle puncture and aspiration. *Ann Surg* 92:169–181, 1930.
4. McGahan JP, Hanson FW: Ultrasonographic aspiration and biopsy techniques. In Dublin AB (ed): *Outpatient Invasive Radiologic Procedures: Diagnostic and Therapeutic*. Philadelphia, W.B. Saunders, 1989, pp 79–113.
5. Holm HH, Kristensen JK: Rasmussen SN et al: Ultrasound as a guide in percutaneous puncture technique. *Ultrasonics* 10:83–86, 1972.
6. Goldberg BB, Pollack HM: Ultrasonic aspiration transducer. *Radiology* 102:187-189, 1972.
7. Holm HH, Torp-Pedersen S, Juul N, Larsen T: Instrumentation for sonographic interventional procedures. In VanSonnenberg E (ed): *Interventional Ultrasound*. New York, Churchill Livingstone, 1987, pp 9–40.
8. McGahan JP: Advantages of sonographic guidance. In McGahan JP (ed): *Controversies in Ultrasound*. New York, Churchill Livingstone, 1987, pp 249–267.
9. McGahan JP: Aspiration and drainage procedures in the intensive care unit: Percutaneous sonographic guidance. *Radiology* 154:531–532, 1985.
10. McGahan JP, Anderson MW, Walter JP: Portable real-time sonographic and needle guidance systems for aspiration and drainage. *AJR* 147: 1241–1246, 1986.
11. Schwimer SR, Marik J, Lebovic J: Percutaneous ovarian cyst aspiration using continuous transvaginal ultrasonographic monitoring. *J Ultrasound Med* 4:259–260, 1985.
12. Lee F, Littrup PJ, Torp-Pedersen ST et al: Prostate cancer: Comparison of transrectal US and digital rectal examination for screening. *Radiology* 168: 389–394, 1988.
13. Rifkin MD, Kurtz AB, Goldberg BB: Sonographically guided transperineal prostatic biopsy: Preliminary experience with a longitudinal linear array transducer. *AJR* 140:745–747, 1983.
14. McGahan JP: Laboratory assessment of ultrasonic needle and catheter visualization. *J Ultrasound Med* 5:373–377, 1986.
15. Buonocore E, Skipper GJ: Steerable real-time sonographically guided needle biopsy. *AJR* 136: 387–392, 1981.
16. Holm HH, Als O, Gammelgaard J: Percutaneous aspiration and biopsy procedures under ultrasound visualization. In Taylor KJD (ed): *Diagnostic Ultrasound in Gastrointestinal Disease*. New York, Churchill-Livingstone, 1979, pp 137-149.
17. Otto R, Deyhle P: Guided puncture under real-time sonographic control. *Radiology* 134:784–785, 1980.
18. Rapaport SI. Preoperative hemostatic evaluation: Which tests, if any? *Blood* 61:229–231, 1983.
19. Ferrucci JT Jr: Surgical and radiological foundations. In Ferrucci JT Jr, Wittenberg J, Mueller PR, Simeone JF (eds): *Interventional Radiology of the Abdomen*, ed 2. Baltimore, Williams & Wilkins, 1985, pp 6–11.
20. Neff CC: Analgesia for abdominal interventional procedures. In Ferrucci JT Jr, Wittenberg J, Mueller PR, Simeone JF (eds): *Interventional Radiology of the*

Abdomen, ed 10. Baltimore, Williams & Wilkins, 1985, pp 12-17.

21. Package insert, Roche Laboratories for Versed Brand of Miconasal. Prepared in March 1988 by Roche Laboratories, a division of Hoffmann-La Roche Inc. 340 Kingsland Street, Nutley, NJ 07110-1199.

22. McGahan JP: Percutaneous biopsy and drainage procedures in the abdomen using a modified coaxial technique. *Radiology* 153:257–258, 1984.

23. Wittenberg J, Mueller PR, Simeone JF: Performing the biopsy. In Ferrucci JT Jr, Wittenberg J, Mueller PR, Simeone JF (eds): *Interventional Radiology of the Abdomen*, ed 2. Baltimore, Williams & Wilkins, 1985, pp 50-85.

24. Reading CC, Charboneau JW, James EM, Hurt MR: Sonographically guided percutaneous biopsy of small (3 cm or less) masses. *AJR* 151:189–192, 1988.

25. Solbiati L, Montali G, Croce F, et al: Parathyroid tumors detected by fine-needle aspiration biopsy under ultrasonic guidance. *Radiology* 148:793–797, 1983.

26. Christensen EE, Curry TS III, Dowdey JE: Ultrasound. In Christensen EE, Curry TS III, Dowdey JE (eds): *An Introduction to the Physics of Diagnostic Radiology*, ed 2. Philadelphia, Lea & Febiger, 1978, pp 361–394.

27. Otto RC, Wellauer J: Principles and technique. In Otto RC, Wellauer J (eds): *Ultrasound-guided Biopsy and Drainage*. New York, Springer-Verlag, 1986, pp 6–42.

28. Heckemann R, Seidel KJ: The sonographic appearance and contrast enhancement of puncture needles. *J Clin Ultrasound* 11:265–268, 1983.

29. Andriole JG, Haaga JR, Adams RB, Nunez C: Biopsy needle characteristics assessed in the laboratory. *Radiology* 148:659–662, 1983.

30. Haaga Jr, LiPuma JP, Bryan PJ, Balsara VJ, Cohen AM: Clinical comparison of small- and large-caliber cutting needles for biopsy. *Radiology* 146:665–667, 1983.

31. Ferrucci JT Jr, Wittenberg J, Mueller PR et al: Diagnosis of abdominal malignancy by radiologic fine-needle aspiration biopsy. *AJR* 134:323–330, 1980.

32. Wittenberg J, Mueller PR, Ferrucci JT Jr et al: Percutaneous core biopsy of abdominal tumor using 22 22 gauge needles: Further observations *AJR* 139:75–80, 1982.

33. Wittenberg J, Mueller PR, Simeone JF: Planning the biopsy. In Ferrucci JT Jr: Wittenberg J, Mueller PR, Simeone JF (eds): *Interventional Radiology of the Abdomen*, ed 2. Baltimore, Williams & Wilkins, 1985, pp 36-49.

34. Ragde H, Aldape HC, Blasko JC: Biopty: An automatic needle biopsy device—its use with an 18-gauge Tru-cut needle. (Biopty-cut) in 174 consecutive prostate core biopsies. *Endosonographique* 3–5, 1987.

35. Parker SH, Hopper KD, Yakes WF, Gibson MD, Ownbey JL, Carter TE: Image-directed percutaneous biopsies with a biopsy gun. *Radiology* 171:663–669, 1989.

APPENDIX 1

Partial List of Biopsy Needle and Catheter Manufacturers

1. Angiomed U.S., Inc.
   Eisenbahnstrasse 36
   71 Karlsruhe 7500
   West Germany
   (49) 72148030
   Needles & Catheters

2. Argon Medical Corp.
   P.O. Box 1970
   Athens, TX 75751
   (800) 527-2983
   Needles & Catheters

3. Bard Interventional Products
   5 Federal Street
   Billerica, MA 01821
   (508) 663-2244
   Catheters

4. Becton-Dickinson
   Rutherford, NJ 07073
   (201) 460-2168
   Needles

5. Cook Incorporated
   P.O. Box 489
   Bloomington, IN 47402
   (812) 339-2235
   Needles & Catheters

6. E-Z-EM, Inc.
   7 Portland Avenue
   Westbury, NY 11590
   (516) 333-8230
   Needles

7. Havel's Inc.
   3726 Lonsdale Avenue
   Cincinnati, OH 45227
   (513) 271-2117
   Needles

8. Ingenor
   70-72 Rue Orfilia
   75020 Paris, FR 210048
   47.97.51.19
   Needles & Catheters

9. Meadox Medicals, Inc.
   112 Bauer Drive
   Oakland, NJ 07436

   (201) 337-6126
   Needles

10. Medi-Tech, Inc.
    480 Pleasant Street
    Watertown, MA 02172
    (617) 923-1720
    Needles & Catheters

11. Namic
    Pruyn's Island
    Glen Falls, NY 12801
    (518) 798-0067
    Needles

12. Picker International, Inc.
    299 Harbor Way
    S. San Francisco, CA 94080
    (800) 824-9235
    Catheters

13. Premiere Biomedical, Inc.
    1440 Lake Front Circle, Suite 180
    The Woodlands, TX 77380
    (800) 662-1777
    Catheters

14. Surgitek
    3037 Mt. Pleasant Street
    Racine, WI 53404
    (414) 639-7205
    Catheters

15. Sherwood Medical
    1831 Olive Street
    St. Louis, MO 63103
    (314) 621-7788
    Catheters & Needles

16. Universal Medical Instrument
    Corporation
    P.O. Box 100
    Ballston Spa, NY 12020
    (518) 587-5095
    Needles

17. X-Ray Marketing Associates, Inc.
    1114 Tower Lane
    Bensenville, IL 60106
    (312) 595-5411
    Catheters & Needles

2 Fine-Needle Aspiration/Cytology for Invasive Ultrasound Techniques

ALBERT SIU
RAYMOND L. TEPLITZ

Cytology

As developed by George Papanicolaou, cytologic examination of cell smears focused upon the female reproductive tract, first of laboratory animals and then of humans (1, 2). This technique involved a staining process that enhanced cytoplasmic and nuclear characteristics. The fundamental impact was the emphasis on cellular, rather than tissue characteristics. This contribution to pathology has become integrated into the daily conduct of microscopy by pathologists world-wide. Such terms as nuclear: cytoplasmic ratio, hyperchromatism, and chromatin clumping are part of the histopathology and cytopathology lexicons.

However, observation of cells from body parts other than the female reproductive tract has shown that the criteria for interpretation of neoplastic, preneoplastic and even nonneoplastic diseases vary from organ to organ and tissue to tissue. Therefore, the criteria used for interpretation must be specific for the organ and tissue under scrutiny. Texts have been filled with these criteria and the reader is directed to them for additional detail. However, it should be emphasized that a considerable body of information must be mastered for interpretative specificity, and experience covering all body parts is desirable when confronted by the demands

of an active cytopathology fine-needle aspiration (FNA) practice. In many institutions, no organ or tissue is far from the probing needle. Thus, the central nervous system, the orbit, the musculoskeletal, endocrine, and lymphoid systems, and retroperitoneal, abdominal and thoracic organs may be targets of needle aspiration. Some hospitals offer FNA interpretation intraoperatively, in association with frozen section, expecially when an area is unsuitable for sharp dissection or time is pressing. This is a procedure in which our laboratory has had early interest and gained wide experience (3, 4).

It is a commonplace that the ease with which a case may be interpreted is largely defined by the adequacy of the specimen, all other things being equal. This is especially true of FNA. A microsection of tissue is being obtained. Will it be representative? In order to make it so, several recommendations are made:

1. Several needle passes should be made on every specimen, whenever possible. Try not to rely on a single specimen attempt no matter how obvious the diagnosis may appear to be clinically.
2. When multiple needle passes are made, use different needle directions.
3. Have the specimen evaluated immediately by a cytotechnologist or cytopathologist as to adequacy. This ensures that if adequate diagnostic material has not been obtained, that the

patient is there and in position (mentally and physically) for another attempt.

Causes of sampling difficulty include:

1. Necrosis. Aspiration of necrotic parts of tumors or other lesions may be nondiagnostic and even obscure the diagnosis.
2. Cyst contents. The cyst wall should be the target of a second aspiration attempt (when possible).
3. Small and moveable targets may be difficult to obtain. Only practice improves results.
4. Fat tissue. Fat or lipoma?

ADENOMA VERSUS CARCINOMA

Morphological criteria, whether applied at the tissue or cellular level, may not meet all of the demands. Notable problems involve the distinction between some benign and malignant processes of the endocrine system. The thyroid gland is an appropriate example. Follicular adenomas are often indistinguishable morphologically from follicular carcinomas of the thyroid. Similar problems of interpretation of microscopic characteristics occur with lesions of parathyroid and adrenals. The source is the lack of strict association between microscopic appearance and biological behavior of the lesion. The graded atypias that are associated with other adenomas or preneoplasias and their malignant counterparts are not reliably present in follicular thyroid and adrenal adenomas and carcinomas. Other criteria are being sought for the resolution of this problem. Among the additional observations that can be made are electron microscopy, immunoperoxidase procedures for specific molecules, quantitative measurements of secretory products, and quantitative morphologic measurements.

QUANTITATIVE DNA AND MORPHOMETRY

DNA quantitation may be accomplished by microspectrophotometry, flow cytometry or image analysis. Microspectrophotometry uses a microscope attached to a photometer and has the advantage of being able to resolve single wavelengths of light. However, it is a slow process. Flow cytometry is the speediest of the methods, measuring fluorescence in cells or nuclei specifically stained, suspended in a droplet of fluid, and illuminated by laser. However, this method requires the suspension of cells from a tissue and inevitably includes normal components and destroys the architecture. Image analysis uses a television camera and optical microscope to measure optical density (OD, gray shades), integrating the OD for each nucleus. Smears are the preferred object of analysis, containing the whole nucleus, but sections may be used. Thus the cells and/or tissues remain available for further studies.

During the past two decades a substantial literature has developed on the nuclear DNA quantitation (QDNA) of many tissues. These studies include examination of the progress from preneoplasia to neoplasia in the lung (5, 6, 7), and of the patterns of DNA in tumors of various organs. In some tumors, a distinct association is apparent between patterns and prognosis. The patterns that have emerged can be simply described as euploid (EUP) or aneuploid/hyperploid (A/H). EUP lesions have DNA quantities that represent diploid or near diploid/or tetraploid amounts of DNA. It is understood that the quantity of DNA does not specify a particular or normal chromosomal complement, which may be quite abnormal. But cytogenetic studies require dividing cells, almost always a minor component of any tissue, and special techniques for obtaining optimum results. Quantitative DNA estimates may be obtained on fixed, stained cells and may be retrospective, contrary to chromosomal analyses. A/H lesions have supradiploid and/or supratetraploid amounts of DNA and often have multiple peaks, indicating multiple clones of tumor cells. The euploid lesions in the breast (8, 9), cervix (10, 11), ovary (12, 13), colon (14, 15), and other organs have been associated with a better prognosis, compared to the A/H lesions.

Image analysis also permits quantitative measurements of nuclear-cytoplasmic areas, their ratios, the chromatin texture, and nuclear curvature. Together with QDNA, morphometry may contribute to the differential interpretation of lesions that visual microscopy alone may abjure. For example, follicular adenoma/carcinoma of the thyroid may be critically examined by these two procedures with benefit. A/H follicular lesions with a nuclear area greater than 90 sq μm and mean nuclear/cytoplasmic (N/C) ratio of 0.77 have a high probability (>95%) of behaving as a malignancy (16). Similar studies of other endocrine and nonendocrine lesions have been reported or are in progress. Our laboratory is engaged in studies of QDNA in a number of organs and diseases, including the parathyroid and osteoblastomas. While data are insufficient for reporting of the former, it is clear that osteoblastomas are consistently diploid or near diploid and may be easily distinguished from osteosarcomas, most of which seem to be A/H (17).

In addition to traditional microscopic criteria for interpretation of cellular atypia, special techniques, including histochemistry, immunoperoxidase stains, QDNA, and morphometry are now available. They aid in final interpretation, increase specificity regarding histogenesis, and add to prognostic capabilities. With respect to QDNA, care must be exercised in interpretation. While aneuploidy is clearly abnormal, it is not exclusively associated with malignancy. Aneuploidy has been identified in various preneoplastic lesions (5, 18, 19). This is an important fact, contributing to greater understanding of neoplasia. But it needs to be emphasized that by itself aneuploidy does not distinguish between preneoplasia and neoplasia.

Fine-Needle Aspiration

CYTOLOGY OF FINE-NEEDLE ASPIRATE SMEARS

Fine-needle aspiration is most commonly used to determine whether a solid mass lesion is benign or malignant. Cytologists apply a number of cellular criteria when examining cells microscopically to designate them as malignant. These criteria involve changes in the nuclei or the cytoplasm of the cells under evaluation. Among the cytologic criteria commonly used are:

1. Cellularity of the smear,
2. Dyscohesion of the cells,
3. Increased nuclear/cytoplasmic (N/C) ratio,
4. Variability of cellular size and shape,
5. Variability of nuclear size and shape,
6. Presence of enlarged, multiple, or abnormally shaped nucleoli,
7. Presence of increased numbers of mitoses and abnormal mitoses,
8. Presence of necrosis.

Many of these characteristic features are illustrated in Figures 2.1 through 2.6.

In general, malignant neoplasms generally have a higher cellularity on the aspirate smears than benign tumors. Due to poor intercellular cohesion among malignant cells, there are more single cells along with clumps of cohesive cells. In benign or normal tissue, the aspirate smears contain flat sheets of cells and few single cells. Necrosis is commonly seen in malignant tumors and is virtually never seen in a benign tumor, so the background resulting from necrotic debris is supportive of a diagnosis of malig-

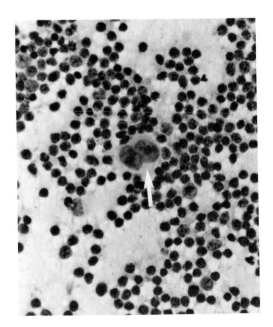

Figure 2.1. Hodgkin's disease in lymph node. A Reed-Sternberg (R-S) cell (*arrow*) is seen in a predominantly lymphoid background. The central R-S cell is large and binucleate. The nuclei have very large nucleoli (X400, Wright).

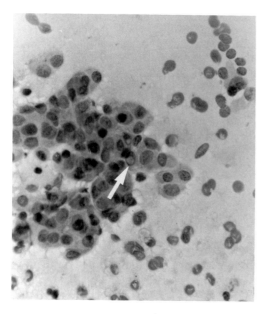

Figure 2.2. Papillary carcinoma of thyroid gland. A sheet of cells with papillary configuration, small clusters and single cells. An intranuclear vacuole (*arrow*) is seen in the large sheet of cells (X400, H&E). Another feature that may be seen is the presence of psammoma bodies.

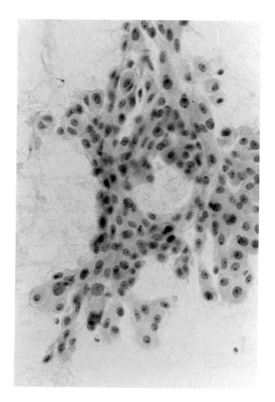

Figure 2.3. Infiltrating ductal carcinoma of breast. Sheet of epithelial cells with variable nuclear size and shape and often large nucleoli (X250, Pap). In the scirrhous type of infiltrating ductal carcinoma, cellularity may be low and the malignant cells tend to be single or in small groups.

nancy in the absence of an inflammatory process.

However, no one of the above diagnostic criteria of malignancy is an absolute, and some of these criteria are more applicable to one organ than another. In some organs, these criteria are insufficient to determine whether a lesion is malignant or not. For example, in the thyroid gland, it is commonly impossible to distinguish cytologically follicular adenoma from follicular carcinoma, and the less specific diagnosis of follicular neoplasm is thus made from the aspirate smear.

History

Physicians from two continents played a major role in the development of the technique of needle-aspiration biopsy. In the late 1920s, Martin and Ellis (20) and Stewart (21) initiated the practice of aspiration of palpable masses and tumors in deeper structures at the Memorial Hospital of New York. Their attempts at interpretation of the aspiration biopsies were enhanced because of their use of cytologic smears along with cell blocks from which histologic sections were obtained. The use of cell blocks to aid in the interpretation of the cytologic smears was of no small importance because virtually all of the pathologists in this country were experienced with tissue biopsy but not with cytologic smears. Furthermore, the general acceptance of the use of cytology in the diagnosis of uterine cancer was yet to be established. This occurred with the 1943 publication by George Papanicolaou of The Diagnosis of Uterine Cancer by Exfoliative Cytology. Despite the rather large experience that was reported in the following years (22), needle-aspiration biopsy continued to see limited use in the United States,

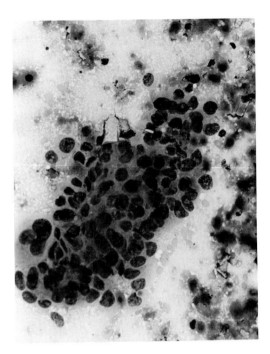

Figure 2.4. Squamous cell carcinoma, lung. Sheet of large epithelial cells with extremely variable nuclei. The nuclei are hyperchromatic and occasionally have irregular contours. The chromatin is coarse. Abundant cytoplasm is eosinophilic (X250, Wright).

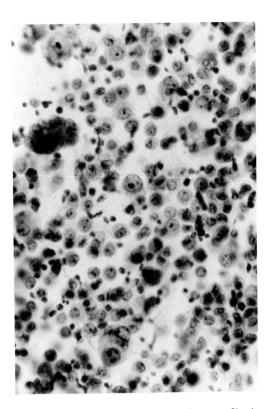

Figure 2.5. Hepatocellular carcinoma. Single or small groups of large cells showing marked variability in size and shape. The large nuclei often have prominent nucleoli (X400, Pap). In better differentiated hepatocellular carcinomas, the tumor cells may resemble hepatocytes of normal or regenerating liver, and bile may be produced.

primarily at Memorial Hospital, until the past twenty years.

Following the acceptance of exfoliative cytology in the diagnosis of cancer, the method of fine-needle aspiration was developed in Europe in the 1940s and 1950s, particularly in Sweden. The names associated with this development include Paul Lopes Cardozo (23) of Holland and Nils Soderstrom (24) and Sixten Franzen (25) of Sweden, all of whom were clinical hematologists. The late Josef Zajicek and Franzen, who were both associated with the Karolinska Hospital, helped formulate diagnostic criteria (26, 27) in the interpretation of the cytology. [Reasons for the strong interest in and development of the application of fine needle aspiration (FNA) cytology in Sweden have been presented by Fox (28).]

Currently, the FNA technique is coupled with fluoroscopy, computed tomography, mammography, and ultrasound imaging to increase the diagnostic yield as well as to allow sampling from internal organs (29, 30).

FINE-NEEDLE ASPIRATION BIOPSY

Definition

FNA biopsy is the diagnostic sampling of lesions by aspiration through a fine-gauge needle (25 to 21 gauge), obtaining cells or small amounts of tissue, which are subsequently examined cytologically. Sufficient material should be aspirated from the lesion in order to allow the cytopathologist to render an adequate evaluation. Obviously, if the needle does not transect the lesion when aspiration biopsy is performed, the

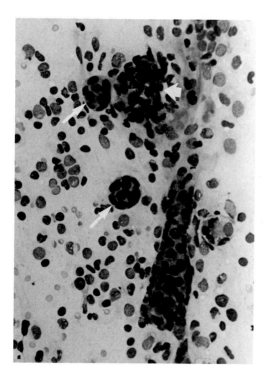

Figure 2.6. Wilm's tumor (nephroblastoma), kidney. Smear contains single as well as small clusters of epithelial and stromal cells. The epithelial cells possess round or oval nuclei and the stromal cells (*broad arrow*) contain elongated or spindled nuclei. Two clusters of epithelial cells forming tubular structures in ball configuration are present (*thin arrows*) (X250, Wright).

cytologic evaluation cannot be representative of the lesion.

Portable Techniques

At our institution a cytotechnologist or a cytopathologist is present during an FNA biopsy performed by the physician under ultrasonic guidance. A microscope mounted on a cart allows transportation of the instrument to the imaging areas or to the patient floors. Other equipment, such as needles, alcohol swabs, syringes, and syringe pistol grip, are transported in a plastic tray (Fig. 2.7). In those cases where the lesion is superficial or palpable, the cytopathologist usually performs the FNA biopsy instead of the clincian. The presence of a microscope at the time of FNA biopsy allows immediate evaluation of smears for adequate cellularity. Furthermore, in unsuspected cases of an infectious nature, material can be obtained and submitted for microbiologic studies during the same procedure. Also, if initial examination suggests that additional investigations may be necessary, for example, malignant lymphoma involving a deep lymph node, more biopsy material may be aspirated to prepare smears suitable for that purpose.

Equipment

The following equipment should be available in order to efficiently perform a FNA biopsy (see Fig. 2.8):

1. Cameco or other adequate syringe pistol,
2. 12.0-ml disposable plastic syringes with Luer Lok tip,
3. 22- to 25-gauge disposable needles, $1^1/_4$ in. and $3^1/_2$ in. long,
4. Alcohol prep sponges,
5. Microscopic glass slides,
6. Glass cover slips,
7. Spray fixative or a jar with 95% ethyl alcohol for fixation of smears,
8. Sterile gauze pads,
9. 1% lidocaine (optional),
10. Dif-Quik or other rapid metachromatic stains.

Aspiration of Palpable or Superficial Masses

The patient to undergo FNA should be in a comfortable position. However, the positioning should also allow the operator to fix the mass with the nonaspirating hand, at which time an estimation of the depth of the mass can be made. We prefer to administer a local anesthetic since at least two passes will be performed in order to ensure that an adequate specimen is obtained. The local anesthetic minimizes the discomfort of introducing the needle through the skin. The anesthetic should not be injected into the lesion, as it may affect the cytology adversely, thus rendering interpretation difficult or impossible. With the skin and subcutis over the mass anesthetized, the skin is swabbed with an alcohol sponge. If the mass is superficial, it is grasped between the thumb and index finger of the free hand. The needle, which

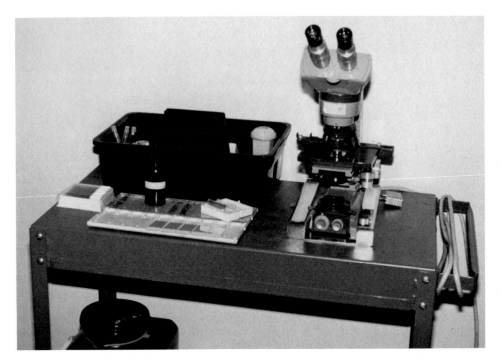

Figure 2.7.   Transportable equipment with microscope for fine-needle aspiration procedures.

has been attached to a syringe on the pistol grip, is guided to the aspiration site. Puncture of the skin should be through the previously anesthetized area. The needle is then advanced into the mass, during which suction is applied so that material will be drawn into the needle. The needle is moved back and forth within the mass in strokes of a few millimeters, which dislodges cells or small fragments of tissue. Constant suction should be maintained during these strokes, and it is recommended that the direction of the needle in the mass be varied with each stroke. This latter tactic ensures representative sampling of the lesion. The aspiration is usually stopped when blood or material are visible in the hub of the needle.

Before withdrawing the needle from the mass, it is critical that the vacuum in the syringe be released to prevent aspiration of material into the syringe, which makes retrieval extremely difficult. Furthermore, the process of attempting retrieval of the material in this eventuality unavoidably introduces air drying artifact. Pressure with a sterile gauze pad is applied over the biopsy site after with-drawal of the needle until hemostasis is attained.

Aspiration of Masses under Sonographic or Computed Tomographic Guidance

Since the 1970s, the diagnostic imaging of body parts has undergone marked improvement due to the availability of ultrasound scanning and computed tomography (CT). Refinements of the two basic technologies have significantly improved the clarity and resolution of the images. Reports of the use of needle aspiration biopsy coupled with ultrasound (31, 32) and CT guidance (33) followed soon after the adoption of these imaging techniques. Initially, the needle aspirations were done with static scanners, but developments in ultrasound scanning soon led to real-time control of aspirations with this modality.

Other factors that led to more generalized adoption of FNA biopsy of deep structures were the acceptance of a cytological diagnosis by clinicians and the development of a

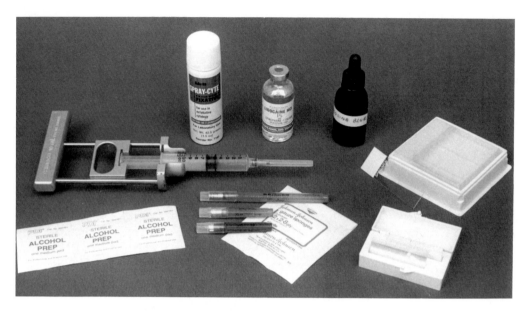

Figure 2.8. The equipment needed for fine-needle aspiration including, among other things, syringes, needles, fixative and toluidine blue stain.

suitable biopsy needle. Franzen developed a fine needle for the aspiration of cellular material from the prostate in 1960 (34). This needle, which is armed with a stylet and which has an outer diameter of 0.7 mm, was adopted in Japan and called the Chiba needle. The Chiba needle with a tip bevel of 45° is preferred for FNA biopsies of deep masses.

Fundamentally, the technique of FNA biopsy of deeply situated masses under image guidance is similar to that for palpable masses. However, in the former case, both hands are free and a pistol grip is not advantageous. In addition, since the needle will likely traverse either pleura or peritoneum and possibly the capsule of an organ, the procedure is somewhat more painful than a superficial aspiration. In any event, the needle is introduced through the skin and subcutaneous tissue with the stylet in place. Both needle and stylet are advanced until the lesion has been entered, at which point the stylet is withdrawn and a 12-ml syringe is attached to the hub of the needle. The plunger of the syringe is pulled back to produce 3 to 5 ml of suction to aspirate the material. With continued suction, the needle and syringe should be moved up and down in strokes of a few millimeters to dislodge additional material to be aspirated. To complete the procedure, the partial vacuum in the syringe is released and the syringe with needle are withdrawn. The material within the needle can be processed in several optional ways, as will be discussed below.

Preparation of Smears and Cell Blocks

After completing the aspiration, the needle is detached from the syringe and air is drawn into the syringe. The needle is then reattached to the syringe and a drop of fluid or material is gently expelled near the center of a glass slide. At this point, one can obtain a cytological preparation by bringing a second glass slide over the first slide at a near perpendicular angle, and gently smearing out the material. The smears can be allowed to air dry or they can be fixed immediately.

Alternatively, prior to smearing, one can apply a drop or two of a temporary stain, such as toluidine blue stain which also fixes the cells in the drop of material. The material can then be prepared as described above. After the slide is coverslipped the smear can be immediately examined to determine if the aspiration is adequate. The toluidine blue stain can be restained with the usual Papanicolaou stain after the coverslip is floated off in 95% ethanol.

Air-dried slides are processed with a Wright stain or the Dif-Quik stain, which is a rapid, modified Wright stain allowing visualization of the cells in a minute or two. The commercially available Dif-Quik stain can be employed to evaluate adequacy of an aspirate. If only blood or debris is present in the aspirate, another aspiration to obtain cells of interest is attempted.

If a smear is designated for Pap staining, then immediate fixation of the still wet smear is required to prevent air drying artifact among the cells. Fixation can be accomplished with a commercial spray fixative or by immersing the smear in 95% ethanol. The slide can then be transported to the laboratory for staining.

After most material in the needle has been expressed for smear preparation, or if visible pieces of the tissue are present with a drop of material on a glass slide, preparation of a cell block should be considered. This means that the material in the needle should be washed out and saved in either a saline or fixative solution. Tissue fragments are plucked from the droplet of material and saved in the same solution used to wash the aspiration needle. If a core of tissue is obtained as a histological specimen, this is usually placed in a fixative such as formalin. More recently, pathologists have placed these specimens in a Lavandowski's fixative of 10% formalin, 95% ethanol, and acetic acid for transport to pathology. Later the cell block is obtained following centrifugation of the wash solution at 2000 rpm for 5 minutes and decantation of the supernatant. The cell block is then processed like a biopsy specimen; fixation, embedding in paraffin, sectioning, and staining are identical.

Permanent Procedures

In our laboratory both air-dried and fixed smears are prepared at the time of aspiration biopsy because we feel that Pap stained and Wright stained smears are complementary. However, the experience of the cytopathologist who is reviewing the cytology will dictate the choice of stain. If the cytopathologist's background is in exfoliative cytology, the Pap stain may be favored. However, if the cytopathologist's background is hematologic, then the Wright stain may be preferred. The prepared smears must be fixed to be suitable for the Pap stain.

Air-dried smears are suitable for staining with the Wright stain or with any of the special histochemical stains, such as mucicarmine, Prussian blue, or Fontana-Masson stains. Furthermore, air-dried smears are usually necessary in the evaluation of a hematologic malignancy as immunoperoxidase techniques employing monoclonal antibodies can now better classify a leukemia or malignant lymphoma (35). In cases where the origin of a malignant neoplasm is not immediately apparent, immunoperoxidase studies on air-dried material may provide an answer (36).

As the cell block often contains small tissue fragments, hematoxylin and eosin (H&E) stained sections from this material may simulate a minibiopsy. Such a cell block complements the cytologic interpretation of the smears and reduces the likelihood of a false-positive or a false-negative diagnosis. Like the usual biopsy specimen, the cell block material can be stained with various histochemical stains as an aid to diagnosis. A number of commercially available antibodies can be applied to formalin-fixed material in the immunoperoxidase technique of staining tissue sections, and their number is increasing rapidly. Thus, the cell block material can also be used for this diagnostic modality should the need arise. As a further diagnostic aid, the cell block can be processed for ultrastructural studies by means of electron microscopy.

It is extremely helpful if ultrastructural studies can be anticipated on clinical grounds, because an aliquot of an aspirate or a whole separate aspirate can be ejected into a 2% or 3% buffered glutaraldehyde solution for fixation and for optimal results. After proper fixation in buffered glutaraldehyde, the material is centrifuged in a conical tube at 1500 rpm for 10 minutes to obtain a cell block, which is subsequently embedded.

At our institution, due to considerations of speed, simplicity, and cost, a hierarchy of further investigative studies is followed:

1. Cytochemical or histochemical stains on air-dried smears or cell block, respectively,
2. Immunoperoxidase staining of air-dried smears or cell block sections,
3. Ultrastructural studies of cell block thin section.

In most cases in which diagnostic difficulties are encountered, the special stains are sufficient to provide the information that is clinically needed to manage the patient. Electron microscopy is reserved for those infrequent cases where other special procedures are equivocal.

DIAGNOSTIC POSSIBILITIES FROM FINE-NEEDLE ASPIRATION BIOPSY BY BODY REGIONS AND SPECIFIC ORGANS

The primary use of FNA biopsy cytology lies in the investigation of lumps or masses that are clinically suspected to be malignant. With optimal aspiration technique and cytologic interpretation, a sensitivity of 80% to 95% can generally be expected in patients with a malignant tumor. The false-negative rate of FNA biopsy is approximately 5% to 20%, even with optimal conditions; if clinical suspicion remains after negative cytologic results, a biopsy for histologic examination should be obtained.

The most common causes of a false negative aspiration are: 1) failure to sample the lesion, particularly if it is less than 1 cm in diameter; 2) an extremely vascular lesion or organ, in which case blood rather than cells of interest is aspirated; and 3) the desmoplastic nature of some tumors, such as pancreatic adenocarcinomas or some ductal carcinomas of the breast, from which few or no neoplastic cells can be aspirated.

In benign or inflammatory conditions, FNA biopsy cytology is more often less specific diagnostically than with malignant disease. However, in the case of benign cystic lesions, aspiration may be therapeutic pro-

vided there is no residual mass. After ascertaining that a lesion is inflammatory in nature, FNA-obtained material may be utilized for microbiologic investigation.

Head and Neck

In the head and neck region, the lesions that have been investigated by fine-needle aspiration have most often been palpable masses occurring in the salivary glands, lymph nodes, or thyroid gland (Fig. 2.1). Occasionally, examination of thyroid lesions can be aided by ultrasonography or CT scanning in the selection of the aspiration site (Fig. 2.2).

However, with intracranial focal lesions intraoperative ultrasound has proved to be extremely useful in guiding placement of a fine needle in order to obtain material for cytologic diagnosis. If the lesion is an abscess or a cyst, ultrasound or CT guidance can allow its aspiration and prove to be therapeutic. Moran and Naidich (37) have described the technique as well as their results. In their group of 15 tumors an accurate diagnosis was provided by CT-guided aspiration in 13 cases (87%).

Recently, ophthalmologists have also adopted the technique of fine-needle aspiration to cytologically diagnose orbital lesions suspected of being malignant. Both ultrasonography and CT scanning are useful for determining the nature and the extent of a mass lesion, selecting the most appropriate direction for the needle's approach to the biopsy site, and verifying that the needle tip is within the lesion prior to aspiration. Dubois and Kennerdell (38) have reviewed the technique, indications, and contraindications of fine-needle aspiration of orbital lesions.

Breast

Palpable breast masses generally have been aspirated successfully and diagnosed cytologically without requiring radiologic imaging. The application of mammography for screening purposes makes possible the detection of a nonpalpable breast lesion, and its location and depth can be estimated from the mammogram. More precise localization of the lesion can be achieved by one of the several methods, which are described by Elyaderani (39). A 22-gauge needle can then be introduced into the localized area for the purpose of aspiration biopsy, which can result in a prompt diagnosis. Ultrasound is very useful in guiding needle placement.

In centers that evaluate large numbers of breast aspirates, the false-positive rate is approximately 1% (40, 41). Most frequently, false-positive diagnosis of malignancy results from technically inadequate smears or artifacts such as air drying. Our experience corresponds to the published literature with respect to accuracy and specificity. Fibrocystic disease is most often associated with a false-positive or false suspicious diagnosis because fibrocystic disease can yield a cellular smear with considerable cellular atypia.

False-negative diagnoses range from a low of 2% (42) to 18% (43). The causes of false-negative diagnoses are failure to pass the needle tip into the tumor, particularly with a small lesion; attempting to aspirate a scirrhous carcinoma, which can lead to a scanty cellularity in the smears; and/or failure to recognize malignant cells. Figure 2.3 shows a scirrhous carcinoma with atypia and prominent nucleoli. Kline (44) has reviewed factors responsible for recognition failure, including inexperience, monomorphism, and the small size of cell or nucleus.

Thorax

The work of Dahlgren and Nordenstrom (45) stimulated the application of transthoracic aspiration biopsy, and there is now widespread acceptance of the method (46, 47). The technique has gained widest acceptance in the investigation of focal pulmonary lesions, particularly tumors. However, pulmonary fine-needle aspiration can provide specimens for culture and for special stains or smears in cases of suspected infectious etiology. Pulmonary aspiration is less useful in establishing a specific disease entity when a pneumoconiosis is strongly suspected. Ultrasound may be used to guide needle placement when the lesion abuts the pleura, thus providing an appropriate acoustic window.

The technique is especially useful in patients who cannot undergo bronchoscopy or who previously have had a negative bronchoscopic biopsy following repeated nondiagnostic sputum examinations. In addition, however, fine-needle aspiration can be a useful diagnostic tool in evaluating mediastinal and pleural lesions. Diagnostic rates of 92% (48) and 96% (49) have recently been reported with intrathoracic fine-needle aspiration (Fig. 6.4). With poorly differentiated squamous cell carcinomas, poorly differentiated adenocarcinomas, and large-cell carcinomas, the cytopathologist may not be able to reliably distinguish these tumors. In general, though, it is possible to distinguish the neoplasms from small-cell carcinomas and from each other when better differentiated lesions are the object of study. In summary, those diagnostic problems that may concern the cytopathologist are the same as those that plague the histopathologist.

Application of FNA intraoperatively has been evaluated and found to be a valuable adjunct to frozen-section diagnosis. It is especially useful when sharp dissection is not possible or is hazardous. In our laboratory, general diagnostic accuracy (cancer or inflammatory) was 100%, while specificity of cell type was 89% (50).

Abdomen

Because disease of the gastrointestinal tract usually can be investigated by endoscopic methods, fine-needle aspiration in the abdomen is commonly restricted to solid abdominal organs; most commonly the liver and intraabdominal lymph nodes. Both ultrasonography and computed tomography can significantly increase the chance of a successful aspiration and reduce the likelihood of complications in intraabdominal procedures.

The most common indication for hepatic fine-needle aspiration is a focal mass lesion, but diffuse disease can also be diagnosed by this technique with reasonable accuracy. Contraindications to the procedure include blood coagulation defects and suspicion of a hydatid cyst or vascular lesion. The highest accuracy with hepatic aspiration is attained with malignant disease (Fig. 2.5). The liver is a very common site of metastatic adenocarcinoma and it may be impossible to differentiate it with certainty from one form of primary carcinoma in the liver, the cholangiocarcinoma. Furthermore, regenerating cells in cirrhosis may closely resemble cells of hepatocellular carcinoma. Recent studies of aspirations of focal liver masses showed that 87% to 91% were correctly diagnosed as malignant with no false positives (51, 52).

Retroperitoneum

Virtually all organs of the retroperitoneum are accessible to the fine needle for aspiration biopsy with radiologic guidance (Fig. 2.6). Diagnostic aspiration of a focal mass in the pancreas, kidney, adrenal gland, and retroperitoneal lymph node can establish whether the mass is malignant or not. The uncommon soft tissue tumors of the retroperitoneum can be evaluated for malignancy by aspiration biopsy, although a specific type may be unrecognizable cytologically or even histologically. Obviously, the size of a retroperitoneal lesion is a major limitation on FNA biopsy. Methods of localization of lesions involving retroperitoneal organs are fully reviewed elsewhere (53).

Ultrasonography or computed tomography may be useful in localizing a space-occupying lesion in the pancreas for a biopsy by the FNA technique. FNA biopsy is most useful in preoperative diagnosis of solid pancreatic neoplasms. Ultrasound localization of a pancreatic lesion, particularly if it is small, is hindered by the presence of gas in the bowel, which is not a difficulty for CT. Recent series of diagnosis of pancreatic malignancies by FNA show a sensitivity between 76% and 81% with a specificity of 100% (54, 55).

Fluoroscopy, ultrasound, or computed tomography can be used for guidance of an FNA procedure to aspiriate solid or cystic renal lesions for diagnostic or management purposes. Ultrasonography is the preferred imaging modality in the diagnostic workup of a renal mass. In general, benign cystic lesions can be diagnosed with confidence, but if not all criteria for a diagnosis of benign re-

nal cyst are met, CT may be a useful adjunct for this purpose. Failure to identify a renal lesion as a benign simple cyst by radiographic means requires further investigation, which may include FNA for cytologic examination. Sensitivities between 73% and 93% and specificities between 96% and 100% are reported in recent FNA diagnosis of renal neoplasms (56, 57).

The adrenal glands are infrequent sites for malignant diseases, which may be metastatic or primary. Because of their small size, the adrenals are preferably imaged by CT rather than ultrasonography for diagnostic FNA. The primary neoplasms in the adrenal glands include adrenal cortical adenoma or carcinoma, pheochromocytoma, and neuroblastoma. Differentiation of adenoma or carcinoma arising in the adrenal cortex may be impossible cytologically.

REFERENCES

1. Papanicolaou GN: Epithelial regeneration in uterine glands and on the surface of the uterus. *Am J Clin Gynecol* 25:30, 1933.
2. Papanicolaou GN, Trout HF, Marchetti AA: *The Epithelial of Women's Reproductive Organs: A Correlative Study of Cyclic Changes.* New York, Commonwealth Foundation, 1948.
3. Pak HY, Yokota S, Teplitz RL, Shaw SL, Werner, TL: Rapid staining techniques employed in fine needle aspirations of the lung *Acta Cytol* 25: 178–184, 1981.
4. Decaro L, Pak HY, Yokota S, Teplitz RL, Benfield JR: Intraoperative cytodiagnosis of lung tumors by needle aspiration. *J Thorac Cardio Surg* 85:404–408, 1983.
5. Pak HY, Ashdjian V, Yokota S, Teplitz RL: Quantitative DNA determinations by image analysis I. Applications to human pulmonary cytology. *Anal Quant Cytol* 4:95–98, 1982.
6. Pak HY, Teplitz RL, Ashdjian V, Yokota S, Hammond W, Benfield JR: Quantitative DNA determination by image analysis II. Application to human and canine pulmonary cytology. *Anal Quant Cytol* 5:263–268, 1983.
7. Teplitz RL, Hill LR: Quantitative DNA in bronchogenic carcinoma. *Anal Quant Cytol* 6:95–98, 1984.
8. Auer GW, Caspersson TO, Wallgren AS: DNA content and survival. *Anal Quant Cytol* 2:161–165, 1980.
9. Auer GW, Eriksson E, Azavedo E, Caspersson TO, Wallgren A: Prognostic significance of nuclear DNA content in mammary Adenocarcinomas in humans. *Cancer Res* 44:394–396, 1984.
10. Welch WR, Fu YS, Robboy SJ, Herbst AL: Nuclear DNA content of clear cell adenocarcinoma of the vagina and cervix and its relationship to prognosis. *Gynecol Oncol* 15:230–233, 1983.
11. Atkins NB: Prognostic significance of ploidy levels

in human tumors. I. Carcinoma of the uterus. *J Nat Cancer Inst* 56:909–912, 1976.

12. Friedlander ML, Taylor IW, Russell P, Tatersall MHN: Cellular DNA content—a stable feature in epithelial ovarian cancer. *Br J Cancer* 49:173–175, 1984.

13. Erkardt K, Auer G, Bjorkholm E, Forsslund G, Moberger B, Silversward C, Wicksell G, Zetterberg A: Prognostic significance of nuclear DNA content in serous ovarian tumor. *Cancer Res* 44:2198–2201, 1984.

14. Kokal WA, Sheibani K, Terz J, Harada JR: Tumor DNA content in prognosis of colorectal carcinoma. *JAMA* 255:3123–3125, 1986.

15. Wooley RC, Schreiber K, Koss LG et al: DNA distribution in human colon carcinomas and its relationship to clinical behavior. *J Nat Cancer Inst* 69:15-19, 1982.

16. Boon ME, Lowhagen T, Cardozo PL, Blonk DI, Kuver PJH, Baak JPA: Computation of preoperative diagnosis probability for follicular adenoma and carcinoma of the thyroid on aspiration smears. *Anal Quant Cytol* 4:1–5, 1982.

17. Teplitz RL, Tesluk H, Unni K: Quantitative DNA values in osteoblastoma (Abstract submitted, 1988).

18. Nasiell M, Kato H, Auer G, Zetterberg A, Roger V, Karlen L: Cytomorphological grading and Feulgen DNA analysis of metaplastic and neoplastic bronchial cells. *Cancer* 41:1511–1515, 1978.

19. Teplitz RL, Butler BB, Min BY, Russell LA, Tesluk H, Jensen H, Hill LR: Quantitative DNA patterns in preneoplastic breast lesions of man and mouse. Abstract presented at the American Society of Cytology. November 1-6, 1988, Kansas City (Submitted for publication).

20. Martin HE, Ellis EB: Biopsy of needle puncture and aspiration. *Ann Surg* 92:169–181, 1930.

21. Stewart FEW: The diagnosis of tumors by aspiration. *Am J Path* 9:801–812, 1933.

22. Martin HE, Ellis EB: Aspiration biopsy. *Surg Gynecol Obstet* 59:578–589, 1934.

23. Lopes-Cardozo P: *Clinical Cytology. Leiden, Staflen, 1954.*

24. Soderstrom N: *Fine Needle Aspiration Biopsy.* Stockholm, Almquist and Wiksell, 1966.

25. Franzen S, Giertz G, Zajicek J: Cytologic diagnosis of prostatic tumors by transrectal aspiration biopsy: A preliminary report. *Br J Urol* 32:193–196, 1960.

26. Zajicek J: Aspiration biopsy cytology. Part 1. Cytology of supra-diaphragmatic organs. *Monographs in Clinical Cytology,* Vol 4. Basel, S Karger, 1974.

27. Zajicek J: Aspiration biopsy cytology. Part 2. Cytology of infra-diaphragmatic organs. *Monographs in Clinical Cytology,* Vol 7. Basel, S Karger, 1979.

28. Fox CH: Innovation in medical diagnosis: The Scandinavian curiosity. *Lancet* 1:1387–1388, 1979.

29. Zornoza J (ed): *Percutaneous Needle Biopsy.* Baltimore, Williams & Wilkins, 1981.

30. Otto RC, Wellauer J: *Ultrasound-guided Biopsy and Drainage.* Berlin, Springer-Verlag, 1986.

31. Goldberg BB, Pollack HM: Ultrasonic aspiration transducer. *Radiology* 102:187–189, 1972.

32. Hancke S, Holm HH, Koch F: Ultrasonically guided percutaneous fine needle biopsy of the pancreas. *Surg Gynecol Obstet* 140:361–364, 1975.

33. Haaga JR, Alfidi RJ: Precise biopsy localization by computed tomography. *Radiology* 118:603–607, 1976.

34. Franzen S, Giertz G, Zajicek J: Cytological diagnosis of prostatic tumours by transrectal aspiration biopsy. A preliminary report. *Br J Urol* 32:193–196, 1960.

35. Levitt S, Cheng L, DuPuis MH, Layfield LJ: Fine needle aspiration diagnosis of malignant lymphoma with confirmation by immunoperoxidase staining. *Acta Cytol* 29:895–902, 1985.

36. Taylor RC: Fixation, processing, special applications. In Taylor RC (ed): *Immunomicroscopy: A Diagnostic Tool for the Surgical Pathologist.* Philadelphia, WB Saunders, 1986, pp 43–69.

37. Moran CJ, Naidich TP: Central nervous system. In Zornoza J (ed): *Percutaneous Needle Biopsy.* Baltimore, Williams & Wilkins, 1981, pp 13–27.

38. Dubois PJ, Kennerdell JS: Orbit. In Zornoza J (ed): *Percutaneous Needle Biopsy.* Baltimore, Williams & Wilkins, 1981, pp 28–36.

39. Elyaderani MK: Aspirations performed for miscellaneous conditions. In Letourneau JG, Elyaderani MK, Castaneda-Zuniga WK (ed): *Percutaneous Biopsy, Aspiration, and Drainage.* Chicago, Year Book, 1987, pp 146–158.

40. Stayric GD, Tevecev DT, Kaftandiiev DR, Novak JJ: Aspiration biopsy cytologic method in diagnosis of breast lesions: A critical review of 250 cases. *Acta Cytol* 17:188–190, 1973.

41. Zajdela A, Ghossein NA, Pilleron JP, Ennuyer A: The value of aspiration cytology in the diagnosis of breast cancer: Experience at the Fondation Curie. *Cancer* 35:499–506, 1975.

42. Schondorf H: *Aspiration Cytology of the Breast.* Philadelphia, WB Saunders, 1978.

43. Rosen P, Hajdu SI, Robbins G, Foote FEW: Diagnosis of carcinoma of the breast by aspiration biopsy. *Surg Gynecol Obstet* 134:837–838, 1972.

44. Kline TS: Breast. In *Handbook of Fine Needle Aspiration Biopsy Cytology.* St. Louis, CV Mosby, 1981.

45. Dahlgren SE, Nordenstrom B: *Transthoracic Needle Biopsy.* Chicago, Year Book, 1966.

46. Arnston TL, Bayd WR: Percutaneous biopsy using a safe, effective needle. *Radiology* 127:265, 1978.

47. Berquist TH, Bailey LB, Cartese DA, Miller WE: Transthoracic needle biopsy: Accuracy in relation to type of lesion. *Mayo Clin Proc* 55:475–481, 1980.

48. Kamholz SL, Pinsker, KL, Johnson J, Schreiber K: Fine needle aspiration biopsy of intrathoracic lesions. *NY State J Med* 82:736–739, 1982.

49. Yazdi, HM, McDonald LL, Hickey NM: Thoracic fine needle aspiration biopsy versus fine needle cutting biopsy. *Acta Cytol* 32:635–640, 1988.

50. Decaro LF, Pak HY, Yokota S, Teplitz RL, Benfield JR: Intraoperative cytodiagnosis of lung tumors by needle aspiration. *J Thorac Cardiovasc Surg* 85:404, 1983.

51. Rosenblatt R, Kutcher R, Moussouris HF, Schreiber K, Koss LG: Sonographically guided fine needle aspiration of liver lesions. *JAMA* 248:1639–1641, 1982.

52. Pinto MM, Avila NA, Heller CI, Crisuolo EM: Fine needle aspiration of the liver. *Acta Cytol* 32:15–21, 1988.

53. Letourneau JG, Elyaderani MK, Castaneda-Zuniga

WR: *Percutaneous Biopsy, Aspiration and Drainage.* Chicago, Year Book, 1987.

54. Pilotti S, Rilke F, Claren R, Milella M, Lombardi L: Conclusive diagnosis of hepatic and pancreatic malignancies by fine needle aspiration. *Acta Cytol* 32:27–38, 1988.

55. Pinto MM, Avila NA, Criscuolo EM: Fine needle aspiration of the pancreas: A five-year experience. *Acta Cytol* 32:39–42, 1988.

56. Dekmezian RH, Charnsangavej C, Rava P, Katz, RL: Fine needle aspiration of kidney tumors in 105 patients: A cytologic and histologic correlation. *Acta Cytol* 29:931, 1985.

57. Pilotti S, Rilke F, Alasio L, Garbagnati F: The role of fine needle aspiration in the assessment of renal masses. *Acta Cytol* 32:1–10, 1988.

3 The Sonographer's Role in Invasive Procedures

SANDRA E. MALESKI
JOHN P. McGAHAN

Introduction

The medical team for an interventional ultrasound procedure consists of a physician, a registered diagnostic medical sonographer, and, occasionally, a registered nurse. As a member of the interventional team, the sonographer's main role is to assist the physician during the procedure. The sonographer is responsible for performing and recording the ultrasound examination, guiding the physician's efforts, and keeping records of the procedure. The sonographer must insure that the patient is prepared and that the appropriate equipment and supplies are available. It therefore cannot be overstated that the ultrasonographer plays a vital role in the successful performance of an ultrasound guided invasive procedure.

Required Background

Depending on the institution, the sonographer's formal training may or may not specifically cover interventional procedures; in any case, considerable practical experience is required to master the delicate methods. Hands-on experience is commonly gained by working closely with an experienced sonologist or sonographer during several procedures. It is best to start with a relatively simple technique, such as fluid aspiration, before advancing to more complex procedures. Since most interventional ultrasound procedures are performed under sterile conditions, a thorough understanding of sterile techniques is essential. In addition, a composed temperament is an asset; the sonographer should exhibit a steady, relaxed demeanor to best assist the physician and the patient.

The Planning Process

The sonographer's role in planning the procedure is extremely important as he/she must fully understand and coordinate the efforts of the interventional team to insure a smooth, trouble-free procedure. The sonographer must thoroughly understand the procedure and any possible alternatives. For instance, a relatively simple procedure such as a paracentesis may reveal an abscess requiring percutaneous drainage with a large-bore catheter. Lack of preparation by the sonographer for this alternative could result in an unacceptable delay. It is vital that the sonographer not only understand the exact nature of the procedure, but also be aware of the pertinent patient information and the type of equipment required, including needle sizes, biopsy guides, and catheters. Clear communication between the sonographer and other members of the medical team is essential.

Initially, the sonographer and the physician should meet to discuss the exact details of the planned procedure. This discussion should focus on the primary approach as well as possible alternatives. Together, the sonographer and the physician should select

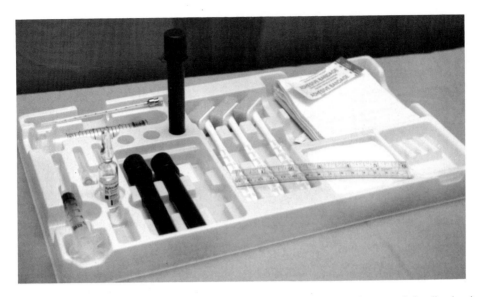

Figure 3.1. A commercially available prepackaged aspiration/biopsy tray contains the basic necessities such as needles, syringes, local anesthesia, for performing any invasive ultrasound technique.

the appropriate equipment and supplies from the ultrasound laboratory. A variety of general purpose items such as acoustic gel, video tapes, and film cassettes must be readily available. In our institution, we use a commercially available prepackaged aspiration/biopsy tray that contains needles, syringes, local anesthetics, and other items needed for sterile, interventional procedures (Figs. 3.1, 3.2)

To further facilitate the selection process, we have dedicated a room in our ultrasound department for guidance of invasive procedures. Here, specialized needles, catheters, guidewires, and dilators are easily accessible (Fig. 3.3). Sterile gloves, bowls, povidone-

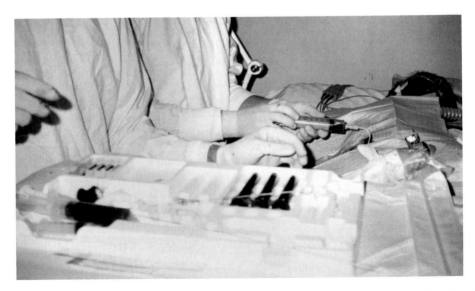

Figure 3.2. Commercially available prepackaged aspiration/biopsy tray placed within the sterile field at the patient's bedside when performing an invasive procedure.

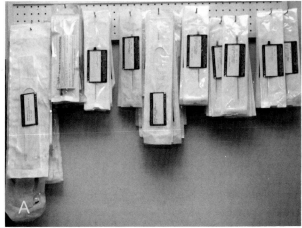
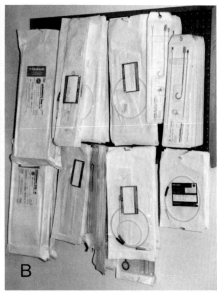

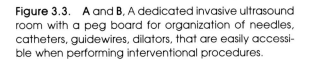

Figure 3.3. **A** and **B**, A dedicated invasive ultrasound room with a peg board for organization of needles, catheters, guidewires, dilators, that are easily accessible when performing interventional procedures.

iodine, suture material, and other supplies are well organized within supply cabinets. All these supplies are within a hand's reach of the sonographer or sonologist so as not to cause any delay if there is an alternative plan with the invasive procedures. To start, we recommend a checklist be used for preparation of each procedure (Table 3.1).

We also keep a large supply bag fully stocked with various items such as povidone iodine, sterile gloves, sterile bowls, specialized needles, catheters, and other materials

so that we are prepared to perform portable ultrasound-guided invasive procedures anywhere in the hospital (Fig. 3.4).

Equipment selected for an invasive procedure may be predetermined by the specific procedure being performed. For instance, a brain biopsy will require a high-resolution probe with a small contact surface. Several commercially available ultrasound units are dedicated to intraoperative ultrasound guidance. Other equipment considerations include system resolution, availability of

Table 3.1.

The following list is intended as a guide for developing a customized checklist* for ultrasound-guided aspiration/biopsy or drainage procedures:

Film	Sterile gauze pads
Video Tape	Sterile bowls
Acoustic gel	Sterile tubes for fluid collection
Biopsy guides	Sterile dressings
Povidone-iodine	Drainage bags
Sterile covering for	Suture material
transducer	Needles (injection & biopsy types)
Sterile gloves	Syringes
Local anesthetic	Dilators
Scalpel	Guidewires
Sterile drapes	Catheters

* Many of these supplies are included in a prepackaged aspiration/biopsy tray.

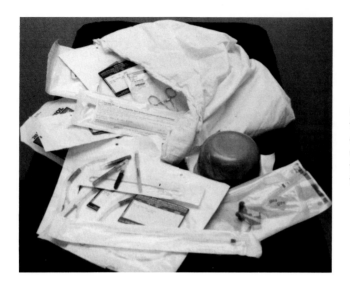

Figure 3.4. A portable supply bag fully stocked with specialized needles, catheters, sterile gloves, allows ultrasound guidance of interventional techniques to be performed throughout the hospital.

guidance attachments, the size, frequency, and focal characteristics of the transducer and the portability of the ultrasound system if the procedure is to be performed elsewhere within the hospital.

After selecting the appropriate supplies and equipment, the sonographer and physician must determine the location within the hospital where the invasive procedure will be performed. We prefer that simple aspiration procedures be performed in the ultrasound department where equipment and accessories are readily available. Simple aspirations such as thoracenteses or paracenteses are easily performed at the patient's bedside when the patient is critically ill. Drainage procedures are best performed in the main radiology department with the combined use of CT, ultrasound, and/or fluoroscopy. However, the patient's condition may determine the location of the procedure. For example, if the patient is on a respirator and other life support devices, it may be more expedient and safer to conduct the procedure at the patient's bedside.

In all situations, the sonographer must inform the patient's nurse and ward team of the procedure to coordinate nursing efforts and to answer questions. Will the patient's nurse be on hand to monitor vital signs and administer drugs or should the department nurse be notified? Should other appropriate hospital personnel such as respiratory ther-

apists or interpreters be needed? In our hospital, the cytologist is always present when a biopsy is performed so that immediate evaluation of the specimen can be conducted. Therefore, informing the cytologist well in advance of any scheduled biopsy is always appreciated. Once again, it is vital that the sonographer effectively communicate with members of the medical team to insure a smooth and successful outcome of the invasive procedure.

Gathering pertinent patient information is yet another responsibility of the sonographer when planning for an ultrasound-guided invasive procedure. Previous diagnostic studies should be reviewed to provide a better understanding of the patient's condition. The sonographer should verify with the attending physician that coagulation studies have been completed and are within an acceptable range (1, 2). He or she should verify that the important legal matter of informed consent has been discussed with the patient prior to initiating the procedure.

In summarizing the planning process, the following items are critical to the success of an ultrasound-guided ainterventional procedure:

- A thorough understanding of the procedure and possible alternatives,
- Clear and concise communication with team members,

- Careful selection of appropriate supplies and equipment,
- Sensible determination of where the procedure is to be performed,
- Complete coordination of the nursing staff and other hospital personnel, and
- Thorough collection of pertinent patient information.

Preparing the Equipment

Even the smallest details, such as optimum positioning of the ultrasound console in relation to the patient and workspace, are important in effectively performing an interventional ultrasound procedure. The ultrasonographer is responsible for room preparation and, therefore, several important points should be emphasized: 1) the ultrasound system console must be positioned so that the power cord can be plugged into a power source; 2) the transducer cable must be able to easily reach the patient, and 3) both physician and the sonographer must be able to see the ultrasound system monitor. We have found that proper positioning of the console is important to allow the physician easy visualization of the monitor with ample working space and simultaneously allow the sonographer clear access to the ultrasound console to optimize and record images.

When preparing the ultrasound probe and accessories for an interventional procedure, slightly different requirements exist depending on the location of the procedure. If the procedure is to be performed in surgery, a sterile sheath covering the transducer as well as the transducer cable is required (3, 4). Many times, we double cover the transducer head to avoid inadvertent contamination. The sonologist or a member of the surgical team handles the sterile transducer while the sonographer, in a sterile cap, gown, mask, and shoe coverings, remains outside the sterile field to optimize system settings and document the procedure on hard copy or video tape. The sonographer also helps in placing sterile coverings over the ultrasound probe so the transducer can be placed into the sterile surgical field (Fig. 3.5). Recently, several manufacturers have introduced gas-sterilized transducers that do not require sterile coverings.

If the interventional procedure is to take place in the ultrasound suite, at the patient's bedside, or in another location, we generally prefer to cover the transducer head with a sterile sheath or glove. This process is a cooperative effort between the physician and the sonographer. To begin, the physician holds a sterile sheath or glove turned partially inside out while the sonographer fills it with acoustic gel. The sonographer then places the transducer into the sheath; the physician pulls the sheath over the probe, completely encasing it (Fig. 3.6). Some hospitals use commercially available sterile probe covers that include sterile ties to hold the sheath snugly in place. We use a sterile glove for this purpose, using the fingers as ties to secure the covering over the probe.

Here, for discussion purposes, it is important to state that the degree of the ultrasound probe's sterility is dependent upon the location of the probe within the sterile field. There are those who do not advocate the use of sterile probe coverings if the transducer is positioned to the side of the entry site and the freehand method of needle guidance is used (5). However, in our hospital, with so many training physicians performing the ultrasound guided procedures, we always use sterile transducer coverings. Povidone-iodine or sterile gel should be used as a transmission medium.

Outside of the surgery suite, the sonographer's role in ultrasound-guided procedures may vary, ranging from optimizing the ultrasound images to scanning and guiding the needle placement. Again, this depends on the institution and the experience of the physician and sonographer. In each situation, the sonographer must be ready to play a major role in the invasive procedure by becoming familiar with the anatomical area of interest and understanding the planned approach as well as the desired outcome.

Preparing the Patient

A well-informed patient who understands the nature of the interventional

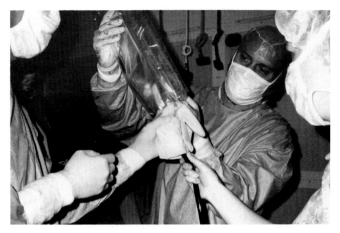

Figure 3.5. In the operating room, the sonographer usually does not scrub for the surgical procedure but instead assists the physician with sterile probe preparation for use in the operative field.

procedure, the reason for it and, most importantly, the benefits derived from it, will most often be a cooperative patient. In turn, a cooperative patient helps facilitate the procedure. Since the sonographer is usually the first person to see the patient prior to the interventional procedure, he or she must be prepared to explain what will take place, answer any questions the patient might have, alleviate apprehensions, and enlist the patient's cooperation. For example, the sonographer should stress the importance of proper suspension of respiration and the necessity of remaining as motionless as possible to insure a successful outcome.

Once the patient has a comfortable knowledge of what will take place, it is the sonographer's duty to position the patient so that optimal access to the anatomical area of interest is achieved. Discussion with the physician is important to determine the most appropriate route of needle access based upon patient comfort and the need to avoid vital intervening structures such as bowel or pleura. It may be necessary to use props such as pillows or angled sponges to help keep the patient immobile during the procedure. In the case of an unconscious patient or an extreme position, several people may be needed to hold the patient in place during the examination. Next, the sonographer must scan the area of interest to locate the specific anatomy and optimize and record the images before starting the interventional procedure.

For expediency, the sonographer should prepare the sterile tray and accessories while waiting for the physician. Once the physician arrives, the sonographer may be asked to re-scan the patient to orient the physician

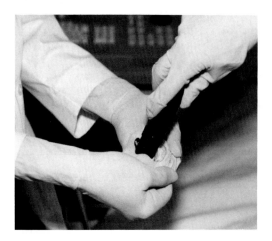

Figure 3.6. The ultrasound probe is prepared for scanning in the sterile field by placing the probe and a small amount of acoustic gel into a sterile glove.

to the area of interest. At this point, the physician is encouraged to scan to get an understanding of the position of the abnormality in relation to other anatomical structures and to more accurately assess the best approach.

Before the procedure begins, it is good practice to check once again that all the necessary supplies are on hand. This step is extremely important since unnecessary delays due to missing supplies could prove detrimental to the patient. For instance, if an aspiration procedure is being performed at the patient's bedside and then it is decided to change this procedure to a catheter drainage, considerable delay may occur if supplies must be retrieved from the main radiology department (6). In our department, we perform approximately one-third of our aspiration/drainage procedures at the patient's bedside (7).

The Interventional Procedure

While the physician performs the actual interventional procedure, the sonographer continues to play a crucial role as a member of the medical team, who may be required to perform a variety of functions during the exam. For example, when direct ultrasound needle guidance is necessary, the physician may ask the sonographer to scan while the physician directs the needle. In addition, the sonographer must control the ultrasound system settings, take appropriate measurements, and record the procedure on film or video tape, as directed by the physician. Once the needle or catheter is in place, the sonographer offers further assistance by providing sterile dressings, drainage bags, suture material, and other necessary supplies.

No procedure is considered complete until follow-up scans are performed immediately after the study. If a biopsy has been performed, it is extremely important to thoroughly check the biopsy site to rule out complications such as hemorrhage. Likewise, if an aspiration or drainage procedure has been done, it is necessary to evaluate the site for adequate fluid drainage. In all cases, the postprocedure sonograms must be documented on hard copy film or video tape.

Postprocedure

Following the interventional procedure it is important that the room is completely cleaned for scanning the next patient. This function must be completed with extreme caution due to the numerous contagious diseases transmitted by body fluids. We always recommend protective gloves for handling contaminated needles, syringes, etc. Needles and other items soiled with blood and/or body fluid should be placed in proper waste containers. Nondisposable items such as biopsy guide attachments must be thoroughly rinsed and prepared for sterilization. Thorough washing of the ultrasound console and transducers with alcohol or germicide is equally important. Usually in our department, after the transducer is cleansed with alcohol it is soaked in a germicide or disinfectant solution for a minimum of 20 minutes if the probe has been used in an invasive, surgical, or intracorporeal procedure. Clean equipment and accessories are necessary when performing any type of ultrasound procedure to inhibit spread of infection and disease.

Equally important is proper record keeping. This may vary among institutions, but will include logging in the procedure within the laboratory records, preparing the hard copy films and matching these with the patient's prior examination, and organizing the patient's file, request form and films for physician interpretation. In most hospitals and outpatient settings, billing forms must also be completed. Accurate record keeping is necessary in any diagnostic laboratory and is especially important when invasive procedures are performed. The records become part of the patient's medical file and serve as a permanent document for not only the patient but the medical team.

ACKNOWLEDGEMENTS

Special thanks to Karen Anderson for preparation of this chapter.

REFERENCES

1. Ferrucci JT Jr: Surgical and radiological foundations. In: Ferrucci JT Jr, Wittenberg J, Mueler PR, Simeone JF (eds): *Interventional Radiology of the Abdomen*, ed 2. Baltimore, Williams & Wilkins, 1985 pp 6–11.

2. Rapaport S: Preoperative hemostatic evaluation: Which tests, if any? *Blood* 61(2):229–231, 1983.
3. Knake JE, Bowerman RA, Silver TM, McCracken S: Neurosurgical applications of intraoperative ultrasound. *Radiol Clin North Am* 23:73–90, 1985.
4. McGahan JP, Boggan JE: Intraoperative ultrasound monitoring. In: McGahan JP (ed): *Controversies in Ultrasound*. New York, Churchill Livingstone, 1987 pp 289–307.
5. Reading CC, Charboneau JW, James EM, Hurt MR: Sonographically guided percutaneous biopsy of small (3 cm or less) masses. *AJR* 151:189–192, 1988.
6. Crass JR, Karl R: Bedside drainage of abscesses with sonographic guidance in the desperately ill. *AJR* 139:183–185, 1982.
7. McGahan JP, Anderson MW, Walter JP: Portable real-time sonographic and needle guidance systems for aspiration and drainage. *AJR* 147:1241–1246, 1986.

4 Intraoperative Cranial and Spinal Sonography

JOHN P. McGAHAN
BERTA M. MONTALVO
ROBERT M. QUENCER
JAMES E. BOGGAN

Recent technological innovations have made possible a variety of new applications for ultrasound guidance of invasive procedures. Ultrasound's role in guiding a number of the newer and specialized invasive procedures has been well described by other authors throughout this text. The emphasis of this chapter deals with the use of ultrasound in monitoring intraoperative neurosurgical procedures. Portable high-resolution equipment has allowed ultrasound to be used in examining patients in various locations throughout the hospital, including the operating room. The major applications of intraoperative cranial sonography (IOCS) include localization of brain tumors and monitoring the extent of surgical resection, guidance of subcortical brain biopsies, shunt-tube placement, and in the evaluation of intraoperative vascular procedures (1). In the spine, intraoperative spinal sonography (IOSS) has been used in detecting, defining extent of, and monitoring resection of spinal tumors; in monitoring surgical reduction of spinal fracture; and in guidance of the surgical approach to spinal stenosis and congenital lesions (2).

Ultrasound has several features that make it well suited for use in the operating room. Portable high-resolution real-time ultrasound units are available that have relatively small and easily maneuverable probes that fit into burr holes and hemilaminec-

tomy sites. Sterile drapes allow the ultrasound probe to be placed in direct contact with tissues being examined so that degradation of detail from intervening structures does not occur. By simply changing the orientation of the ultrasound probe, sonographic anatomy can be displayed in any orientation the surgeon desires. Structures are viewed in real time, that is, the image displayed on the video monitor is a precise reproduction of the tissue being scanned with the transducer at that instant. These features facilitate the use of ultrasound to define and localize disease precisely and help decrease complications by avoiding unnecessary surgical dissection (3). The use of ultrasound shortens the surgical procedure and helps to make it safer and more accurate. This chapter will outline the important technical considerations necessary when performing intraoperative sonography (IOS), briefly review the normal sonographic appearance of the intracranial and intraspinal contents and describe the important applications of ultrasound in the neurosurgical suite.

Ultrasound Advantages

There are certain features of real-time ultrasound that allow for its wide application in guidance of neurosurgical procedures (3). For instance, in most hospitals a high-resolution ultrasound scanner is already available (4). Almost any portable real-time unit with a sector transducer operating at frequencies from 5 MHz to 7.5 MHz is appropriate for use in the operating room. Unlike fixed stereotaxic computed tomography (CT) systems, the ultrasound units are easily moved to the operating room and the patient does not have to be placed into a headframe.

Intraoperative ultrasound has the advantage of displaying intracranial and spinal anatomy in real time. One can observe any change in the lesion, such as decreased size of the brain cyst or abscess during aspiration, during closed biopsy or instrumentation. This is not possible with CT, magnetic resonance imaging (MRI) or angiography. In closed brain biopsies the needle can be seen easily and verification of needle placement is immediate.

Unlike other imaging procedures IOS provides significant flexibility in that the anatomical plane of scan (coronal, sagittal, axial, or oblique) can be changed by simply rotating or tilting the transducer to locate masses less than 1 cm in diameter (5). This is particularly important when one considers the differences between the operating room position of the patient and the various radiological imaging scan planes.

The diameter, distance, or measurement of different regions of the imaged lesion of the brain can be obtained with the electronic digital calipers that are incorporated into the ultrasound machine. After the resection of lesions, ultrasound can be used to check for complications such as hemorrhage and to document the completeness of resection.

IOS usually requires little additional time commitment if there is proper notification of the sonographer on the day of examination. The average time actually spent scanning the patient is ten minutes, but may vary from ten minutes to two hours, depending on the length of the surgical procedure and the familiarity of the physician with IOS (6).

Technical Considerations

In general, ultrasound equipment is selected according to the exact applications for which sonography will be used. Most dedicated intraoperative ultrasound probes operate at frequencies between 5.0 to 10.0 MHz. Occasionally, lower frequency transducers (that is, 3.0–3.5 MHz) will be required in localizing deep-seated intracranial lesions or to assess a large area of brain in establishing relationships with other structures. High-frequency transducers provide higher resolution and improved image quality but have poor tissue penetration. A transducer with a frequency of 5 MHz is usually adequate for guidance of most brain biopsy procedures or shunt-tube placement, providing a good balance between sonographic resolution and tissue depth penetration. However, in detection of superficial cortical lesions, in the examination of the spinal cord, and for study of vascular structures, higher-frequency transducers (7.5 MHz or greater) provide the best anatomical detail (7).

Sterile technique is essential when using the ultrasound probe in the operating room. Gas sterilization is not used. The probe is cleansed thoroughly before each use. After cleansing, sterile scanning gel is placed in a sterile sheath or in the thumb of a surgical glove, and the probe is fitted into this covering. Occasionally, we have utilized double sheaths or gloves as added protection against inadvertent contamination of the operative field. If a glove is used, a sterile covering such as a stockinette or arthroscopic sleeve is placed over the cable of the ultrasound probe. Commercially available sterile sheaths are long enough to cover the cable. The sterile coverings are fastened into place with rubber bands or sterile ties, and any air bubbles are expressed away from the transducer face as they will degrade the image (Figs. 4.1, 4.2).

The brain is examined after craniotomy; the spinal cord after laminectomy. The size of the burr hole, craniotomy, or laminectomy will be determined by the planned surgical procedure and the size of the ultrasound probe. The footprint (tip) of most real-time sector probes is approximately 3 cm in diameter, and while it is possible to image the region of interest through small laminectomies or enlarged burr holes, opti-

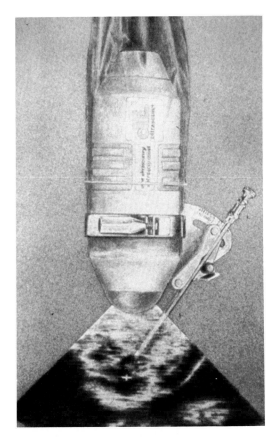

Figure 4.1. Image of ATL real-time sector scanner with biopsy guide and needle superimposed over ultrasound image showing the echogenic needle being placed into the lesion. (Courtesy of Advanced Technology Laboratories, Inc.; Bothell, Washington).

mal imaging is achieved with craniotomy or full laminectomy. Newer smaller ultrasound probes may fit into a burr hole.

Because the ultrasound beam is not transmitted by air, a coupling agent between the probe and the tissue to be examined is required. In the spine, the patient is prone and sterile saline is placed into the operative field. In the brain, continuous gentle irrigation of saline will usually maintain acoustical coupling between the probe and the brain. Having the exposed surface of the brain parallel to the floor will help maintain the saline-filled waterpath within the cranial opening (8). The brain can be imaged through closed or open dura with the transducer placed di-

rectly on the exposed surface; the spinal cord is usually imaged with the transducer suspended in a saline-filled water path without touching the closed dura.

The ultrasound image of superficial brain lesions may be obscured by near-field artifact caused by echoes originating from the surface of many transducers (5). This artifact is seen on the video screen as a 1- to 2-cm region of bright echoes adjacent to the transducer head. This obscuration of superficial anatomical detail may be avoided by placing a Lucite cylinder filled with saline over the area to be scanned (9,10). The distance of the probe from the cortical surface allows the brain to be scanned in the optimal focal plane of the transducer. However, newer high-frequency transducers operating at 10.0 MHz are better focused to allow good near-field imaging.

Adjustment of the ultrasound instrumentation ensures good tissue penetration, uniform intensity, and brightness. This is achieved by proper setting of different controls of the ultrasound equipment, the most important of which is the Time Gain Compensator (TGC). The TGC will determine the amplification of different portions of the ultrasound image. As the ultrasound beam penetrates into the target tissue, it is attenuated by intervening structures. Therefore, the sound reflected from deep structures must be amplified to a greater amount than the returning echoes from superficial structures if uniform image brightness is to be obtained. Increase in the overall gain may amplify the brightness of the entire ultrasound image. If these technical factors are not optimized, obscuration of lesions or misinterpretation of the image can occur.

Brain

NORMAL ANATOMY

Once the image is optimized, the brain appears hypoechoic while landmarks such as dural coverings, sulcal spaces, ventricular walls, choroid plexus, and bone appear brightly echogenic (11, 12; Fig. 4.3). Identification of arterial pulsations in major vessels is helpful for anatomical orientation. Cere-

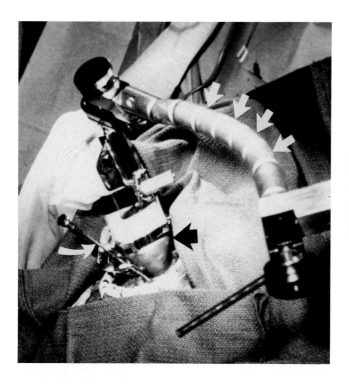

Figure 4.2. Real-time sector scanner (*black arrow*) fixed in place with surgical clamps (*white arrows*) after craniotomy. A biopsy needle (*curved arrow*) is fixed in guidance attachment for brain biopsy.

bral spinal fluid within the cisterns or ventricles is anechoic with ventricular walls appearing as well-demarcated echogenic lines. Scanning in at least two different anatomical planes is often necessary for orientation and to identify abnormal masses and their relationship to surrounding structures (11, Fig. 4.3). Ultrasound images may be recorded on videotape and/or hard copy.

BRAIN BIOPSY

Sonography may be used for guidance of intraoperative needle placement in the performance of brain biopsy, or for guidance of the transcortical surgical approach for open resection of lesions. After a craniotomy or placement of a burr hole, the ultrasound transducer is placed on the closed dura or

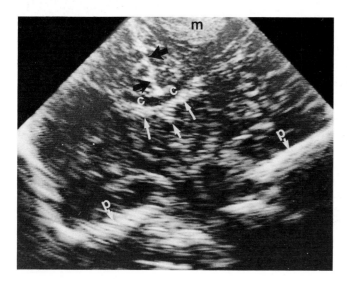

Figure 4.3. Normal Anatomy/Meningioma. Coronal sonogram depicting some of the normal landmarks of the brain, such as the interhemispheric fissure (between *black arrows*), the choroid plexus (*white arrows*) in the collapsed lateral and third ventricles, and the petrous bones (*p*). Mass (*m*) on the edge of the film represents a meningioma. (Reproduced with permission from Quencer RM, Montalvo BM: Intraoperative cranial sonography. *Neuroradiology* 28:528–550, ©1986, Springer-Verlag.)

cortical surface. Biopsy may be performed using the freehand method or one of the biopsy guidance systems discussed in Chapter 1 (Fig. 4.4). Alternatively, a calibrated guide may be attached to the ultrasound transducer to stabilize the biopsy needle relative to the transducer and ensure an appropriate needle trajectory to the desired target (3, 9, 10, 13; Fig. 4.5). Ultrasound transducers may also attach to self-retaining retractor arms that maintain the probe's position and eliminate unwanted movements that can occur when the probe is hand held (3, 10; Fig. 4.2).

Special biopsy needles have been designed to optimize sonographic visualization of the needle tip (14, 15). After needle biopsy of the brain, the biopsy track is visualized as an echogenic trail. This echogenic trail is thought to represent minor postbiopsy hemorrhage or residual air within the needle tract (9; Fig. 4.6). Following removal of the biopsy needle cannula, the transducer should be maintained in position for several minutes to check for hemorrhage at the biopsy site. The incidence of hemorrhage with closed needle biopsy is small and occurs in fewer than 5% of cases (5).

When 15-mm diameter burr hole ultrasound probes are used, the probe is usually removed and the biopsy needle placed in the desired trajectory without visualization of the needle on the video output screen (16; Fig. 4.7). A probe guide attached to the burr hole is locked into a fixed position after visualization of the target lesion determined during ultrasound imaging. The needle trajectory and the depth are determined by ultrasound. The ultrasound probe is then removed and replaced with a biopsy needle-guidance system. Although this is a "blind" biopsy without real-time imaging during

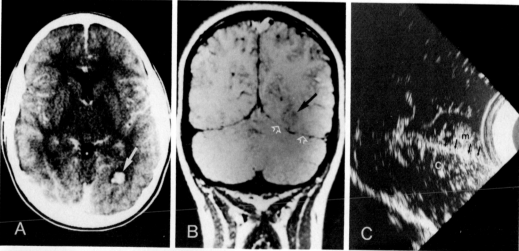

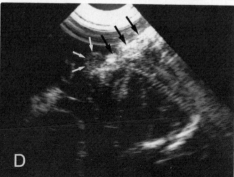

Figure 4.4. Freehand biopsy. Neuroectodermal tumor in the occipital lobe. **A,** Axial CT showing enhancing lesion (*arrow*) in the left occipital lobe. **B,** Coronal MR demonstrating the relationship of the mass (*black arrow*) to the tentorium cerebelli (*open arrows*). **C,** Left parasagittal sonogram. Mass (*m*), tentorium cerebelli (*arrows*), and cerebellum, (*C*). **D,** The surgeon had been unable to biopsy the lesion successfully because of its unusual position. By noting the relationship of the mass to the tentorium on the sonographic views, the surgeon directed the needle in the appropriate direction, and the biopsy was monitored with real-time. Left oblique view showing needle (*black arrows*) entering the mass (*white arrows*).

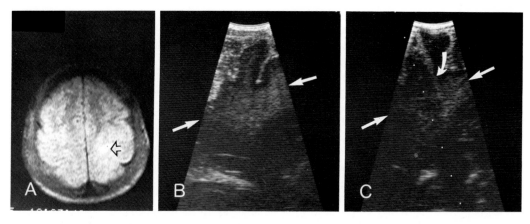

Figure 4.5. Closed brain biopsy of Grade II astrocytoma. **A,** Magnetic resonance scan shows an area of increased signal intensity in the posterior parietal region (*open arrow*). **B,** Intraoperative ultrasound performed through a small craniotomy defect shows ill-defined echogenic tumor (*arrows*). **C,** Echogenic biopsy needle (*curved arrow*) being placed into tumor (*arrows*). Biopsy demonstrated grade II astrocytoma. (Reproduced by permission from McGahan JP, Boggan JE: Intraoperative ultrasound monitoring. In McGahan JP (ed): *Controversies in Ultrasound*. New York, Churchill Livingstone, 289–307, 1987.)

needle placement, the needle follows the exact plane and preset depth as selected by the guidance system after it has been locked into place during sonographic imaging (17).

SHUNT CATHETER PLACEMENT

Placement of ventricular shunt catheters in infants is monitored by ultrasound performed through the anterior fontanel. Occasionally, the posterior fontanel may be used for sonographic monitoring. The shunt tube may be placed via the posterior parietal or the frontal approach under sonographic control. If the anterior fontanel is not placed within the sterile field, then the transducer probe need not be draped (9, 10, 18). The catheter tip should be placed within the frontal horn of the lateral ventricle anterior to the foramen of Monro. Malposition of the shunt and perforation of the septum pellucidum can be readily identified on sonography. If the catheter is seen coursing towards an improper location, it can be redirected easily. When the septum pellucidum is absent, the shunt tube may float freely from one lateral ventricle to the other (Fig. 4.8). Complications of ventricular catheter placement include brain parenchymal or in-

traventricular hemorrhage in the region of catheter insertion (19).

Sonographic monitoring of catheter placement for the purpose of draining fluid-filled cysts, either alone or in conjunction with shunting dilated ventricles, can ensure optimal drainage (11; Fig. 4.9).

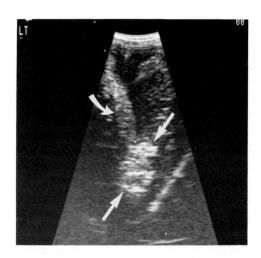

Figure 4.6. Glioma postbiopsy. Echogenic tract site identified (*curved arrow*) after biopsy of glioma (*arrows*). Echogenicity is thought to represent hemorrhage or air in needle tract.

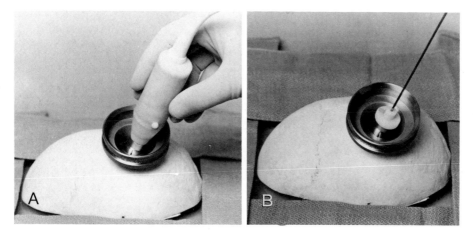

Figure 4.7. Burr hole biopsy. **A,** Diasonics burr hole transducer placed into Berger ring-type biopsy device. This device may be screwed into the skull and then fixed in position to a preselected angle for biopsy. **B,** After the ultrasound probe is removed, the needle attachment with a needle stop, set at a desired depth, is placed into the prefitted guidance device for lesion biopsy. (Courtesy of Mitchell Berger, M.D. of San Francisco, California, and Diasonics, Inc., Sunnyvale, California).

OTHER APPLICATIONS (BRAIN)

There are numerous other future intraoperative neurosurgical applications. For instance, Brown et al have reported the use of ultrasound stereotaxy to guide the precise placement of periaqueductal gray electrodes in dog brains, a procedure that previously relied on traditional stereotaxic techniques (20).

Ultrasound has also been used to monitor neurovascular applications. Arteriovenous malformations are fairly echogenic lesions, presumably due to the reflections of multiple vascular channels within the mass (8). Real-time and Doppler ultrasound may be helpful in mapping out the arterial and venous feeders in these lesions (21). The pulsations of the hyperechoic blood vessel walls are easily

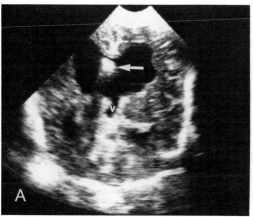
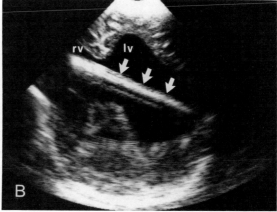

Figure 4.8. Guidance of ventriculoperitoneal shunt (in Arnold-Chiari syndrome). **A,** Axial view showing the tip of the shunt catheter (*arrow*) in the frontal horn, at midline. Note the position of the third ventricle (*v*). **B,** Oblique view, showing the longitudinal axis of the catheter (*arrows*). The catheter was introduced through a left posterior parietal burr hole into the left ventricle (*lv*) with the catheter tip in the right frontal horn (*rv*). There is absence of the septum pellucidum.

seen with ultrasound. The use of color flow imaging, in which velocity information derived from the Doppler signal is presented as color information added to the conventional two-dimensional image, has been helpful in intraoperative neurovascular applications (22). Flow within arteries or veins is usually displayed as either a red or blue pattern, depending on whether the flow is towards or away from the transducer face. Therefore, color flow may be helpful in rapid appreciation of arteriovenous malformation and also in determining flow within cerebral aneurysms that are to be resected. Ultrasound may be used to image the aneurysm and its feeding vessel and to demonstrate clotted thrombus or calcium within the aneurysm. Ultrasonography may also be used to evaluate any surrounding hematoma.

Other recent applications of Doppler sonography include assessment of superficial temporal artery to middle cerebral artery bypass operations (23). Combined real-time scanning with either pulsed Doppler techniques or color Doppler may be used in assessment of carotid endarterectomies (5, 24). Other potential applications of IOS include transdural laser ablation of specific areas of the brain.

TUMOR CHARACTERISTICS

While most tumors cannot be specifically characterized by intraoperative ultrasound, sonography is helpful in showing various components of the tumor. In general, cerebral neoplasms are sonographically echogenic (8, 12, 25, 26, 27) and only a few cases of hypoechoic or isoechoic low-grade neoplasms have been reported (8). For instance, intracranial gliomas are generally hyperechoic. Low-grade gliomas usually have a well-defined tumor margin and may contain areas of calcifications or cysts that are well characterized by ultrasound (12, 28). Calcifications within the tumors are highly echogenic and often exhibit acoustic shadowing. Intracranial cysts are anechoic with accompanying distal acoustic enhancement and are similar in sonographic appearance to other cerebrospinal fluid-containing spaces.

More invasive gliomas have rather serpiginous margins and a peripheral boundary of intermediate echogenicity (12). In general, the more anaplastic the astrocytoma, the more serpiginous the tumor margins and the greater the inhomogeneity of the internal architecture of the tumor. High-grade neoplasms often have central areas of necrosis or hemorrhage that are usually echogenic (12). Even though this central portion of the high-grade gliomas is often necrotic, this region may appear echogenic rather than cystic on ultrasound, which may cause confusion in selecting a site for possible biopsy. Compared to normal brain, even areas of edema in the brain tend to be relatively hyperechoic (12). Mass lesions and surrounding edema can cause obliteration of sulcal markings, which may be an important clue in localizing small tumors (9).

In contrast to primary malignant tumors, such as astrocytomas, metastatic lesions are often quite discrete. These lesions are usually echogenic with well-defined borders (8, 9, 10). However, rapidly growing metastatic lesions may contain areas of central necrosis or may be surrounded by intermediate echogenicity, probably secondary to surrounding edema (1). Metastatic lesions are well suited for sonographic interrogation as they are often subcortical, small (1–3 cm) and may be otherwise difficult to locate during surgical exploration.

Meningiomas are usually highly echogenic, with the dense echogenicity often accompanied by acoustic shadowing when there are internal calcifications. These lesions may be poorly visualized if they are small or superficial. Dural meningiomas adjacent to the superficial cortex may be difficult to evaluate with ultrasound but are usually readily apparent by visual inspection during operation. Other intracranial neoplasms have a variety of appearances but are generally echogenic compared to the surrounding brain. For instance, lymphomas are uniformly echogenic, poorly marginated with a similar acoustic architecture throughout (11, 29).

Intracerebral abscesses are well-demarcated masses accompanied by a thick hyperechoic rim. Abscesses contain anechoic

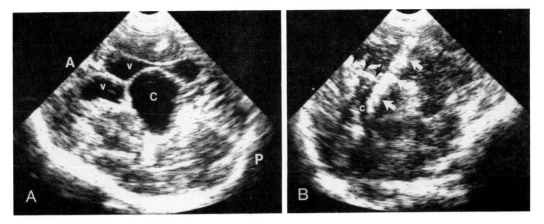

Figure 4.9. Guidance of shunt into midline subarachnoid cyst. **A,** Axial sonogram performed through temporal lobe demonstrating dilated lateral ventricles (*v*) and a midline cyst (C) (*A = Anterior, P = Posterior*). **B,** Coronal sonogram. Catheter (*white arrows*) within partially collapsed cyst (c). Note the interhemispheric fissure (*black arrows*).

or hypoechoic centers separated by hyperechoic septations if loculations are present (3, 8). Ultrasound may be used for needle aspiration or drainage of these lesions, especially when the brain abscess is deeply seated or in a critical area (3, 4).

Spine

NORMAL ANATOMY

Intraoperative ultrasound of the spinal canal is performed in both the longitudinal and transverse plane (30). The entire procedure may be recorded on video tape and/or film. Since almost all patients are scanned prone, the transverse sonograms are labeled so that the patient's left will be on the viewer's left and, on longitudinal sonograms, the cephalad portion of the image is on the viewer's left.

The spinal cord gray and white matter is uniformly hypoechoic (Figs. 4.10, 4.11, 4.12). The linear, highly reflective structure in the mid to ventral part of the cord is the central echo. While this central echo has long been regarded as representing the central canal, some authors contend that it represents the central aspect of the anterior median fissure (31; Fig. 4.12). The dural coverings, pial surface, dentate ligaments, and dorsal arachnoid septations are highly reflective structures. The bony margins are highly reflective with no through transmission of the ultrasound. Disc material is visualized as an area of mid-echogenicity. On sagittal scans, characteristic tapering of the conus medullaris is seen (29). The dorsal and ventral nerve roots can be identified with high resolution instrumentation (8; Figs. 4.11 & 4.12).

When saline initially fills the operative field, small microbubbles will be visualized as highly reflective echoes within the fluid. Other than microbubbles, highly reflective echoes may be secondary to small amounts of tissue, cottonoid pledgets, gel foam, or powder. Surgical instruments will appear echogenic with accompanying acoustic shadowing or reverberation artifact.

IOSS can demonstrate several types of periodic motion of the dura, the spinal cord and nerve roots (32). The spinal cord and nerve roots float freely in the CSF and undulate with respiration. The anterior spinal artery pulsates within the subarachnoid space. The spinal cord and nerve roots also pulsate with the same periodicity as the cardiac cycle. These periodic motions may have important diagnostic and therapeutic implications. While, in the past, neurosurgeons interpreted the presence of dural pulsations as indirect evidence that the spinal cord was free from compression, the dura and the spi-

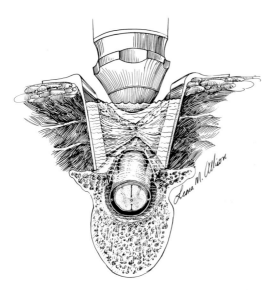

Figure 4.10. Diagram of the position of the probe during spinal sonography. The tip of the probe is within the water bath. (Reproduced by permission from Montalvo BM, Quencer RM, Green BA et al.: Intraoperative sonography in spinal trauma. *Radiology* 153:125–134, 1984.)

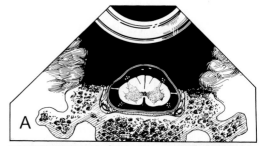

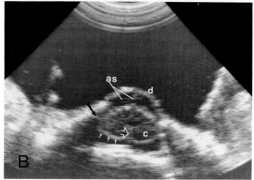

Figure 4.11. Normal cervical anatomy. **A,** Diagram, axial view of cervical cord. **B,** Axial sonogram, cervical cord. Dura (*d*), cord surface (*small white arrows*), arachnoid septations (*as*) in the subarachnoid space, cord substance (c), anterior median fissure (*open arrow*), denticulate ligament (*black arrow*). (Reproduced by permission from Quencer RM, Montalvo BM: Normal intraoperative sonography. *AJNR* 5: 501–505, ©American Roentgen Ray Society.)

nal cord can be seen to move independently of each other during IOSS. Thus, the presence of dural pulsations does not exclude the diagnosis of spinal cord compression (32).

One of the most important attributes of intraoperative sonography is the ability to monitor the progress of surgery. Many spinal lesions compress the cord or cauda equina. Criteria for decompression help determine the endpoint of surgery. Decompression is considered adequate when the spinal cord and the cauda equina are not deviated from their normal course. Other helpful signs of decompression include a normal or near normal shape of the spinal canal, a normal shape of the thecal sac, the absence of mass in the canal, and sufficient subarachnoid fluid in the thecal sac.

SPINAL MASSES

Masses located within the spinal cord or canal are usually operated upon to obtain tissue for diagnosis, to extirpate them completely, or to effect partial removal in order to decompress the spinal cord or cauda equina. These masses may be degenerative, inflammatory, or neoplastic in origin.

Metastases account for 30% of masses within the canal. Meningioma and neurinoma each account for 25% of the neoplasms that affect the spinal cord. Gliomas constitute 10% of the masses that affect the spinal cord (33). Dermoids, vascular malformation and lipomas are unusual. Primary epidural tumors, infections and hemorrhage can also compress the spinal cord and cauda equina (34–36).

Sonography is invaluable in the surgical

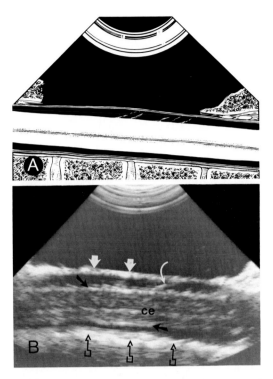

Figure 4.12. Normal anatomy, sagittal view. **A,** Diagram, sagittal view of cervical cord. **B,** Sagittal sonogram of cervical cord. Dura (*white arrows*), cord surface (*black arrows*), central echo of the cord (*ce*), arachnoid septations within the subarachnoid space (*curved white arrow*) and bony spine (*open arrows*). (Reproduced by permission from Quencer RM, Montalvo BM: Normal intraoperative sonography. *AJNR* 5:501–505, 1984, ©American Roentgen Ray Society.)

management of tumors of the spinal cord or canal since IOSS:

1. Accurately depicts the craniocaudal and ventral extent of tumors.
2. Localizes the tumor and helps choose the optimal site for biopsy by showing one or more of the following:
   a. Area of maximal cord enlargement,
   b. Transition zone or boundary between intramedullary mass and normal cord,
   c. Boundary of demarcation between mass and normal cord,
   d. Solid component of complex masses.
3. May show the necessity of extending the laminectomy.
4. Immediately evaluates the adequacy of tumor resection.

We believe that sonography is essential in the surgery of soft tissue masses of the spinal cord and spinal canal and we strongly recommend its use in those cases where tumor biopsy or resection is planned (30).

INTRAMEDULLARY LESIONS

Intramedullary lesions arise from the substance of the cord and expand the cord as they grow. They may be localized but typically they involve long segments of the spinal cord, and occasionally the entire cord. Intramedullary lesions enlarge the cord and obliterate the central echo (36, 3). Most solid intramedullary masses appear iso-echoic or subtly hyperechoic when compared to normal cord (Fig. 4.13). Some tumors, most commonly ependymomas, appear homogeneously hyperechoic with well-delineated, smooth boundaries (37). Metastases are echogenic and cause cord enlargement (38). Astrocytomas and ependymomas often have internal cystic degeneration or are associated with an adjacent cyst (39, 40). Ultrasound helps differentiate cystic tumors from benign cystic lesions of the cord.

At surgery, ultrasound delineates cystic intramedullary lesions such as syringohydromyelia and posttraumatic cystic myelopathy and differentiates them from solid lesions such as myelomalacia or solid components of tumors; finds intracystic loculations that may have to be lysed or separately shunted; and localizes the optimal site for catheter introduction. The surgical procedure to decompress benign intramedullary cysts involves shunting them to the subarachnoid space, and this procedure should be monitored sonographically to ensure adequate decompression (2, 41; Fig. 4.14).

EXTRAMEDULLARY MASSES

Extramedullary noncystic masses (meningiomas, neurofibromas, neurilemomas and dropped metastases) are always more echogenic than the normal cord and easily visualized by intraoperative ultrasound through the closed dura. Similarly, intradural lipomas have been identified and appear more echogenic than the adjacent

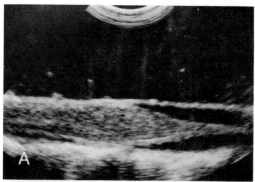

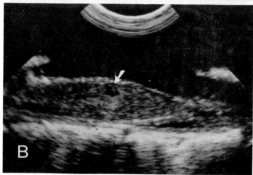

Figure 4.13. Biopsy of intramedullary mass (metastasis). **A,** Longitudinal sonogram prior to opening the dura shows local conal enlargement with obliteration of the central echo of the cord. **B,** The dura is opened and a small fluid collection (*arrow*) remains at the site of the biopsy. (Reproduced by permission from Quencer RM, Montalvo BM, Green BA, Eismont FJ: Intraoperative spinal sonography of soft tissue masses of the spinal cord and spinal canal. *AJNR* 5:507–515, 1984, ©American Roentgen Ray Society.)

spinal cord (35, 42, 43). Large tumors cause marked compression of the spinal cord and obliteration of the central spinal canal. Sonography is helpful in delineating the cephalad and caudal tumor extent, the distortion of the cord by tumor, and the adequacy of surgical resection.

EXTRADURAL LESIONS

Extradural lesions usually displace the dura eccentrically or concentrically, and narrow the subarachnoid space. They may be smoothly bordered or irregular. Their

configuration depends on their origin and extent. They may be well circumscribed, as in the case of epidural hematomas (37) or metastases (35); or extensive, as in the case of spinal infections (44), large bone tumors (35), or lymphomas (42). Sonography has been proven to be superior to magnetic resonance imaging in assessing the extent of epidural abscesses (44). If very extensive and concentric, extradural lesions can obliterate the central echo of the cord. Intradural extent of tumor not suspected at surgery may be revealed by sonography (35). In general, extradural lesions tend to be homogeneous and to be more echogenic than the spinal cord itself but lower in echogenicity than the lumbar epidural fat.

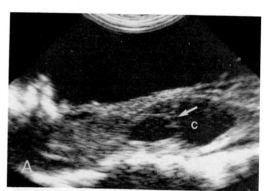

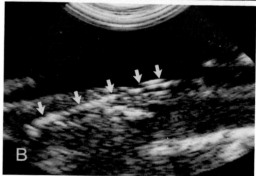

Figure 4.14. Posttraumatic spinal cord cyst: shunt guidance. **A,** Longitudinal sonogram depicts a bilobed cyst (c) with a septation (*arrow*) in the spinal cord in this patient who had suffered a cervical fracture. **B,** after a myelotomy, the catheter (*arrows*) is seen coursing from the subarachnoid space into the spinal cord, and the cyst has collapsed.

SPINAL FRACTURES

Intraoperative ultrasound is particularly useful in the surgical management of thoracolumbar spinal fractures. Operative treatment may vary but often includes decompression and metallic rod stabilization (45–48). Sonography of the spinal canal is performed after laminectomy, hemilaminectomy, or removal of the pedicle when a lateral approach is used. Real-time sonography delineates the relationship between the spinal cord or nerve roots and displaced elements of the fractured bony spinal canal. The position of the posterior portion of the vertebral body is ascertained before placement of rods or as distraction is applied (Fig. 4.15). If ultrasound determines that canal decompression is not adequate after distraction, the surgeon may elect to perform posterolateral decompression and either impact the compressing bone fragment or remove it. IOSS confirms the adequacy of vertebral fracture reduction. Because sonography has been shown to significantly alter surgical management in patients undergoing metallic rod instrumentation for spinal fractures, we recommend its use in all such operative cases (46, 48).

HERNIATED DISKS

Following a complete one-level laminectomy or a hemilaminectomy (at least 1.5 cm in length), IOSS can easily visualize the structures that lie ventral to the laminectomy. IOSS cannot successfully image the lateral recesses of the spinal canal but smaller pencil-like probes may prove helpful in these cases. Most degenerative disk herniations appear homogeneous and of medium echogenicity, whereas acute, post-traumatic disk herniations appear hypoechoic. Degenerative disks are more echogenic than spinal cord but less echogenic than epidural fat. Peripherally calcified disks may "shadow," while disks with internal calcification show bright punctate echoes. Herniated disks displace the ventral dura, distort the shape of the thecal sac and may compress nerve roots of the cauda equina (2).

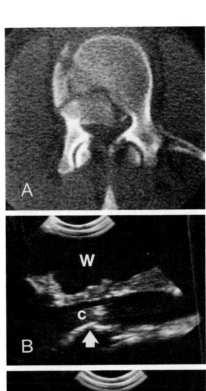

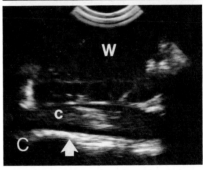

Figure 4.15. Burst fracture. **A,** CT scan showing burst fracture of T 12 with bony displacement into spinal canal. **B,** IOSS with spinal cord (c) scanned through saline (w) showing displaced fracture of posterior part of T 12 (*arrow*). **C,** postreduction sonogram after placement with Harrington rods and bony impactions showing good reduction of fracture (*arrow*) (W = saline, C = cord). (Reproduced with permission from McGahan JP, Benson D, Chehrazi B, Walter JP, Wagner FC Jr: Intraoperative sonographic monitoring of reduction of thoracolumbar burst fractures. *AJR* 145:1229–1232, 1985, ©American Roentgen Ray Society.)

OTHER INDICATIONS

Ultrasonography is useful in assessing adequacy of decompression following laminectomy and medial facetectomies in symptomatic lumbar canal stenosis and is helpful in evaluating concomitant abnormalities such as herniated disks.

In spinal dysraphism, sonography can identify and locate the lesion and all associated abnormalities. In the tethered cord syndrome, sonography will show the relationship of the tethering mass to the cord and will demonstrate the completeness of removal of the mass. Shunting of syrinxes under sonographic control will ensure adequacy of drainage (49).

Summary

Knowledge of ultrasound instrumentation, sterile surgical technique, and neurosurgical anatomy is needed for proper utilization of intraoperative neurosurgical ultrasonography. This unique application of ultrasound in guidance of intraoperative neurosurgical procedures that can shorten the surgical procedure and make the operation safer and more accurate, is now regarded as invaluable in many specific indications.

ACKNOWLEDGMENTS

Special thanks to Lou McHugh and Karen Anderson for their help in the preparation of this manuscript.

REFERENCES

1. McGahan JP, Boggan JE, Gooding GA: Intraoperative use of ultrasound. In Youmans JR (ed): *Neurological Surgery*, ed 3. Philadelphia, W. B. Saunders (in press).
2. Montalvo BM, Quencer RM: Intraoperative sonography in spinal surgery: Current state of the art. *Neuroradiology* 28: 551–590, 1986.
3. McGahan JP, Boggan JE: Intraoperative ultrasound monitoring. In McGahan JP (ed): *Controversies in Ultrasound*. New York, Churchill Livingstone, 289–307, 1987.
4. Lee LL, McGahan JP, Wagner FC: Percutaneous ultrasound guided needle aspiration of the brain. *Br J Radiol* 58: 1123–1125, 1985.
5. Rubin JM, Dohrmann GJ: Intraoperative neurosurgical ultrasound in the localization and characterization of intracranial masses. *Radiology* 148: 519–524, 1983.
6. Quencer RM, Montalvo BM: Time requirements for intraoperative neurosonography. *AJNR* 7: 155–158, 1986.
7. Sigel B, Flanigan DP, Schuler JJ, Machi J, Beitler JC, Coelho JC: Imaging ultrasound in the intraoperative diagnosis of vascular defects. *J Ultrasound Med* 2: 337–343, 1983.
8. Rubin JM, Dohrmann GJ: Efficacy of intraoperative US for evaluating intracranial masses. *Radiology* 157: 509–511, 1985.
9. Knake JE, Bowerman RA, Silver TM, McCracken S: Neurosurgical applications of intraoperative ultrasound. *Radiol Clin North Am* 23: 73–90, 1985.
10. Merritt CR, Voorhies RM, Connolly E, Coulon R: Intraoperative neurosurgical ultrasound. *Semin Ultrasound, CT MR* 6:31–47, 1985.
11. Quencer, RM, Montalvo BM: Intraoperative cranial sonography. *Neuroradiology* 28: 528–550, 1986.
12. McGahan JP, Ellis WG, Budenz RW, Walter JP, Boggan JE: Brain gliomas: Sonographic characterization. *Radiology* 159:485–492, 1986.
13. Dohrmann GJ, Rubin JM: Dynamic intraoperative imaging and instrumentation of brain and spinal cord using ultrasound. *Neurol Clin* 3:425–437, 1985.
14. McGahan JP: Laboratory assessment of ultrasonic needle and catheter visualization. *J Ultrasound Med* 5:373–377, 1986.
15. Rubin JM, Dohrmann GJ: A cannula for use in ultrasonically guided biopsies of the brain, *J Neurosurg* 59:905–907, 1983.
16. Enzmann DR, Irwin KM, Marshall WH, Silverberg GD, Britt RH, Hanbery JW: Intraoperative sonography through a burr hole: guide for brain biopsy. *AJNR* 5:243–246, 1984.
17. Berger MS: Ultrasound guided stereotactic biopsy using the diasonics neurobiopsy device for deep seated intracranial lesions. [Proceedings] Annual Meeting of the American Association of Neurological Surgeons, Atlanta, Georgia, 1985.
18. Shkolnik A, McLone DG: Intra-operative real-time ultrasonic guidance of intracranial shunt tube placement in infants. *Radiology* 144:573–576, 1982.
19. Mahoney BS, Gross BH, Callen PW et al.: Intraventricular hemorrhage following ventriculoperitoneal shunt placement: real-time ultrasonic demonstration. *Ultrasound Med* 3:143–145, 1983.
20. Brown FD, Rachlin JR, Rubin JM, Fessler RG, Smith LJ, Schaible KL: Ultrasound-guided periventricular stereotaxis. *Neurosurgery* 15:162–164, 1984.
21. Nornes H, Grip A, Wikeby P: Intraoperative evaluation of cerebral hemodynamics using directional doppler technique. Part 1: Arteriovenous malformations. *J Neurosurg* 50:145–151, 1979.
22. Nelson TR, Pretorius DH: The Doppler signal: Where does it come from and what does it mean? *AJR* 151:439–447, 1988.
23. Gilsbach JM, Hassler WE: Intraoperative Doppler and real-time sonography in neurosurgery. *Neurosurg Rev* 7:199–208, 1984.
24. Zierler RE, Bandyk DF, Thiele BL: Intraoperative assessment of carotid endarterectomy. *J Vasc Surg* 1:73–83, 1984.
25. Gooding GAW, Boggan JE, Powers SK, Martin NA, Weinstein PR: Neurosurgical sonography: Intraoperative and postoperative imaging of the brain. *AJNR* 5:521–525, 1984.
26. Knake JE, Chandler WF, Gabrielsen TO, Latack JT, Gebarski SS: Intraoperative sonography in the nonstereotaxic biopsy and aspiration of subcortical brain lesions. *AJNR* 4:672–674, 1983.

27. Merritt CR, Coulon R, Connolly E: Intraoperative neurosurgical ultrasound: transdural and transfontanelle applications. *Radiology* 148:513–517, 1983.

28. Knake JE, Chandler WF, Gabrielsen TO, Latack JT, Gebarski SS:. Intraoperative sonographic delineation of low-grade brain neoplasms defined poorly by computed tomography. *Radiology* 151:735–739, 1984.

29. Enzmann DR, Wheat R, Marshall WH, Bird R et al.: Tumors of the central nervous system studied by computed tomography and ultrasound. *Radiology* 154:393–399, 1985.

30. Quencer RM, Montalvo BM: Normal intraoperative spinal sonography. *AJR* 143:1301–1305, 1984.

31. Nelson MD Jr, Sedler JA, Gilles FH: Spinal cord central echo complex: Histoanatomic correlation. *Radiology* 170:479–481, 1989.

32. Jokich PM, Rubin JM, Dohrmann GJ: Intraoperative ultrasonic evaluation of spinal cord motion. *J Neurosurg* 60:707–711, 1984.

33. Taveras JM, Wood EH: Diseases of the spinal cord. In Taveras JM, Wood EH (eds): *Diagnostic Neuroradiology*, ed 2 Baltimore, Williams & Wilkins, 1976; pp 1168–1180.

34. Dohrmann GJ, Rubin JM: Intraoperative ultrasound imaging of the spinal cord: Syringomyelia, cysts, and tumors—a preliminary report. *Surg Neurol* 18:395–399, 1982.

35. Knake JE, Chandler WF, McGillicuddy JE, Gabrielson TO, Latack JT, Gebarski SS, Yang PJ: Intraoperative sonography of intraspinal tumors: Initial experience. *AJNR* 4:1199–1201, 1983.

36. Quencer RM, Montalvo BM, Green BA, Eismont FJ: Intraoperative spinal sonography of soft-tissue masses of the spinal cord and spinal canal. *AJR* 143:1307–1315, 1984.

37. Post MJD, Quencer RM, Green BA, Montalvo BM, Eismont FJ: Radiologic evaluation of spinal cord fissures. *AJNR* 7:329–335, 1986.

38. Post MJ, Quencer RM, Green BA, Montalvo BM, Tobias JA, Sowers JJ, Levin IH: Intramedullary spinal cord metastases, mainly of non-neurogenic origin. *AJNR* 8:339–346, 1987.

39. Enzmann DR, Murphy-Irwin K, Silverberg GD, Djang WT, Golden JB: Spinal cord tumor imaging with CT and sonography. *AJNR* 6:95–97, 1985.

40. Raghavendra BN, Epstein FJ, McCleary L: Intramedullary spinal cord tumors in children: Localization by intraoperative sonography. *AJNR* 5: 395–397, 1984.

41. Quencer RM, Morse BM, Green BA, Eismont FJ, Brost P: Intraoperative spinal sonography: Adjunct to metrizamide CT in the assessment and surgical decompression of posttraumatic spinal cord cysts. *AJR* 142:593–601, 1985.

42. Chadduck WM, Flanigan S: Intraoperative ultrasound for spinal lesions. *Neurosurgery* 16:447–483, 1985.

43. Rubin JM, Dohrmann GJ: Intraoperative sonography of the spine and spinal cord. *Semin Ultrasound CT, MR* 6:48–67, 1985.

44. Post, MJ, Quencer RM, Montalvo BM, Katz BH, Eismont FJ, Green BA: Spinal infection: Evaluation with MR imaging and intraoperative US. *Radiology* 169:765–771, 1988.

45. Dickson JH, Harrington PR, Erwin WD: Results of reduction and stabilization of the severely fractured thoracic and lumbar spine. *J Bone Joint Surg* 60:799–805, 1978.

46. McGahan JP, Benson D, Chehrazi B, Walter JP, Wagner FC Jr: Intraoperative sonographic monitoring of reduction of thoracolumbar burst fractures. *AJR* 145:1229–1232, 1985.

47. Montalvo BM, Quencer RM, Green BA, Eismont FJ, Brown MJ, Brost P: Intraoperative sonography in spinal trauma. *Radiology* 153:125–134, 1984.

48. Quencer RM, Montalvo BM, Eismont FJ, Green BA: Intraoperative spinal sonography in thoracic and lumbar fractures: Evaluation of Harrington rod instrumentation. *AJNR* 6:353–359, 1985.

49. Quencer RM, Montalvo BM, Naidich TP, Post MJD, Green BA, Page LK: Intraoperative sonography in spinal dysraphism and syringohydromyelia. *AJNR* 8:329–337, 1987.

5 Neck and Parathyroid

MARILYN J. MORTON
J. WILLIAM CHARBONEAU
CARL C. READING

Introduction

The use of high-frequency (7.5 to 10 MHz) real-time ultrasonography in the examination of the neck allows excellent visualization of the thyroid gland and surrounding structures. The superior resolution of this imaging method permits detection and morphologic characterization of thyroid nodules with a high degree of sensitivity and permits accurate localization of enlarged parathyroid glands and cervical lymph nodes. (1–4).

In the evaluation and management of the patient with a palpable thyroid nodule, the clinical challenge is to establish the likelihood of malignancy. Although sonography is highly sensitive in the detection of thyroid nodules, it is not capable of differentiating benign from malignant lesions. Fine-needle aspiration biopsy(FNAB) by direct palpation has proven to be a highly reliable and cost-effective technique to differentiate benign from malignant thyroid nodules and it is the initial diagnostic procedure used in our practice to evaluate a clinically palpable thyroid nodule. In this group of patients with nodular thyroid disease, sonography can be used to provide continuous real-time guidance for biopsy of thyroid nodules when FNAB by direct palpation is unsuccessful. In the patient with a known thyroid malignancy, sonography has a two-fold purpose: 1) detecting nonpalpable occult neck masses postoperatively and 2) providing guidance for biopsy of these masses to confirm or exclude tumor recurrence.

The diagnosis of primary hyperparathyroidism is relatively straightforward and is based on clinical and chemical criteria. Because enlarged parathyroid glands are rarely palpable and can lie in various locations in the neck or mediastinum, the difficulty presented to the surgeon is one of localization. In many practices, high-frequency sonography has become the imaging procedure of choice for the preoperative localization of enlarged parathyroid glands in the neck. Aspiration biopsy under sonographic guidance can increase the accuracy of localization by providing histologic confirmation of the presence of a parathyroid adenoma. This is particularly important in the patient undergoing reoperation for persistent or recurrent hypercalcemia after the initial neck exploration.

In this chapter we present our biopsy technique, review the anatomy of the neck as it relates to the thyroid and parathyroid glands, and present diagnostic as well as therapeutic applications of sonographically guided biopsy in patients with known or suspected thyroid and parathyroid disease.

Technique of Sonographically Guided Aspiration Biopsy

Sonographic examination of the thyroid and parathyroid glands is performed with the patient in the supine position. A small

59

pad is placed under the shoulders to hyper-extend the neck. The thyroid gland and lower neck are examined thoroughly in both transverse and longitudinal planes using a high-frequency (7.5- to 10-MHz) trans-ducer. Subsequent aspiration biopsies of so-nographically detected thyroid nodules, cervical lymph nodes, and suspected para-thyroid adenomas are performed under con-tinuous real-time sonographic guidance using a 5- or 7.5-MHz linear phased-array transducer (Acuson, Mountainview, CA). The advantage of the linear-array trans-ducer for biopsy purposes is that it provides high-quality images of the superficial soft tissues in the near field. This allows visual-ization of the needle during the beginning of the biopsy as it enters the subcutaneous tis-sues. Consequently, early adjustments in needle trajectory can be made if needed.

Before the biopsy is performed, the trans-ducer is thoroughly cleaned with isopropyl alcohol and povidone iodine solution. Ster-ile gel is used as a coupling agent. A separate sterile transducer cover is not used because the cover can degrade the quality of the im-age. We have had no complications from in-fection with this method of transducer sterilization.

After the skin is cleaned with povidone io-dine solution, the needle is introduced in a freehand manner adjacent to the edge of the linear-array transducer and parallel to the center beam (Fig 5.1). In our experience, at-tachable biopsy guides and special biopsy transducers have been more awkward to use and may limit the access route for biopsy of these superficial structures. We prefer the freehand technique because it allows greater flexibility and maneuverability. The needle enters the image obliquely from the side. Vi-sualization of the biopsy needle is aided by an in-and-out jiggling motion of the needle during insertion. If the needle tip echo is lost within the image field, it can be relocated by slightly angling the transducer to one side or the other of the needle. Once the needle tip is positioned within the lesion, suction is ap-plied and several up-and-down movements are made with a rotary motion. When aspi-ration cytologic sampling is performed, suc-tion is released prior to withdrawal of the needle from the lesion, thereby avoiding as-piration of the sample into the syringe bar-rel. The aspirated material is placed on slides and immediately fixed in 95% alcohol. Al-ternatively, a cytologist may be available for immediate handling and/or staining of the specimen.

To obtain optimal material from thyroid nodules, fine-needle cytologic rather than histologic sampling is routinely performed. For this purpose we begin the aspiration bi-opsy with a 1¹/₂-inch, 25-gauge, noncutting, bevel-edged needle (Becton Dickinson, Rutherford, NJ). We find the smaller needle to be less traumatizing to the tissue, with less contamination of the aspirate by blood.

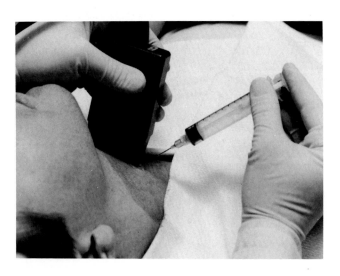

Figure 5.1. Freehand technique. Needle puncture is made at end of long axis of transducer at an oblique angle. Needle path is par-allel to ultrasound beam.

The needle is attached to a vacuum syringe that has a self-locking plunger (Cook Inc., Bloomington, IN) that maintains a continuous negative pressure in the needle without the need for a second hand to apply suction. The other hand is free to hold the transducer to continuously monitor the needle position during the aspiration biopsy.

If an adequate cell sample is not obtained initially, repeat cytologic aspiration can be performed with a larger 21-gauge needle. A histologic core sample can be obtained with a 25- or 23-gauge modified Menghini cutting needle (Surecut, Meadox, Surgimed, Oakland, NJ).

Aspiration biopsy of cervical lymph nodes and suspected parathyroid adenomas is performed as described above for thyroid nodules. In most cases a cytologic aspirate can confirm or exclude the presence of para-thyroid cells in a suspected parathyroid mass, or malignant cells in a cervical lymph node. However, at times it may be necessary to obtain a histologic core specimen as well. In addition to the evaluation of cytologic and histologic specimens, the presence of hyperfunctioning parathyroid tissue can be verified by measuring the concentration of parathyroid hormone (PTH) levels in the aspirate (5).

Thyroid Gland

ANATOMY

The thyroid gland is easily identified in the lower portion of the neck with its characteristic sonographic appearance of homogenous medium level echoes. The right and left lobes of the thyroid gland lie along

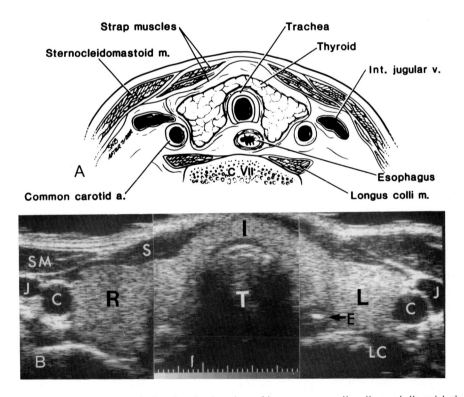

Figure 5.2. Normal anatomy. **A,** Anatomic drawing of transverse section through thyroid gland, **B,** Composite transverse sonogram of normal thyroid gland and surrounding anatomy. *L,* left thyroid lobe; *R,* right thyroid lobe; *I,* thyroid isthmus; *T,* trachea; *E,* esophagus; *C,* carotid artery; *J,* jugular vein; *LC,* longus colli muscle; *S,* strap muscle; *SM,* sternocleidomastoid muscle. (Reproduced with permission from James EM: High-frequency (10 MHz) thyroid ultrasonography. *Semin Ultrasound CT MR* 6:295, 1985.)

either side of the trachea and are joined across the midline by the isthmus (Fig. 5.2). The common carotid arteries and jugular veins lie immediately lateral to the lobes of the thyroid and can serve as useful anatomic landmarks. The sternocleidomastoid muscles and strap muscles (Sternohyoid and sternothyroid muscles) lie anterior to the thyroid and are visualized as hypoechoic bands. Posterior and slightly lateral to each thyroid lobe are the longus colli muscles, which appear as hypoechoic wedge-shaped structures adjacent to the anterolateral aspect of the cervical vertebrae in the transverse image. The air-filled trachea gives a characteristic sonographic appearance of a curvilinear reflecting surface with reverberation echoes and acoustic shadowing posteriorly. Occasionally, the esophagus may be seen posterior to the thyroid, usually on the left side. This laterally located segment of esophagus should not be mistaken for a thyroid or a parathyroid mass. Generally, the esophagus is easily identified by the characteristic sonographic appearance of bowel ("target" appearance). In addition, movement can be visualized within the esophagus when the patient swallows.

CLINICAL PROBLEM

The discovery of a nodule in the thyroid gland gives rise to concern because of the potential for malignancy. Nodules of the thyroid gland are common: a palpable thyroid nodule is estimated to exist in about 4% to 7% of the population in the United States (6, 7). In contrast, thyroid carcinoma is rare, with an estimated overall incidence of 5 per 100,000 population per year or 0.0005% (8). Thyroid carcinoma accounts for less than 1% of all malignancies (9). These data indicate that the overwhelming majority of thyroid nodules are benign. For each newly diagnosed thyroid carcinoma, approximately 2,000 benign nodules are estimated to exist (7). The clinical challenge is to identify the patient at risk for malignancy.

High-frequency real-time ultrasonography provides the most detailed analysis of the anatomy and pathology of the thyroid gland currently available. The sensitivity of sonography in detecting thyroid nodules is quite high. Cystic and solid masses as small as 2 to 3 mm are readily visualized (1, 2). However, the specificity of the findings is low. The sonographic appearances of benign and malignant thyroid nodules frequently overlap and no specific sonographic characteristic can reliably differentiate benign from malignant nodules (1, 10–12).

FNAB of Thyroid Nodules by Direct Palpation

Fine-needle (21- to 25-gauge) aspiration biopsy performed by direct palpation is the first and usually the only diagnostic procedure performed on a clinically palpable thyroid nodule in many practices. It is generally recognized that FNAB of the thyroid is the most accurate and cost-effective method for diagnosing or excluding malignancy in a thyroid nodule (13–15). FNAB allows precise cytologic evaluation of thyroid nodules with an accuracy that compares favorably with that of thick-core biopsy (16). In most large series, the overall accuracy rate in differentiating benign from malignant nodules exceeds 90% (13–16).

FNAB by palpation is a simple and safe procedure that is usually performed on an outpatient basis. Hematomas and mild local discomfort may occur but no serious complications have ever been reported despite its widespread use (13, 15–17). Needle biopsy rarely gives false-positive diagnostic information and there has been no documented case of seeding of the needle tract after FNAB of thyroid nodules (13–18). The main limitations of FNAB by palpation include the following.

1. Nondiagnostic and false-negative cytologic results because of incorrect location of sampling. A certain percent of aspiration biopsies performed by direct palpation will be nondiagnostic because of an inadequate cell sample. In our practice, approximately 20% of specimens obtained by aspiration biopsy by direct palpation are cytologically indeterminate (8). Approximately one-half of these unsatisfactory aspirates are attributable to cystic lesions from which an adequate cell sample was not obtained. This occurs because of placement of

the needle into the cystic rather than the solid portion of the nodule.

2. Inability to distinguish between benign and malignant follicular neoplasms. Cytologic examination usually does not permit distinction between well-differentiated follicular carcinoma and benign follicular adenoma (14, 16). This is detailed in Chapter 2, dealing with cytological techniques. The distinction between the two conditions usually requires surgical excision of the mass for histologic demonstration of capsular or vascular invasion.

Sonographically Guided FNAB of Thyroid Nodules

Percutaneous FNAB by sonographic guidance is well recognized as a safe, highly accurate, and widely applicable method of obtaining tissue specimens for pathologic diagnosis (19, 20). Traditionally, aspiration biopsy under sonographic guidance has been limited to biopsies of large, superficial, or cystic masses. Recently, improvements in image resolution and biopsy methods have resulted in a high level of accuracy for biopsy of small, deeply located masses (21). Sonographically guided FNAB has become an integral part of the diagnostic evaluation of selected thyroid nodules and other neck masses in our practice. Some current indications for sonographically guided FNAB of the thyroid and cervical region include:

1. Nondiagnostic (cytologically indeterminate) FNAB by direct palpation. As mentioned previously, when FNAB by direct palpation is nondiagnostic, it is often because the needle is placed into a cystic rather than solid component of the nodule. Under continuous sonographic guidance, the needle can be directed into the more solid portion of the nodule where the diagnostic yield is greater (Fig. 5.3). Continuous needle monitoring also decreases the chance of a geographic miss when aspirating small lesions.

2. The indeterminate mass detected in a patient with a history of thyroid carcinoma. After surgical removal of the thyroid gland, scarring and fibrosis in the neck can make palpation a difficult and unreliable method of detecting tumor recurrence. Recent studies have shown that high-frequency ultrasonography can detect occult residual, recurrent, or locally metastatic thyroid cancer with a high degree of sensitivity (22, 23).

The normal postoperative bed shows ab-

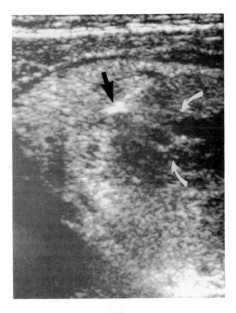

Figure 5.3. Mixed solid/cystic thyroid nodule. Longitudinal sonogram shows large thyroid nodule with cystic component centrally (*curved arrows*). Needle (*straight arrow*) is directed into solid, peripheral component.

sence of the thyroid tissue, close approximation of the strap muscles and cervical vessels to the trachea, and a uniform echo texture. A solid hypoechoic mass within the thyroid bed is the typical sonographic appearance of locally recurrent thyroid cancer (Fig. 5.4) (23, 24).

Normal cervical lymph nodes are oval to slender in shape, usually have a maximum anteroposterior diameter of 5 mm, and have an echogenic central hilum (24, 25). In contrast, larger, rounded lymph nodes lacking an echogenic hilum are usually abnormal and potentially malignant (Fig. 5.5; 24). However, size and appearance of cervical lymph nodes cannot reliably differentiate benign from malignant disease.

In addition to lesion detection, sonography can be used as a guide for biopsy of clinically occult enlarged cervical lymph nodes or thyroid bed masses in patients with a history of thyroid malignancy (Fig. 5.6). In our recent experience with over 300 postoperative patients with a history of thyroid malignancy, 52 underwent sonographically guided needle biopsy of a mass in the thyroid bed or for an enlarged cervical lymph node. Forty-four of these masses were nonpalpable. In 49 (94%) patients an accurate diagnosis of either positive or negative for malignancy was made

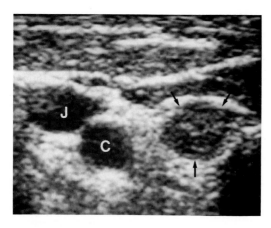

Figure 5.4. Recurrent papillary carcinoma. Transverse sonogram of right side of neck after thyroidectomy shows occult, nonpalpable 8-mm nodule (*arrows*) in right thyroid bed. Biopsy was positive for papillary carcinoma. *J*, internal jugular vein; *C*, common carotid artery. (Reproduced with permission from Reading CC: Sonographically guided percutaneous biopsy of small (3 cm or less) masses. *AJR* 151:191, 1988, © American Roentgen Ray Society.)

(24). There were no complications and biopsy results were indeterminate in only three patients.

3. Cytologic configuration of occult nonpalpable thyroid tumors in patients at high risk for carcinoma. Patients who have a history of head and neck irradiation during childhood as well as patients with a history of MEN type II syndrome have a known increased risk of developing thyroid malignancy. If clinically impalpable thyroid nodules are detected sonographically in these patients, biopsy under sonographic guidance can be performed to document or exclude malignancy. Similarly, patients with clinically occult papillary carcinoma of the thyroid gland who present with cervical lymph node metastasis but no palpable thyroid abnormality may undergo guided FNAB of a sonographically visible thyroid nodule. Sonographically guided needle biopsy of occult thyroid nodules in such patients is a reliable technique to document the presence of thyroid cancer.

Parathyroid

ANATOMY

The normal parathyroid gland measures 5 × 3 × 1 mm and weighs 35 to 40 mg (26).

Although other structures of this size can be resolved, the normal parathyroid gland is not routinely visualized sonographically. A likely explanation for this is that most normal glands are in close apposition to the posterior surface of the thyroid and have a similar echotexture.

To localize abnormal parathyroid glands, it is essential to have an understanding of the anatomic distribution of normal parathyroid glands. Parathyroid glands usually number four: two superior and two inferior glands, although supernumerary glands occur in about 3% to 4% of individuals (26, 27). The superior parathyroid glands are invariably found in close proximity to the posterior surface of the upper pole and midportion of the thyroid gland. In about 1% of individuals, the superior gland may be located in the retropharyngeal or retroesophageal space or may descend into the posterior superior mediastinum (26). The inferior glands are less consistent in location. In one series of 160 autopsy cases, 42% of inferior glands were found adjacent to the lower pole of the thyroid. An equal number were located lower in the neck within the thymic tongue at the thoracic inlet (26). Some inferior glands may descend with the thymus into the anterior superior mediastinum. Rarely, parathyroid glands can be located within the thyroid gland, within the carotid sheath, and in an undescended position high in the neck superior to the carotid bifurcation.

When attempting to locate abnormal parathyroid glands, it is important to remember these variations in gland location. If primary hyperparathyroidism is suspected and no adenoma can be found posterior to the thyroid, scanning the other areas of the neck is essential. It is important to angle the transducer behind the clavicles, maximally hyperextend the neck, and have the patient swallow during the scan. This allows visualization of adenomas caudal to the thyroid in the thoracic inlet. The region of the carotid sheaths should be examined and, to detect abnormal glands that lie in the retroesophageal or retrotracheal position, it is important to angle the transducer as far medially behind these structures as possible.

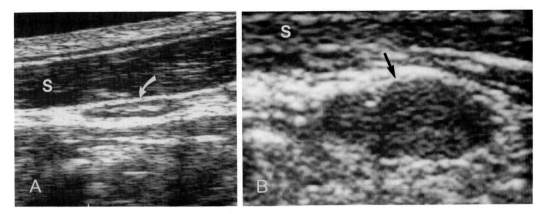

Figure 5.5. **A,** Longitudinal sonogram of normal cervical lymph node (*arrow*) shows oval shape and linear echogenic hilum, a good indicator of benign nature of this node. Maximum anteroposterior (AP) diameter is 3 mm. *S*, sternocleidomastoid muscle. **B,** Longitudinal sonogram of enlarged, rounded lymph node (*arrow*) that was not palpable. Maximum AP diameter is 1 cm. Sonographically guided biopsy was positive for medullary carcinoma of thyroid, *S*, sternocleidomastoid muscle.

Clinical Problem

The diagnosis of primary hyperparathyroidism is relatively straightforward and is based on biochemical abnormalities: persistent hypercalcemia and elevated levels of serum parathyroid hormone (28). Surgical treatment is usually indicated to prevent the progressive damaging consequences of renal dysfunction, urolithiasis, and bone disease. With the widespread use of routine biochemical screening profiles, the diagnosis of primary hyperparathyroidism has been made with increasing frequency. In the United States, it is estimated that the annual age-adjusted incidence is approximately 30 cases per 100,000 population or about 35,000 to 85,000 newly diagnosed cases each year (29).

Primary hyperparathyroidism is the result of a solitary parathyroid adenoma in over 85% of patients, whereas multiple gland enlargement (multiple adenomas or hyperplasia) accounts for about 10% to 15% of cases (30, 31). The well-known exceptions to single-gland disease are the multiple endocrine neoplasia syndromes, chronic renal insufficiency, and familial hyperparathyroidism. The incidence of parathyroid hyperplasia with multiple gland involvement is much higher in this group of patients. Parathyroid carcinoma is found in less than 1% of all cases of primary hyperparathyroidism (31).

Sonographic Parathyroid Localization

The ability of high-frequency real-time sonography to identify enlarged parathyroid glands in the neck has been well documented (3, 4, 32–36). The results of several prospective clinical trials indicate a moderately high degree of sensitivity (69% to 88%) and an accuracy of greater than 80% for parathyroid localization (3, 4, 32–34). We initiate the search for an abnormal parathyroid gland with high-frequency sonography because it combines a moderate degree of accuracy with noninvasiveness, relatively low cost, and same day availability. If the sonographic examination is negative, then computed tomography, magnetic resonance imaging, or thallium-201/technetium-99m scintigraphy is performed.

The indications for preoperative parathyroid localization in patients with primary hyperparathyroidism vary among practitioners. Many initial cervical explorations are performed without preoperative localization (30, 31, 37). When surgical treatment is performed by an experienced parathyroid surgeon, a cure rate of 95% or greater can be expected (30, 31, 37, 38). Preoperative local-

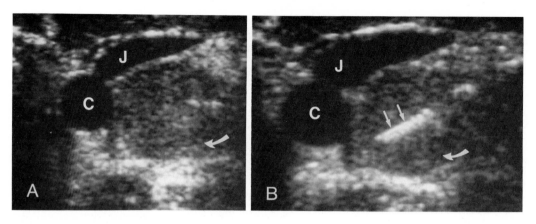

Figure 5.6. Sonogram of positive cervical lymph node biopsy. **A,** Transverse sonogram shows 1.3 × 1.5 cm nonpalpable lymph node (*arrow*) lateral to common carotid artery (*C*) and posterior to the internal jugular vein (*J*). **B,** Transverse sonogram shows biopsy needle (*straight arrows*) within enlarged lymph node (*curved arrow*). Biopsy was positive for papillary carcinoma. (Reproduced with permission from Sutton, RT. US-guided biopsy of neck masses in postoperative management of patients with thyroid cancer. *Radiology*, 168:770, 1988.)

ization by any imaging method is unlikely to improve this rate of surgical success. However, preoperative parathyroid localization may help to direct neck surgery. Preoperative parathyroid localization studies are helpful in patients undergoing reoperation for persistent or recurrent hypercalcemia, the most common cause of which is inadequate resection of abnormal parathyroid tissue at the initial cervical exploration. The most common location for the missing parathyroid adenoma is still within the neck, accessible to sonographic localization (38–43). Because of the scarred surgical field, repeat cervical exploration has a lower rate of success and a higher incidence of complication (39–41). Preoperative localization with sonography has been shown to increase the surgical success rate and to significantly decrease the operating time (39).

Sonographically Guided FNAB of Parathyroid Masses

High-frequency sonography can be used as a guide in needle biopsy of suspected abnormal parathyroid glands in selected patients. Several reports in recent years have found sonographically guided FNAB to be a highly accurate technique to confirm the presence or absence of parathyroid tissue in suspicious neck masses (5, 44, 45). In our practice, aspiration biopsy is not performed on patients who have not had an initial neck exploration. As mentioned above, an experienced surgeon can successfully treat about 95% of these patients without preoperative localization. However, in the patient undergoing reoperation for persistent or recurrent hypercalcemia, surgical localization can be a more difficult problem. After the initial cervical exploration, postoperative scarring and adhesions can distort the operative field and complicate the surgical technique. Consequently, reoperation is technically more difficult and has a lower success rate (36, 38–40). Moreover, morbidity is higher than in the primary cervical exploration, with a higher incidence of permanent postoperative hypocalcemia and recurrent laryngeal nerve damage (38–40). Aspiration biopsy under sonographic guidance is often performed in the reoperative patient to confirm or exclude the presence of parathyroid tissue in a visualized mass (Fig. 5.7). Histologic confirmation of parathyroid tissue lends considerable reassurance to the patient and is of significant value to the surgeon at the time of cervical reexploration.

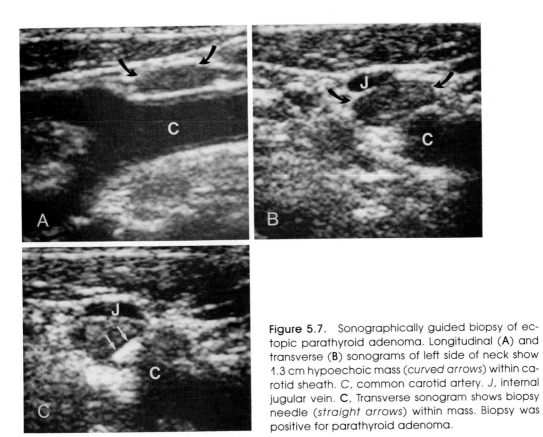

Figure 5.7. Sonographically guided biopsy of ectopic parathyroid adenoma. Longitudinal (**A**) and transverse (**B**) sonograms of left side of neck show 1.3 cm hypoechoic mass (*curved arrows*) within carotid sheath. *C*, common carotid artery. *J*, internal jugular vein. **C**, Transverse sonogram shows biopsy needle (*straight arrows*) within mass. Biopsy was positive for parathyroid adenoma.

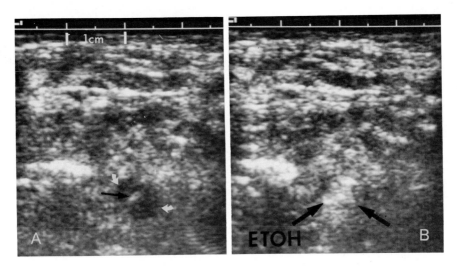

Figure 5.8 **A**, longitudinal sonogram of lower pole of right thyroid lobe, shows heterogeneous parenchyma containing a 0.8 cm round hypoechoic nodule (*curved white arrows*). Within this nodule is a bright echogenic focus representing tip of needle (*black arrow*). **B**, Hypoechoic nodule shown in *A* became hyperechoic at moment of injection of alcohol (*ETOH*) (*arrows*). From Charboneau, JW. Persistent primary hyperparathyroidism: successful ultrasound-guided percutaneous ethanol ablation of an occult adenoma. (Reproduced with permission from *Mayo Clinic Proceedings*, 63:915, 1988.)

Therapeutic Ablation by Alcohol Under Sonographic Guidance

Percutaneous ablation by alcohol of enlarged parathyroid glands under sonographic guidance has been shown to be a successful means of decreasing gland mass in patients with secondary hyperparathyroidism (46). In our own experience, this procedure was a successful therapeutic alternative to reoperation in a high-risk patient who had persistent hyperparathyroidism after previous cervical explorations (47).

With the freehand technique described previously, aspiration biopsy is first performed to confirm histologically the presence of a parathyroid adenoma. Then a 22-gauge spinal needle is inserted into the lesion under continuous sonographic guidance. When the tip of the needle is visible within the mass, absolute alcohol is injected via a 1-ml syringe. One-half milliliter of alcohol is injected per 1 cm of gland size. The alcohol is injected into the center as well as the peripheral portions of the mass. As the alcohol is being injected, the normally hypoechoic adenoma will become highly echogenic as a result of microbubbles in the alcohol solution (Fig. 5.8).

To achieve normal levels of serum calcium and PTH, serial injections are usually required at 2- to 3-day intervals. Reported complications of this technique have been limited to transient local pain and mild transient dysphonia (46).

REFERENCES

1. Scheible W, Leopold GR, Woo VL, Gosink BB: High Resolution real-time ultrasonography of thyroid nodules. *Radiology* 133:413–417, 1979.
2. Katz JF, Kane RA, Reyes J, Clarke MP, Hill TC: Thyroid nodules: Sonographic-pathologic correlation. *Radiology* 151:741–745, 1984.
3. Reading CC, Charboneau JW, James EM et al.: High-resolution parathyroid sonography. *AJR* 139:539–546, 1982.
4. Simeone JF, Mueller PR, Ferrucci JT Jr et al.: High-resolution real-time sonography of the parathyroid. *Radiology* 141:745–751, 1981.
5. Doppman JL, Krudy AG, Marx SJ et al.: Aspiration of enlarged parathyroid glands for parathyroid hormone assay. *Radiology* 148:31–35, 1983.
6. Stoffer RP, Welch JW, Hellwig CA, Chesky VE, McCusker EN: Nodular goiter: Incidence, morphology before and after iodine prophylaxis, and clinical diagnosis. *Arch Intern Med* 106:10–14, 1960.
7. Brown CL: Pathology of the cold nodule. *Clin Endocrinal Metab* 10:235–245, 1981.
8. Hay ID: Malignant thyroid nodules: A clinician's perspective. *Current Med* 23–28, 1988.
9. Rossi RL, Nieroda C, Cady B, Wool MS: Malignancies of the thyroid gland: The Lahey Clinic experience. *Surg Clin N Am* 65:211–230, 1985.
10. Simeone JF, Daniels GH, Mueller PR et al.: High resolution real-time sonography of the thyroid. *Radiology* 145:431–435, 1982.
11. James EM, Charboneau JW: High-frequency (10 MHz) thyroid ultrasonography. *Semin Ultrasound CT MR* 6:294–309, 1985.
12. Solbiati L, Volterrani L, Rizzatto G et al.: The thyroid gland with low uptake lesions: Evaluation by ultrasound. *Radiology* 155:187–191, 1985.
13. Walfish PG, Hazani E, Strawbridge HTG, Miskin M, Rosen IB: A prospective study of combined ultrasonography and needle aspiration biopsy in the assessment of the hypofunctioning thyroid nodule. *Surgery* 82:474–482, 1977.
14. Gershengorn MC, McClung MR, Chu EW, Hanson TAS, Weintraub BD, Robbins J: Fine-needle aspiration cytology in the preoperative diagnosis of thyroid nodules. *Ann Intern Med* 87:265–269, 1977.
15. Hamberger B, Gharib H, Melton LJ III, Goellner JR, Zinsmeister AR: Fine-needle aspiration biopsy of thyroid nodules: Impact on thyroid practice and cost of care. *Am J Med* 73:381–384, 1982.
16. Suen KC, Quenville NF: Fine needle aspiration biopsy of the thyroid gland: A study of 304 cases, *J Clin Pathol* 36:1036–1045, 1983.
17. Gobien RP: Aspiration biopsy of the solitary thyroid nodule. *Radiol Clin N Am* 17:543–554, 1979.
18. Clark OH: Thyroid nodules and thyroid cancer: Surgical aspects. *West J Med* 133:1–8, 1980.
19. Holm HH, Pedersen JF, Kristensen JK, Rasmussen SN, Hancke S, Jensen F: Ultrasonically guided percutaneous puncture. *Radiol Clin Am* 13:493–503, 1975.
20. Grant EG, Richardson JD, Smirniotopoulos JG, Jacobs NM: Fine-needle biopsy directed by real-time sonography: Technique and accuracy. *AJR* 141:29–32, 1983.
21. Reading CC, Charboneau JW, James EM, Hurt MR: Sonographically guided percutaneous biopsy of small (3 cm or less) masses. *AJR* 151:189–192, 1988.
22. Gorman B, Charboneau JW, James EM, et al.: Medullary thyroid carcinoma: role of high-resolution US. *Radiology* 162:147–150, 1987.
23. Simeone JF, Daniels GH, Hall DA, et al.: Sonography in the follow-up of 100 patients with thyroid carcinoma. *AJR* 148:45–49, 1987.
24. Sutton RT, Reading CC, Charboneau JW, James EM, Grant CS, Hay ID: US-guided biopsy of neck masses in postoperative management of patients with thyroid cancer. *Radiology* 168:769–772, 1988.
25. Marchal G, Oyen R, Verschakelen J, Gelin J, Baert AL, Stessens RC: Sonographic appearance of normal lymph nodes. *J Ultrasound Med* 4:417–419, 1985.
26. Wang C-A: The anatomic basis of parathyroid surgery. *Ann Surg* 183:271–275, 1976.

27. Gilmour JR. The gross anatomy of the parathyroid glands. *J Pathol* 46:133–147, 1938.

28. Austin CW. Ultrasound evaluation of thyroid and parathyroid disease. *Semin Ultrasound* 3:250–262, 1982.

29. Heath H III, Hodgson SF, Kennedy MA. Primary hyperparathyroidism: incidence, morbidity, and potential economic impact in a community. *N Engl J Med* 302:189–193, 1980.

30. van Heerden JA: Aspects of primary hyperparathyroidism—a clinical review based on the John Hellström lecture, Stockholm 1985. *Acta Chir Scand* 152:161–167, 1986.

31. van Heerden JA, Beahrs OH, Woolner LB. The pathology and surgical management of primary hyperparathyroidism. *Surg Clin N Am* 57:557–563, 1977.

32. Sample WF, Mitchell SP, Bledsoe RC: Parathyroid ultrasonography. *Radiology* 127:485–490, 1978.

33. Duffy P, Picker RH, Duffield S, Reeve T, Hewlett S: Parathyroid sonography: A useful aid to preoperative localization. *J Clin Ultrasound* 8:113–116, 1980.

34. Scheible W, Deutsch AL, Leopold GR: Parathyroid adenoma: Accuracy of preoperative localization by high-resolution real-time sonography. *J Clin Ultrasound* 9:325–330, 1981.

35. van Heerden JA, James EM, Karsell PR, Charboneau JW, Grant CS, Purnell DC: Small-part ultrasonography in primary hyperparathyroidism: Initial experience. *Ann Surg* 195:774–779, 1982.

36. Reading CC, Charboneau JW, James EM, et al.: Postoperative parathyroid high-frequency sonography: Evaluation of persistent or recurrent hyperparathyroidism. *AJR* 144:399–402, 1985.

37. Russell CF, Edis AJ. Surgery for primary hyperparathyroidism: Experience with 500 consecutive cases and evaluation of the role of surgery in the asymptomatic patient. *Br J Surg* 69:244–247, 1982.

38. Satava RM Jr, Beahrs OH, Scholz DA: Success rate of cervical exploration for hyperparathyroidism. *Arch Surg* 110:625–628, 1975.

39. Grant CS, van Heerden JA, Charboneau JW, James EM, Reading CC: Clinical management of persistent and/or recurrent primary hyperparathyroidism. *World J Surg* 10:555–565, 1986.

40. Edis AJ, Sheedy PF II, Beahrs OH, van Heerden JA: Results of reoperation for hyperparathyroidism, with evaluation of preoperative localization studies. *Surgery* 84:384–393, 1978.

41. Brennan MF, Marx SJ, Doppman J, et al.: Results of reoperation for persistent and recurrent hyperparathyroidism. *Ann Surg* 194:671–675, 1981.

42. Martin JK Jr, van Heerden JA, Edis AJ, Dahlin DC: Persistent postoperative hyperparathyroidism. *Surg Gynecol Obstet* 151: 764–767, 1980.

43. Wang C-A: Parathyroid re-exploration: A clinical and pathological study of 112 cases. *Ann Surg* 186: 140–145, 1977.

44. Gooding GAW, Clark OH, Stark DD, Moss AA, Montgomery CK: Parathyroid aspiration biopsy under ultrasound guidance in the postoperative hyperparathyroid patient. *Radiology* 155:193–196, 1985.

45. Solbiati L, Montali G, Croce F, Bellotti E, Giangrande A, Ravetto C. Parathyroid tumors detected by fine-needle aspiration biopsy under ultrasonic guidance. *Radiology* 148:793–797, 1983.

46. Solbiati L, Giangrande A, De Pra L, Bellotti E, Cantù P, Ravetto C: Percutaneous ethanol injection of parathyroid tumors under US guidance: Treatment for secondary hyperparathyroidism. *Radiology* 155:607–610, 1985.

47. Charboneau JW, Hay ID, van Heerden JA: Persistent primary hyperparathyroidism: Successful ultrasound-guided percutaneous ethanol ablation of an occult adenoma. *Mayo Clin Proc* 63:913–917, 1988.

6 Interventional Ultrasound of the Breast

BRUNO D. FORNAGE

Fine-needle aspiration biopsy (FNAB) of palpable breast masses is routinely performed by palpation using a technique that has not significantly changed since it was first reported in 1930 (1–7). On the other hand, demonstration of nonpalpable lesions by mammography has fostered the development of a number of techniques, including stereotaxic methods for preoperative FNAB and localization of lesions (8–18). These mammographic techniques have two basic limitations, namely, the lack of real-time imaging and the display of planar projections. They require step-by-step mammographic confirmation and repositioning and can be time-consuming. Recently, sonography has been used to guide FNAB and preoperative or intraoperative localization of nonpalpable breast masses (19–25).

Mammography and sonography are fully complementary imaging techniques for the breast, the limitations of one technique being compensated by the advantages of the other. Sonography has proved effective for dense breasts, for which mammography is of limited value (26–32). Because it involves no radiation exposure, sonography can be performed on pregnant patients and is the modality of choice for adolescents and young adults. Peripheral breast lesions, small breasts, and breasts with augmentation prostheses, which are difficult to evaluate with mammography, can easily be assessed by real-time sonography. In addition, the axilla and infraclavicular areas are systematically evaluated during breast so-

nography. On the other hand, because it can demonstrate isolated microcalcifications and carcinomas less than 5 mm, mammography is employed for mass screening of breast cancer.

Ultrasound-guided Fine-needle Aspiration Biopsy of Breast Masses

Ultrasound guidance is more accurate than palpation guidance for biopsy of palpable masses, but the most significant indication for ultrasound guidance is biopsy of nonpalpable tumors. Nonpalpable lesions may be visible on both mammograms and sonograms or on sonograms only. Ultrasound-guided FNAB should be performed after mammography to avoid false-positive interpretations of postbiopsy hematomas (33) and mammograms must be carefully reviewed before the procedure is undertaken.

TECHNICAL CONSIDERATIONS

Instrumentation

FNAB can be performed using 20- to 25-gauge needles. We use 20-gauge, 1.5-inch (3.8-cm) hypodermic needles. Small cutting needles can also be used for needle core biopsies. The biopsy tray includes a 20-ml syringe (two if a pneumocystogram is to be done), sterile gauze or gauze pads, and a cup filled with alcohol.

State-of-the-art real-time equipment with

71

high-frequency hand-held transducers is mandatory to delineate small lesions. Linear-array electronic transducers have proven superior to sector scanners in imaging superficial organs because of the great width and high resolution of the tissue within their near-field. A 7.5-MHz linear-array transducer is most effective for this application. The transducer is soaked for 3 to 5 minutes in a sterilizing solution (see Chapter 1). If soaking is contraindicated by the manufacturer, is wrapped in a sterile covering. In the latter case, a small amount of coupling medium is placed on the transducer.

Technique of Biopsy

The procedure is explained to the patient and informed consent obtained. Depending on the location of the tumor, the patient is then placed in a dorsal decubitus or oblique position, to spread the breast on the chest wall. The skin is cleaned with alcohol, which also serves as an acoustic coupling medium. The probe is then placed in direct contact with the skin in such a manner that the lesion lies on the midline of the scan. Local anesthetization is optional.

Two different techniques are available for needle insertion (22, 23). In the first, the needle is inserted perpendicularly to the long axis of the transducer and obliquely so that the tip of the needle will reach the scan plane at the level of the lesion, where it appears as a distinct bright echo (Fig. 6.1). The obliquity of the needle is determined by the depth of the lesion; the more superficial the lesion, the more oblique the needle. With this technique, only the tip of the needle is visualized, and it is not seen until it has reached the scan plane.

In the second technique, the needle is inserted obliquely from one end of the transducer within the scan plane (Fig. 6.2). With this technique, both the tip and the distal portion of the needle are continuously visualized, which guarantees absolute safety when the lesion is close to the chest wall or in a very small breast (Fig. 6.2C). The successful placement of the needle requires coordination of the respective positions of the scan plane and the needle. Therefore, the procedure is performed most effectively when the transducer and the needle are manipulated by a single operator.

When the needle has reached the target, the position of the tip is documented. In the case of a cyst, the fluid is evacuated. An x-ray pneumocystogram can then be performed after insufflation of air through the needle. The air will resorb in 1 to 2 weeks.

FNAB of solid lesions is performed using strenuous suction; thorough sampling of the lesion is obtained with to-and-fro and fan-like movements of the needle under continuous real-time monitoring. The negative

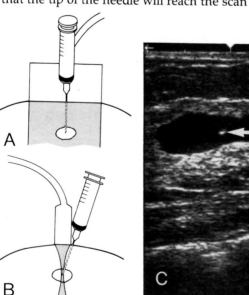

A

B

C

Figure 6.1. Technique of ultrasound-guided FNAB. The needle is inserted perpendicularly to the long axis of the transducer and obliquely. **A,** Diagram shows the linear-array transducer and the needle and syringe. **B,** Side-view shows the obliquity of the needle in relation to the transducer. **C,** Sonogram demonstrates the needle tip as a bright echo (arrow) at the center of a cyst.

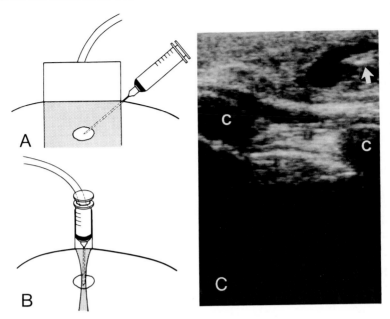

Figure 6.2. Technique of ultrasound-guided FNAB. The needle is inserted obliquely from the end of the linear-array probe along the scan plane. **A,** Diagram of the front of the transducer shows the obliquity of the needle relative to the transducer. **B,** End-on diagram shows the needle within the scan plane. **C,** Sonogram demonstrates the echogenic distal portion of the needle (*arrow*) penetrating a 0.8-cm cyst. Note the small size of the breast and the proximity of the lesion to the chest wall. c = costal cartilage.

pressure in the syringe can be created by several methods outlined in Chapter 1, including use of vacuum test tubes (Vacutainer 34). Rotation of the needle (corkscrew maneuver) increases dissociation of the tumor tissue. The suction is released before the needle is withdrawn. Fine cutting needles with automatic biopsy devices are currently under evaluation at our institution.

Preparation of Smears

The aspirate is expelled onto glass slides and the smears are prepared. If possible, the smears are stained immediately and checked by the cytopathologist to ensure the adequacy of the specimen, so that a repeat aspiration can be performed if the specimen is inadequate. Papanicolaou stain is routinely used at our institution. The smears must be fixed without delay by dipping the slides in the appropriate medium or by using a spray fixative to avoid air-drying artifacts. Different staining techniques are reviewed in Chapter 2.

Because of the accuracy of ultrasound-guided needle placement in the breast, only one pass is needed in most cases. Our policy is to limit needle passes to three. Multiple biopsies occasionally have been necessary with fibroadenomas. Ultrasound-guided FNAB of a breast mass rarely takes more than 5 minutes.

FIBROCYSTIC DISEASE

Cysts

Cysts smaller than 1 cm can be aspirated under sonographic guidance.

FIBROADENOMA

Fibroadenomas usually appear as hypoechoic, well-circumscribed, elongated masses (Fig. 6.3) (36). A few fibroadenomas are isoechoic or hyperechoic. A moderate sound through transmission can be seen, although a few fibroadenomas are associated with marked shadowing. Infrequently, a fibroadenoma particularly when surrounded

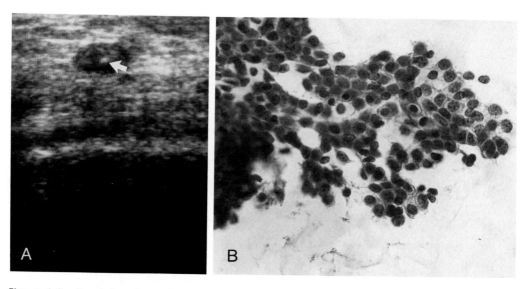

Figure 6.3. Small (less than 1 cm) fibroadenoma. **A,** Sonogram shows the small oval-shaped hypoechoic mass. The needle tip is clearly visualized inside the lesion (*arrow*). **B,** Cytologic smear shows antler horn cluster of benign cells.

by fat, cannot be identified on sonograms (37).

Strict cytologic criteria are required when diagnosing fibroadenomas (38). In our experience, a definite cytologic diagnosis of fibroadenoma has been obtained from ultrasound-guided FNAB specimens in only 62% of cases (Fig. 6.3), while inadequate specimens were obtained in 16% of cases (39). Even with strenuous aspiration, it is difficult to lower the failure rate of FNAB, which is related to the histologic composition of the tumor rather than to the aspiration technique. Whenever the specimen is inadequate, the procedure must be repeated. However, after a repeated failure, it is unlikely that subsequent passes will be more productive, and we therefore routinely limit the number of passes to three. An alternative is the use of newly developed fine cutting needles with automatic biopsy devices.

Cystosarcoma phyllodes, which may be benign or malignant, is a rare variant of fibroadenoma with a highly cellular, sarcoma-like stroma containing fluid-filled clefts. Differentiation between benign and malignant cystosarcoma phyllodes may not be possible from cytologic examination.

OTHER BENIGN CONDITIONS

Abscess

Abscesses are sonolucent, hypoechoic, or of mixed echogenicity with echogenic debris. Margins are irregular and often blurred on sonograms. Occasionally, an abscess cannot be differentiated from an inflammatory carcinoma. Diagnosis is readily confirmed by an ultrasound-guided FNAB.

Fat Necrosis

Fat necrosis develops after trauma, including surgery. The lesion may resemble carcinoma on physical, mammographic, and sonographic examinations. Ultrasound-guided FNAB (Fig. 6.4) can confirm the diagnosis by showing amorphous and inflammatory material interspersed with fat cells containing large vacuoles.

Postsurgical Collections

Hematoma. Excision of breast tumors is often associated with a residual hematoma at the site of the excised lesion that generally resolves within a few weeks. It may persist or grow and then mimic tumor recurrence. Ultrasound-guided FNAB confirms the di-

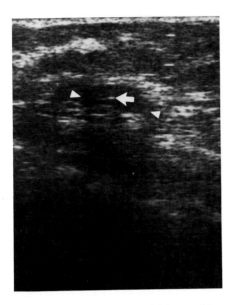

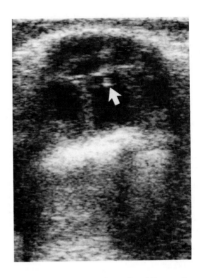

Figure 6.4. Patient with a history of breast cancer and reconstructed breast. Sonogram shows an ill-defined hypoechoic mass (*arrowheads*). The *arrow* points to the needle tip. Cytology confirmed fat necrosis.

Figure 6.5. Large postsurgical hematoma of the breast. Sonogram shows an organized hematoma with fibrinous septa. The needle tip is clearly documented (*arrow*). Because of the septa, the hematoma could not be completely evacuated. Follow-up sonograms confirmed progressive resolution.

agnosis and allows complete evacuation unless the hematoma is clotted or organized with fibrin septation (Fib. 6.5).

Lymphocele. Lymphoceles develop as a complication of axillary lymph node dissection. Small collections are effectively treated by percutaneous aspiration under ultrasound guidance. Large collections, however, require surgical drainage.

CARCINOMA

The sonographic appearances of benign and malignant solid masses in the breast overlap (36, 37, 40, 41). In most cases, the sonographic pattern of carcinoma is characteristic. A carcinoma appears as a focal hypoechoic mass disrupting the smooth architecture of breast tissue planes. The margins are irregular, and echotexture is nonhomogeneous. Acoustic shadowing is found in fewer than 50% of cases. A desmoplastic reaction of fibrosis and edema can be seen as an ill-defined echogenic rim surrounding the hypoechoic malignant core. Unlike fibroadenomas, carcinomas are spheric or even grow anteroposteriorly with a length to anteroposterior diameter ratio of less than 1. About 10% to 15% of carcinomas appear as well-circumscribed nodules on both mammograms and sonograms. Of this group, medullary carcinomas are markedly hypoechoic with occasional distal acoustic enhancement and can mimic cysts (32, 42, 43). Twenty to thirty per cent of breast cysts have an atypical ultrasound appearance with low-level internal echoes, irregular margins, or lack of distal sound enhancement. As a result, some cysts may appear as indeterminate hypoechoic masses. Sonography may be helpful in diagnosis of indeterminate masses on mammograms. Ultrasound can demonstrate the cystic nature of the mass and ultrasound-guided FNAB spares the patient an unnecessary surgical biopsy (Figs. 6.6 & 6.7).

Pneumocystography is useful for precise and objective correlation of sonographic and mammographic findings (Fig. 6.7D). It is also the best technique for demonstrating small intracystic tumors that may not be visible on sonograms. A pneumocystogram is mandatory when hemorrhagic fluid has

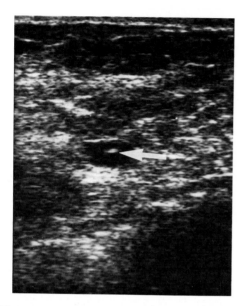

Figure 6.6. Ultrasound-guided FNAB of a small cyst. Sonogram shows a deep 0.8 × 0.5-cm cyst. The needle tip is clearly visualized (*arrow*).

been aspirated or when the sonogram suggests the presence of an intracystic lesion. Pneumocystography has been claimed to have some therapeutic value, the mechanism of which is unclear (35).

Inspissated cysts are characterized by the presence of viscid contents. Internal echoes can be present, although a typical cystic pattern may also be found. At the most, only a few drops of thick material can be aspirated. Infected cysts may also contain a viscid fluid that cannot be easily evacuated.

Cytologic and microbiological examinations of the aspirate are performed when an infected cyst is suspected. Cytologic examination is considered unnecessary by some authors when the aspirated fluid is clear and straw-colored in a patient with a low risk of cancer.

Occasionally, some difficulties may occur in puncturing cysts. A thickened wall may resist needle passage. Cysts that are not under tension may show a significant deformation under the needle's pressure; penetration of the wall requires a brief and firm forward thrust of the needle. Also, small cysts in a fatty environment may move significantly under the needle. Increasing the

pressure of the transducer on the skin may help keep lesions stationary.

Cysts that require aspiration include those that do not have a typical pattern on sonograms and those that appear as indeterminate densities on mammograms. Symptomatic cysts are aspirated for a therapeutic purpose. Asymptomatic typical cysts in a patient with fibrocystic disease do not require aspiration unless they demonstrate growth on repeat examination.

Proliferative Fibrocystic Disease

Proliferative fibrocystic disease comprises papillomatosis, ductal epithelial hyperplasia, lobular hyperplasia, and sclerosing adenosis. Clinically, it often results in lumpy areas within the breast. Sonographic abnormalities are mostly diffuse with occasional ill-defined, rather echogenic areas poorly demarcated from the rest of the breast parenchyma. FNAB yields benign epithelial cells; on occasion, the cytologic diagnosis of florid hyperplasia leads to surgical biopsy. Papillomas are a well-known cause of false-positive cytologic results because of the hypercellularity of such lesions (23).

Infrequently, sonography can demonstrate carcinomas not seen on mammograms, particularly in dense breasts (Fig. 6.8, 44), breasts with postsurgical and/or postirradiation changes (Fig. 6.9), or breasts with prostheses. However, it is well known that isolated microcalcifications cannot be visualized on sonography (32, 45) and any attempt at identifying clusters of microcalcifications not associated with a mass by sonography would yield deceptive results (21). Biopsy of such lesions must be performed under mammographic (stereotaxic) guidance.

In the vast majority of cases, ultrasound-guided FNAB is performed to confirm or exclude a diagnosis of breast cancer when an indeterminate solid mass is seen on sonograms or mammograms. In our experience, this technique has proved highly effective in the early diagnosis of nonpalpable carcinomas as small as 0.7 to 0.8 cm in diameter (Fig. 6.10), and it represents an effective alternative to follow-up mammograms (46).

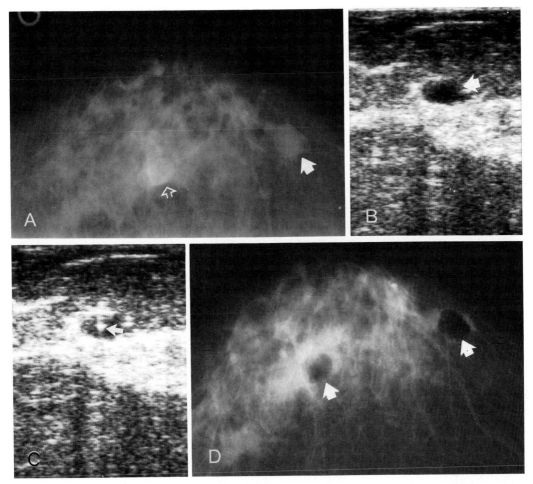

Figure 6.7. A 65-yr-old patient referred for preoperative needle localization of a nonpalpable suspicious mass on mammograms. **A,** Craniocaudal mammogram shows a suspicious density with a poorly defined posterior wall (*arrow*). A well-circumscribed, benign-appearing mass is also noted in the mid portion of the breast (*open arrow*). **B,** Sonogram of the region of the suspicious density demonstrates a cyst (*arrow*). **C,** Sonogram obtained during FNAB shows the bright needle tip (*arrow*) in the cyst. **D,** Pneumocystogram obtained after aspiration of the two mammographic abnormalities confirms two cysts (*arrows*) with smooth internal walls.

ACCURACY OF ULTRASOUND-GUIDED FNAB

Because of the unique real-time continuous visualization of the tip of the needle within the mass, ultrasound-guided FNAB is extremely accurate, and lesions as small as 5 mm can be successfully aspirated. As a rule, the cytologic diagnosis of malignancy is easily made by an expert cytopathologist. In addition, some types of carcinomas (including medullary and colloid tumors), lymphomatous involvement, and some metastatic deposits can be characterized on cytology. It must be kept in mind that results of ultrasound-guided FNAB of breast masses reflect the combination of a) the accuracy of the guiding technique, b) the success rate of tissue extraction, and c) the expertise of the cytopathologist. In a 1982–1987 series of ultrasound-guided biopsies of 325 breast masses, 44% of which were not palpable, the sensitivity, specificity, and overall accuracy of the technique

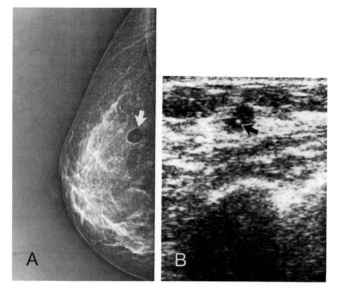

Figure 6.8. A 33-year-old patient after excision of a left axillary lymph node metastasis. No breast mass could be palpated. **A,** Lateral mammographic projection obtained after aspiration and insufflation of a 0.9-cm cyst seen on sonogram in the upper breast (*arrow*). No other discrete mass can be visualized, particularly in the inferior breast. **B,** Ultrasound-guided FNAB of a suspicious 0.7-cm hypoechoic mass detected on sonograms in the 6 o'clock region. Note the jagged margins. The needle tip is distinctly visualized (*arrow*). Cytologic diagnosis was infiltrating ductal carcinoma. Pathological examination demonstrated a 0.9-cm medullary carcinoma.

were 90%, 91%, and 91%, respectively (Table 6.1). However, these values would increase to 92%, 98%, and 97%, respectively, if inadequate specimens were excluded and to 100%, 98%, and 99%, respectively, if, in addition, suspicious findings were assimilated with positive ones.

A cytologic result is considered negative

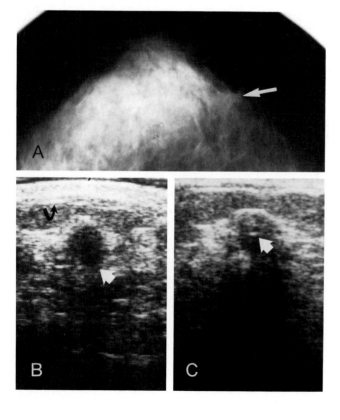

Figure 6.9. A 32-year-old patient with an infiltrating lobular carcinoma treated by segmental mastectomy and radiation therapy. Nine months later, ultrasound examination detects a nonpalpable local recurrence. **A,** Craniocaudal mammographic projection shows minor distortion at the site of previous surgery (*arrow*). No masses can be delineated. **B,** Sonogram clearly demonstrates a suspicious, 0.9-cm, hypoechoic mass (*arrow*) with an anteroposterior growth axis. Note the postirradiation thickening of the skin (*curved arrow*). **C,** Sonogram obtained during FNAB shows the needle tip (*arrow*) in the center of the mass. Cytology was positive for malignancy; at pathology, a 1-cm recurrent lobular carcinoma was found.

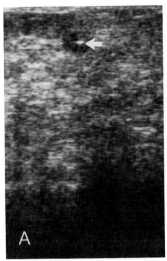
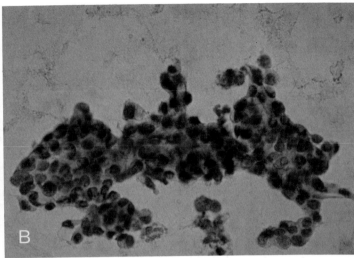

Figure 6.10. Ultrasound-guided FNAB of a small, nonpalpable breast carcinoma in an 81-year-old patient. **A,** Sonogram shows the bright tip of the needle (*arrow*) in a 0.6-cm rounded mass. **B,** Cytologic diagnosis was adenocarcinoma.

when the specimen is adequate in quantity and quality and does not show any malignant cells. It is widely admitted that with palpation guidance, a negative cytologic result is clinically irrelevant because the needle may have missed the target. With continuous sonographic guidance, however, the needle tip is clearly identified and documented within the mass during the procedure, providing evidence that the tissue specimen has been accurately extracted from the questionable mass. Therefore, a negative cytologic result taken from a solid mass under continuous real-time ultrasound guidance is now a strong indication (if not evidence) of a benign lesion.

On the other hand, an inadequate specimen should be considered a complete failure of the procedure and should prompt a repeat aspiration. A high rate of inadequate specimens has been associated with fibroadenomas, whereas needle aspirations of carcinomas usually provide abundant material because of the loose intercellular adhesion of these tumors.

ULTRASOUND VERSUS MAMMOGRAPHIC GUIDANCE

A new and simple strategy for FNAB of nonpalpable breast masses has emerged. For lesions seen exclusively on mammograms, including isolated microcalcifications and solid masses less than 0.7 to 0.8 cm, needle biopsies must be performed using stereotaxic mammographic guidance. In contrast, ultrasound guidance is the technique of

Table 6.1.
Results of Ultrasound-Guided Fine-Needle Aspiration Biopsy of 325 Breast Masses

Final Diagnosis	No. of Biopsies	Cytologic Diagnosis			
		Positive	Suspicious	Negative	Inadequate Specimen
Malignant	78	70	6	0	2
Benign	247	1	3	225	18
Total	325	71	9	225	20

choice for lesions visualized on both sonograms and mammograms or on sonograms only, including cysts and solid masses greater than 0.7 to 0.8 cm. As a general rule, whenever a discrete mass is apparent on sonograms, FNAB can be performed under real-time ultrasound guidance. Ultrasound guidance can also be used for FNAB of lymph nodes in the axillae and infra- or supraclavicular areas.

A mass can be poorly seen or obscured on mammograms in patients with dense breasts (including adolescent and young adult patients and patients with fibrocystic disease, inflammatory carcinomas, or irradiated breasts). Sonography usually demonstrates the lesion in those circumstances and therefore provides accurate guidance for FNAB. Ultrasound-guided FNAB can be performed in pregnant patients (Fig. 6.11) and in those who refuse radiation exposure.

Real-time continuous monitoring of the tip of the needle also makes the technique safe and ultrasound guidance can be used to aspirate lesions close to the chest wall (Fig. 6.2C) or adjacent to an augmentation prosthesis.

Strong cooperation between the sonologist and the cytopathologist is mandatory for the successful application of ultrasound-guided FNAB of the breast. Communication with the cytopathologist will help improve the beginner's aspiration technique. With such a team effort, a cytologic diagnosis of (nonpalpable) breast cancer should be possible in about 90% of cases.

Ultrasound-guided Localization of Nonpalpable Breast Masses

PREOPERATIVE LOCALIZATION

Real-time sonography can also be used to guide the insertion of localizing needles or hookwires that are routinely manipulated under mammographic guidance (Fig. 6.12) (9, 12–16). For lesions that are seen equally well on mammograms and sonograms, ultrasound guidance is faster and less traumatic to the patient than mammographically guided techniques because only one pass is generally needed. Mammographic confirmation of correct placement of the localizer is strongly recommended.

The injection of dye into nonpalpable lesions (spot localization) is a fast and effective alternative to metal localizer insertion and can be readily performed under ultrasound guidance. Of the vital dyes whose presence does not affect pathological analysis of the specimen, methylene blue is the most popular (47, 48). After proper placement of the needle under ultrasound guid-

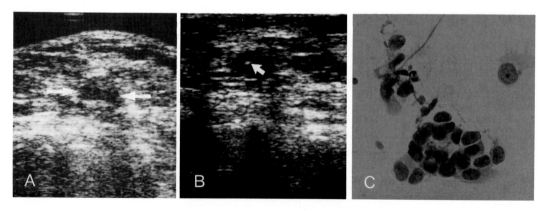

Figure 6.11. Ultrasound-guided FNAB of a nonpalpable breast carcinoma in a 32-year-old pregnant patient presenting with axillary lymph node metastases. **A,** Sonogram shows a deeply located, ill-defined mass about 2 cm in diameter (*arrows*). **B,** Sonogram obtained during FNAB shows the needle tip (*arrow*) inside the suspicious mass. **C,** Cytologic diagnosis was adenocarcinoma.

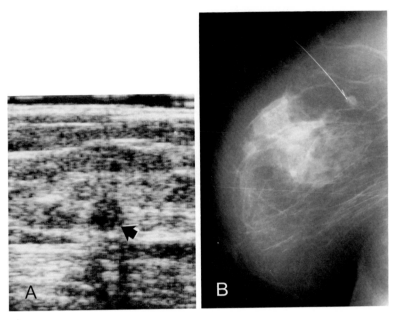

Figure 6.12. Ultrasound-guided preoperative insertion of a Kopans hookwire into a nonpalpable breast carcinoma. **A,** Sonogram clearly delineates a rounded, hypoechoic, 0.6-cm tumor (*arrow*). **B,** The Kopans hookwire has been inserted under sonographic guidance. A mammographic view confirms the accurate placement of the wire adjacent to the tumor. Pathologic examination showed a 0.5-cm carcinoma.

ance, a small amount (0.1–0.2 ml) of dye is injected by tuberculin syringe at the periphery of the lesion with or without a small amount of radiopaque water-soluble contrast medium for optional mammographic control. Continuous injection of dye while the needle is withdrawn has been proposed to identify the needle track (47). Surgery should be performed within a few hours after dye injection to minimize the risk of diffusion.

INTRAOPERATIVE LOCALIZATION AND IN VITRO SCANNING OF SPECIMEN

Intraoperative ultrasound localization of nonpalpable solid breast masses is a recent technique (25). A 7.5-MHz linear-array transducer is used to localize the mass while the patient is on the operating table. The projection of the lesion is marked on the skin and the depth of the lesion is determined from the sonogram. If necessary, a hypodermic needle can be inserted into the mass under ultrasound guidance to aid the surgeon in the surgical approach. Further real-time guidance is also available by placing the sterile probe in the open wound.

After excision, the surgical specimen is placed in a cup filled with saline, and sonography is performed using the same transducer. The definite demonstration of the mass within the specimen confirms the successful excision (Fig. 6.13).

Intraoperative ultrasound localization of nonpalpable breast masses requires the presence of a well-trained sonographer/sonologist in the operating room, but the patient is spared the anxiety and discomfort of the insertion of a metal localizer, with its potential risk of migration (49, 50).

ACKNOWLEDGMENTS

The author thanks Marie-José Faroux for providing the cytopathologic illustrations, Rose Salazar for her secretarial support, and Melissa G. Burkett for editorial assistance.

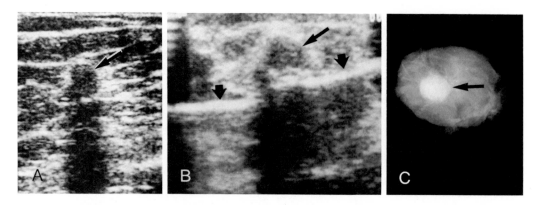

Figure 6.13. Intraoperative localization of a nonpalpable breast fibroadenoma. A Sonogram obtained with the patient lying on the operating table shows a rounded 0.8-cm mass (*arrow*) with marked shadowing. The projection of the lesion is easily marked on the skin. The lesion lies at a depth of 1.5 cm. **B**, Sonogram of the excised specimen demonstrates the tumor (*Long arrow*). *Short arrows* indicate the bottom of the saline-filled container. **C**, Radiograph of the specimen confirms the successful excision of the lesion (*arrow*).

REFERENCES

1. Martin HE, Ellis EB: Biopsy by needle puncture and aspiration. *Ann Surg* 92:169–181, 1930.
2. Palombini L, Fulciniti F, Vetrani A et al.: Fine-needle aspiration biopsies of breast masses. A critical analysis of 1956 cases in 8 years (1976–1984). *Cancer* 61:2273–2277, 1988.
3. Kline TS, Joshi LP, Hunter SN: Fine-needle aspiration of the breast: diagnoses and pitfalls. A review of 3545 cases. *Cancer* 44:1458–1464, 1979.
4. Zajdela A, Ghossein NA, Pilleron JP, Ennuyer A: The value of aspiration cytology in the diagnosis of breast cancer: experience at the Foundation Curie. *Cancer* 35:499–506, 1975.
5. Frable WJ. Needle aspiration of the breast. *Cancer* 53:671–676, 1984.
6. Griffith CN, Kern WH, Mikkelsen WP. Needle aspiration cytologic examination in the management of suspicious lesions of the breast. *Surg Gynecol Obstet* 162:142–144, 1986.
7. Bell DA, Hajdu SI, Urban JA, Gaston JP: Role of aspiration cytology in the diagnosis and management of mammary lesions in office practice. *Cancer* 51:1182–1189, 1983.
8. Löfgren M, Andersson I, Bondeson L, Lindholm K: X-ray guided fine-needle aspiration for the cytologic diagnosis of nonpalpable breast lesions. *Cancer* 61:1032–1037, 1988.
9. Dodd GD: Preoperative radiographic localization of nonpalpable lesions. In Gallager HS (ed): *Early Breast Cancer: Detection and Treatment.* New York, John Wiley & Sons, 1975, pp 151–153.
10. Threatt B, Appelman H, Dow R, o'Rourke T: Percutaneous needle localization of clustered mammary microcalcifications prior to biopsy. *AJR* 121:839–842, 1974.
11. Hall FM, Frank HA: Preoperative localization of nonpalpable breast lesions. *AJR* 132:101–105, 1979. (num12. Kopans DB, Meyer JE. Versatile spring hookwire breast lesion localizer. *AJR* 138:586–587, 1982.
13. Libshitz HI, Feig SA, Fetouh S: Needle localization of nonpalpable breast lesions. *Radiology* 121:557–560, 1976.
14. Kalisher L: An improved needle for localization of nonpalpable breast lesions. *Radiology* 128:815–817, 1978.
15. Sitzman SB: A new needle for pre-operative localization of nonpalpable breast lesions. *Radiology* 131:533, 1979.
16. Homer MJ: Nonpalpable breast lesion localization using a curved-end retractable wire. *Radiology* 157:259–260, 1985.
17. Bolmgren J, Jacobson B, Nordenström B: Stereotaxic instrument for needle biopsy of the mamma. *AJR* 129:121–125, 1977.
18. Svane G. Silfverswärd C: Stereotaxic needle biopsy of nonpalpable breast lesions: cytologic and histopathologic findings. *Acta Radiol [Diagn.](Stockh)* 24:283–288, 1983.
19. Kopans DB, Meyer JE, Lindfors KK, Bucchianeri SS: Breast sonography to guide cyst aspiration and wire localization of occult solid lesions. *AJR* 143:489–492, 1984.
20. Laing FC, Jeffrey RB, Minagi H: Ultrasound localization of occult breast lesions. *Radiology* 151:795–796, 1984.
21. Weber WN, Sickles EA, Callen PW, Filly RA: Nonpalpable breast lesion localization: limited efficacy of sonography. *Radiology* 155:783–784, 1985.
22. Fornage BD, Faroux MJ, Simatos A: Breast masses. US-guided fine-needle aspiration biopsy. *Radiology* 162:409–414, 1987.
23. Fornage B, Peetrons P, Djelassi L et al.: # Ultrasound guided aspiration biopsy of breast masses. *J Belge Radiol* 70:287–298, 1987.
24. Rizzatto G, Solbiati L, Croce F, Derchi LE: Aspiration biopsy of superficial lesions: Ultrasonic guid-

ance with a linear-array probe. *AJR* 148:623–625, 1987.

25. Rifkin MD, Schwartz GF, Pasto ME et al.: Ultrasound for guidance of breast mass removal. *J Ultrasound Med* 7:261–263, 1988.

26. Fleischer AC, Muhletaler CA, Reynolds VH, et al.: Palpable breast masses: Evaluation by high frequency, hand-held real-time sonography and xeromammography. *Radiology* 148:813–817, 1983.

27. Fornage B, Touche D, Deshayes JL: L échographie du sein: Revue et expérience personnelle. *Journal d'Echographie et de Médecine Ultrasonore* 5: 113–122, 1984.

28. Rosner D, Blaird DL: What ultrasonography can tell in breast masses that mammography and physical examination cannot. *J Surg Oncol* 28:308–313, 1985.

29. Rubin E, Miller VE, Berland LL, Han SV, Koehler RE, Stanley RJ: Hand-held real-time breast sonography. *AJR* 144:623–627, 1985.

30. Egan RL, Egan KL: Automated water-path full-breast sonography: Correlation with histology of 176 solid lesions. *AJR* 143:499–507, 1984.

31. Walsh P, Baddeley H, Timms H, Furnival CM: An assessment of ultrasound mammography as an additional investigation for the diagnosis of breast disease. *Br J Radiol* 58:115–119, 1985.

32. McSweeney MB, Murphy CH: Whole-breast sonography. *Radiol Clin North Am* 23:157–167, 1985.

33. Klein DL, Sickles EA: Effects of needle aspiration on the mammographic appearance of the breast: A guide to the proper timing of the mammography examination. *Radiology* 145:44, 1982.

34. Fornage BD: Fine-needle aspiration biopsy with a vacuum test tube. *Radiology* 169:553–554, 1988.

35. Tabar L, Pentek Z, Dean PB: The diagnostic and therapeutic value of breast cyst puncture and pneumocystography. *Radiology* 141:659–663, 1981.

36. Cole-Beuglet C, Soriano RZ, Kurtz AB, Goldberg BB: Fibroadenoma of the breast: Sonomammography correlated with pathology in 122 patients. *AJR* 140:369–375, 1983.

37. Jackson VP, Rothschild PA, Kreipke DL, Mail JT, Holden RW: The spectrum of sonographic findings of fibroadenoma of the breast. *Invest Radiol* 21: 34–40, 1986.

38. Bottles K, Chan JS, Holly EA, Chiu S, Miller TR: Cytologic criteria for fibroadenoma. A step-wise logistic regression analysis. *Am J Clin Pathol* 89: 707–713, 1988.

39. Fornage BD: Sonographic appearance of fibroadenoma of the breast. Presented at the Annual Meeting of the American Institute of Ultrasound in Medicine, Washington, DC, October 17-21, 1988.

40. Heywang SH, Lipsit ER, Glassman LM, Thomas MA: Specificity of ultrasonography in the diagnosis of benign breast masses. *J Ultrasound Med* 3: 453–461, 1984.

41. Hilton SvW, Leopold GR, Olson LK, Willson SA: Real-time breast sonography: Application in 300 consecutive patients. *AJR* 147:479–486, 1986.

42. Meyer JE, Amin E, Lindfors KK, Lipman JC, Stomper PC, Genest D: Medullary carcinoma of the breast: Mammographic and US appearance. *Radiology* 170:79–82, 1989.

43. Cole-Beuglet C, Soriano RZ, Kurtz AB, Goldberg BB: Ultrasound analysis of 104 primary breast carcinomas classified according to histopathologic type. *Radiology* 147:191–196, 1983.

44. Lambie RW, Hodgden D, Herman EM, Kopperman M: Sonomammographic detection of lobular carcinoma not demonstrated on xeromammography. *J Clin Ultrasound* 11:495–497, 1983.

45. Jackson VP, Kelly-Fry E, Rothschild PA, Holden RW, Clark SA: Automated breast sonography using a 7.5-MHz PVDF transducer: Preliminary clinical evaluation. *Radiology* 159:679–684, 1986.

46. Fornage BD: Real-time ultrasound-guided fine-needle aspiration of nonpalpable breast carcinoma (abstract). *J Ultrasound Med* 7(suppl): 170, 1988.

47. Egan JF, Sayler CB, Goodman MJ: A technique for localizing occult breast lesions. *CA* 26:32–37, 1976.

48. Hermann G, Janus C, Schwartz IS, Krivisky B, Bier S, Rabinowitz JG: Nonpalpable breast lesions: Accuracy of prebiopsy mammographic diagnosis. *Radiology* 165:323–326, 1987.

49. Bristol JB, Jones PA: Transgression of localizing wire into the pleural cavity prior to mammography. *Br J Radiol* 54:139–140, 1981.

50. Davis PS, Wechsler RJ, Feig SA, March DE: Migration of breast biopsy localization wire. *AJR* 150: 787–788, 1988.

7 Interventional Procedures in the Thorax

WILLIAM E. BRANT

Despite the sonographic barriers of air-filled lung and bony thorax, ultrasound has proven extremely useful in directing interventional procedures in the pleural space, pulmonary parenchyma, and mediastinum. Fluid in the pleural cavity, parenchymal masses and consolidation abutting the chest wall, and the heart, liver, and spleen provide sonographic windows to disease within the thorax. Ultrasound offers convenience, portability, and the capability to continuously monitor interventional procedures in the thorax. Interventional procedures can be performed with the patient in an upright position, allowing optimal access to gravity-layered free pleural fluid, an advantage not possible with computed tomography. Ultrasound usually provides differentiation between pleural fluid and pleural thickening, a distinction often difficult with plain films or computed tomography. Procedures can be performed portably within intensive care units saving critically ill patients potentially hazardous and manpower-intensive transport to the radiology department (1, 2). Needle and catheter placement, as well as adequacy of fluid drainage, can be monitored continuously while the procedure is performed, assuring maximum safety and benefit. This chapter will examine applications of ultrasound in the guidance of interventional procedures in the pleural space, pulmonary parenchyma, and mediastinum.

Pleural Space

Uses of interventional ultrasound in the pleural space include: a) diagnostic thoracentesis, b) therapeutic drainage of effusions, c) catheter drainage of empyema, d) pleural sclerotherapy, and e) pleural biopsy (3–6). Effective intervention in the pleural space combines accurate ultrasound diagnosis with knowledge of the specialized techniques of aspiration, biopsy, and catheter drainage.

ULTRASOUND DIAGNOSIS

Normal Pleural Space

The normal pleural space can best be appreciated by use of a linear-array transducer applied directly to the chest (Fig. 7.1). The broad near-field view of a high-frequency (5 MHz) linear transducer allows visualization of both the parietal and visceral pleura. A sector scanner may also suffice, but there is often near field artifact especially with mechanical sector transducers (Fig. 7.2). The normal pleural surfaces are seen as bright echogenic lines separated by a thin dark line representing normal fluid within the pleural space. Ribs are seen as rounded echogenic interfaces with prominent posterior acoustic shadowing. The highly reflective interface of the air-filled lung causes echogenic reverberation, the so-called dirty air shadow. Identification of the pleural surfaces is aided by observing the location and depth of the ribs. The thickness of the subcutaneous tissues and intercostal muscles can then be determined. The parietal pleural is approximately 1 cm deep to the rib interface. Observing movement of the lung and visceral pleura with real-time scanning during respiration confirms the identity of the pleural surfaces.

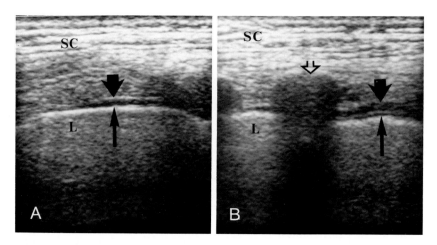

Figure 7.1. Normal pleural space. **A,** Transverse scan in an intercostal space using a linear transducer demonstrates the normal pleural space containing a minimal amount of pleural fluid. The parietal pleura is indicated by the *short arrow*. The visceral pleura is indicated by a *long arrow*. Pleural fluid is seen as the anechoic zone between the two pleural surfaces. Air-containing lung (*L*) causes a highly reflective interface that produces dense reverberation artifact deep to the visceral pleura (*SC* = subcutaneous tissue). **B,** Longitudinal scan using a linear transducer demonstrates ribs and intercostal space. A rib (*open arrow*) causes a strong echogenic interface and casts a dense acoustic shadow. Parietal pleura (*short arrow*) is found at a level approximately 1 cm deep to the rib interface. Visceral pleura (*long arrow*) is best identified by observing its movement relative to parietal pleura during respiration. (*SC* = subcutaneous tissue, L = lung)

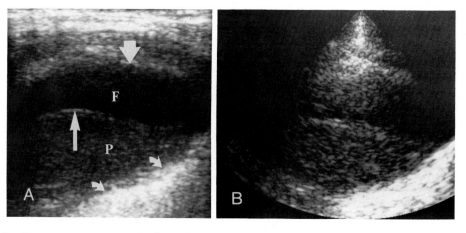

Figure 7.2. Linear array versus sector transducer. **A.** An image from a linear-array transducer demonstrates a small pleural effusion (*F*) 2 cm from the skin surface. The parietal pleural is indicated by the *short arrow*. The visceral pleura is indicated by the *long arrow*. An infiltrate within the lung (*P*) allows sound to penetrate through the lung until an air interface (*curved arrows*) is encountered. **B,** Artifact in the near field of this sector transducer image obtained in the same area as **A** obscures the near field anatomy and makes interpretation difficult.

An upwardly directed subcostal or low intercostal approach through the liver or spleen using a sector transducer will demonstrate the diaphragm as a bright, curved interface (Fig. 7.3). When the lung above the diaphragm is air filled, the strong, curved specular reflection of the diaphragm-lung interface will often produce a mirror image of the liver or spleen above the diaphragm (7). While this is well recognized as an artifact, it can also be interpreted as definitive evidence of the absence of pleural fluid (8, 9).

Appearance of Pleural Fluid and Lung Consolidation

Fluid within the pleural space will separate the visceral and parietal pleura with a band of echolucency (Fig. 7.4 **A**). Transudative effusions are anechoic. Effusions containing cells or cellular debris show internal particulate matter that can be observed to move or "float" with respiration. Viscous effusions and hemothorax may be quite echogenic. However, it should be noted that even empyemas may be anechoic and that diagnostic thoracentesis is required to determine the nature of the pleural fluid. Even echo-free pleural lesions may not always yield free fluid (10). This may be due to

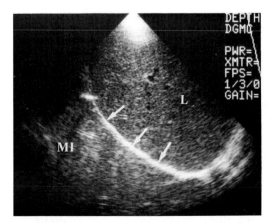

Figure 7.3. Normal pleural space. Subcostal scan through the liver (*L*) using a sector transducer demonstrates the diaphragm as a brightly echogenic interface (*arrows*). A mirror image pattern (*MI*) of the liver parenchyma is displayed above the diaphragm giving evidence of the absence of pleural fluid.

pleural thickening or pleural edema, which is echolucent, or may be caused by viscosity of the pleural fluid being too high to aspirate through a small-gauge needle. Ultrasound observations that reliably indicate that fluid can be aspirated from the pleural space include: a) change in shape of a pleural lesion with respiration, b) presence of septations within the pleural lesion which demonstrate motion (11), and c) floating echodensities within the pleural lesion.

The signs of pleural effusion using a subcostal abdominal approach include: a) visualization of a hypoechoic area above the diaphragm, b) visualization of the inside of the bony thorax through the fluid collection, and c) absence of the mirror image reflection of the liver or spleen above the diaphragm (Fig. 7.4 **B**). Care must be taken not to mistake artifactual duplication of the diaphragm for the inner aspect of the bony thorax (Fig. 7.4 **C**). Note that the inside of the thorax forms a straight line while the artifactual reflection of the diaphragm is curved.

Replacement of alveolar air with fluid due to parenchymal disease allows transmission of sound through the lung instead of the lung acting as a totally reflective interface. Consolidated or atelectatic lung may be seen as a wedge-shaped density suspended in pleural fluid and serves as an acoustic window to visualize other portions of the thorax (Fig. 7.5). Ultrasound signs that help to differentiate diseased lung from echogenic pleural fluid, pleural thickening, or solid pleural masses include: a) sonographic air bronchogram, b) sonographic fluid bronchogram, c) visualization of pulmonary vessels radiating toward the hilum, and d) movement corresponding to respiration. The sonographic air bronchogram is the visualization of air filled bronchi within consolidated lung as linear high amplitude branching echoes that converge toward the hilum (12; Fig. 7.6). Posterior acoustic shadowing and reverberation artifacts may be seen with larger bronchi. Sonographic fluid bronchograms are seen as anechoic branching tubular structures representing fluid-filled bronchi within consolidated lung (13). Pulmonary vessels may be differentiated from fluid bronchograms by visualization of pulsations or demonstration

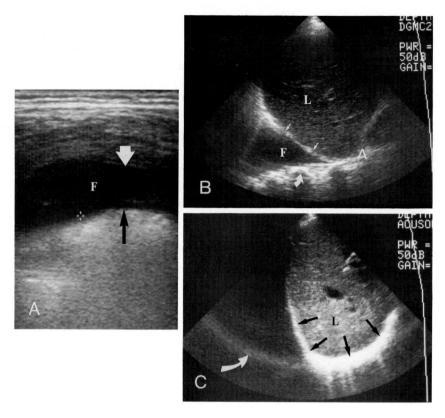

Figure 7.4. Pleural fluid. **A,** Intercostal scan using linear transducer displays pleural fluid (*F*) as an area of echolucency between the parietal pleura (*white arrow*) and the visceral pleura (*black arrow*). The plus sign (+) marks the depth of the lung surface in preparation for thoracentesis. **B,** Subcostal sagittal sector scan through the liver (*L*) reveals pleural fluid (*F*) between the diaphragm (*arrows*) and the inner aspect of the bony thorax (*curved arrow*). Fluid fills the posterior costophrenic angle. **C,** A subcostal sagittal scan through the liver (*L*) in another patient demonstrates artifactual duplication (*curved arrow*) of the diaphragm. This can be recognized as an artifact by observing its curving course duplicating the curve of the true diaphragm (*arrows*). The artifact is accentuated by high-gain settings.

of Doppler flow within the tubular structures. Consolidated lung that is not fixed to the parietal pleura by adhesions will move appropriately with inspiration and expiration. Lung abscess has been reported to demonstrate expansion of the walls of its entire circumference with inspiration, while empyema will only show slight motion of the wall adjacent to the lung (8).

Pitfalls

Pleural Space Septations. Septations extending across the pleural space between visceral and parietal pleura may pose a significant obstacle to aspiration and drainage

of fluid within the pleural space (14; Fig. 7.7). The septations may be fibrin strands or fibrous adhesions. Complex patterns of septation may produce multiple loculations that require multiple catheter placements to drain. Septations will commonly occlude needles or single-hole catheters during aspiration or drainage. For this reason, catheters with multiple side holes are preferred. Passage of a guidewire into the pleural space using the Seldinger technique for catheter placement may break these septations.

Pleural Thickening. Pleural thickening may, at times, be indistinguishable from loculated pleural fluid on routine chest radiographs even with decubitus views. Similar

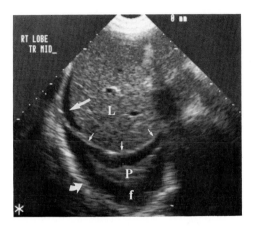

Figure 7.5. Consolidated Lung. Consolidated lung is seen as a wedge-shaped density (*P*) suspended within pleural fluid (*f*) on this transverse image through the liver using a subcostal approach. This patient also has ascites (*large arrow*) seen as an anechoic region between the liver (*L*) and the diaphragm (*small arrows*). The *inside* of the bony thorax (*curved arrow*) is visualized through the pleural effusion and consolidated lung.

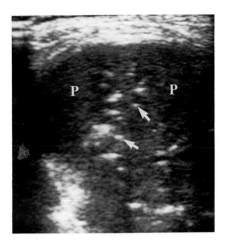

Figure 7.6. Sonographic air bronchogram. Transverse image in an intercostal space demonstrates consolidated lung (*P*) with sonographic air bronchograms (*arrows*) seen as high-amplitude linear echodensities.

difficulties may be encountered with ultrasound. On ultrasound examination, pleural fluid may be echogenic and mimic pleural thickening, or pleural thickening may be relatively echolucent and mimic pleural fluid (15; Fig. 7.8). The differentiation can usually be made by careful real-time ultrasound examination. The key to correct diagnosis is positive identification of the pleural surfaces by observing relative movement during exaggerated respiration. Even a severely diseased lung will show some motion relative to the thorax and allow identification of the visceral pleura. The parietal pleura can then be identified relative to the visceral pleura by its reflective interface.

Viscous Pleural Fluid. Occasionally, pleural fluid may be too viscous to aspirate through small (22-gauge) needles. When the ultrasound examination shows evidence of pleural fluid, yet none can be aspirated despite accurate needle placement, larger needles (18- to 20-gauge) should be tried. Rarely, catheters that are relatively stiff, with multiple large side holes may be necessary for simple aspiration.

Anechoic Empyema. Demonstration of anechoic pleural fluid by ultrasound does not prove the absence of infection within the pleural space. Pleural fluid must be aspirated for laboratory analysis to demonstrate its nature and exclude infection.

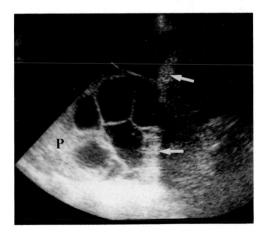

Figure 7.7. Pleural space septations. Longitudinal image at the level of the diaphragm shows multiple septation suspended in fluid extending between lung (*P*) and diaphragm (*arrows*). The septations pose an obstacle to fluid aspiration and drainage.

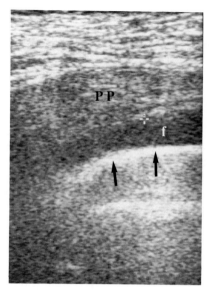

Figure 7.8. Pleural thickening versus pleural fluid. Thickening of the parietal pleura is seen as hypoechoic band (*PP*) extending from the inside of the bony thorax on this sonogram obtained through an intercostal space. A small pleural effusion (*f*) is also present. The lung surface and visceral pleura (*arrows*) are seen as a bright interface positively identified by observation of appropriate motion with respiration during real-time scanning.

TECHNIQUE

Diagnostic Thoracentesis

Diagnostic thoracentesis precedes most other interventional procedures within the pleural space. Aspiration of fluid with a fine needle will demonstrate the nature of the pleural fluid and help determine if further intervention is indicated. The optimal technique is to have the patient sit on an examination table facing away from the sonologist. The patient's arms are placed in a comfortable position resting upon a bedside table adjusted to the appropriate height. Patients who are unable to sit are placed in a lateral decubitus position with the diseased lung up. Diagnostic ultrasound examination is performed to confirm the presence of fluid and to select and mark the puncture site. The largest portion of the collection abutting the chest wall is selected for

puncture. The depth of the collection and the distance from skin surface to lung are measured. The puncture site and surrounding area are cleaned with povidone-iodine solution. Standard aseptic technique is used, but draping is generally not necessary or practical when the patient is in an upright position. The puncture site is anesthetized with local anesthetic (1% lidocaine) attempting to infiltrate both rib periosteum and parietal pleura. Actual puncture is made in the intercostal space just superior to the lower rib to avoid injury to the neurovascular bundle that courses along the inferior aspect of the rib. Once the puncture site has been chosen and marked by ultrasound examination, the probe is removed and the puncture made with careful attention paid to the depth of the collection and the location and depth of the lung. If the fluid collection is small or difficulty with aspiration is encountered, a glove may be placed over the transducer. The transducer can then be used within the sterile field for precise localization. Puncture can also be made using an attached biopsy guide with continuous sonographic monitoring (see Chapter 1). A 22-gauge needle attached to a 12-ml syringe is generally used for diagnostic aspiration. The pleural fluid obtained is inspected grossly for color and clarity and sent to the laboratory for Gram stain, cell count, aerobic and anaerobic culture, cytology, and any special studies warranted by the patient's clinical condition.

Therapeutic Drainage of Effusions

Large or loculated effusions may be a cause of chest pain or dyspnea. Drainage of these collections for relief of patient symptoms can generally be performed in one operation without leaving an indwelling catheter, provided that the pleural space is not infected. Diagnostic thoracentesis is performed in the manner described above. If a large amount of fluid is to be withdrawn, the aspiration needle is replaced with a flexible catheter to decrease the possibility of pneumothorax. (Pharmaseal thoracentesis catheter, American Pharmaseal Company, Valencia, CA) The catheter is attached to a three-way stopcock that is connected to a syringe for aspiration and to a drainage bag for fluid collection. This provides a closed system to limit the possibility of contaminating the pleural space. Contact with the lung by the catheter will produce pain or cause the patient to cough, often indicating that fluid drainage is nearly complete. Ultrasound can be used to monitor the amount of fluid remaining and provide guidance for catheter manipulation into additional pockets of fluid. Aspiration is continued until fluid removal is complete, then the catheter is removed. An immediate and a 4-hour follow-up chest x-ray are obtained to check for pneumothorax and document adequacy of fluid drainage.

Catheter Drainage of Empyema

Empyema is considered to be present when pleural fluid aspiration yields: a) gross pus, b) bacteria on Gram-stained smears, c) pH less than 7.0, d) glucose less than 40 mg/ 100 ml, e) positive cultures (5, 16). Image-directed percutaneous catheter drainage of empyema was originally used as a supplement to failed surgically placed thoracostomy tube drainage (3, 4, 17) but has recently been advocated as a primary treatment method (5). Thoracostomy tube drainage fails most frequently due to tube malposition and undrained loculations. Image-guided catheter placement can effectively overcome these problems. Smaller percutaneously placed catheters offer a lower complication rate and are considerably more comfortable for the patient than surgically placed large chest tubes. Both percutaneous catheters and surgically placed chest tubes have a successful empyema treatment rate of 70% to 88% (3–5, 17, 18). Persistent fibrous pleural peel encasing the lung remains a cause of failure for both techniques and usually requires thoracotomy for removal. Ultrasound is preferred over computed tomography and fluoroscopy as the guidance modality of choice for most patients because of its ease of use and capability of continuously monitoring the procedure (5). This procedure can also be performed using portable ultrasound in the

intensive care unit (Fig. 7.9). Computed tomography is used when sonographic visualization is inadequate, usually due to the presence of air within the collection.

The procedure is preceded by fine-needle image-guided thoracentesis to confirm the diagnosis of empyema. The drainage catheter is placed at the same site as the thoracentesis, usually directed at the largest portion of the collection abutting the chest wall. The Seldinger technique, using guidewire exchange and dilators, was initially employed for catheter placement, but direct catheter placement with a trocar system is now usually preferred (3–5). The trocar method overcomes problems with catheter buckling as it is advanced through thickened pleura. A variety of one-step placement trocar catheter systems are available for empyema drainage (Fig. 7.10). The Sacks catheter

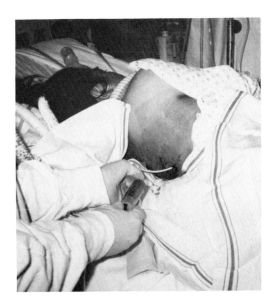

Figure 7.9. Portable empyema drainage. Portable ultrasound was used to direct catheter placement for drainage of empyema in this victim of multiple trauma who was septic and too ill to be moved to the radiology department. A 12-French catheter was placed in the right-sided empyema using the trocar method. (Reproduced by permission from McGahan JP, Anderson MW, Walter JP: Portable real-time sonographic and needle guidance systems for aspiration and drainage. *AJR* 147:1241–1246, 1986.)

(Electro-Catheter Corporation, Rahway, NJ) is a multiple-hole pigtail catheter available in 5.5, 7.0, 8.2 and 9.4 French sizes. The relatively rigid 10–12 French Mueller catheter (Cook, Bloomington, IN) with a soft curved tip and multiple distal side holes was specially designed for empyema drainage (5). The McGahan catheter (6.7F and 8.4F, Cook) is a softer pigtail catheter with a string system designed to form a tight pigtail loop. All catheter systems have an inner cannula used to straighten the catheter for insertion. A trocar pointed stylet is inserted through the cannula to provide a 3- to 4-mm pointed tip for puncture and insertion.

For one-step catheter placement into the pleural space, a small skin incision is made with a number 11 blade at the site of diagnostic thoracentesis after use of local anesthesia. A small hemostat is used to spread the skin and subcutaneous tissue. While the thumb stays on the hub of the trocar, the catheter assembly is advanced into the collection at the angle previously determined by ultrasound. The trocar is removed and fluid aspiration is attempted through the cannula. If no fluid is aspirated, the trocar can be reinserted and the catheter assembly re-positioned. When fluid has been entered, the cannula is held firmly while the catheter is advanced over the cannula into the collection. The cannula is then removed, and the catheter is attached to a three-way stopcock with syringe and drainage bag to complete initial drainage. The fluid collection is aspirated completely and irrigated with 10 to 15 cc of sterile saline. The catheter is sutured to the skin and connected to a standard three-bottle underwater seal pleural drainage system (Pleur-evac, Queensville, NY). The patient is reexamined sonographically to determine if any additional undrained fluid pockets are present. Additional fluid collections will usually require placement of additional drainage catheters. Contrast sonography using propyliodone oil suspension (Dionosyl) should be performed after catheter placement to detect unsuspected bronchiopleural fistula. Propyliodone oil suspension is used as a contrast agent to prevent pulmonary edema possible with standard water-soluble contrast agents if bronchiopleural fistula is present and the lungs are exposed to the agent.

Postprocedure care includes continuous negative suction (–20-cm water pressure), irrigation of the drainage catheter with 10 to 15 ml of saline every 6 to 8 hours, routine wound care, and measurement of the volume of pleural fluid drained. Drainage is considered complete when the drainage from the catheter is less than 10 cc for a 24-hour period and chest radiograph or ultrasound examination shows no residual

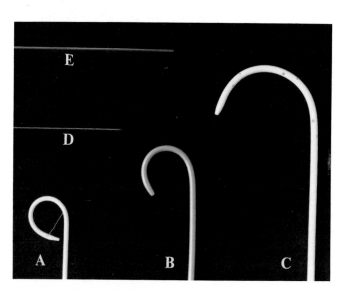

Figure 7.10. Pleural space drainage catheters. **A,** The McGahan drainage catheter. **B,** The Sacks drainage catheter. **C,** The Mueller empyema drainage catheter. **D,** Trocar pointed inner stylet. **E,** Inner cannula.

collection. The catheter is then disconnected from active suction and placed to water seal. If no pneumothorax or pleural effusion is evident after 12 to 24 hours, the catheter is removed.

Pleural Sclerotherapy

Chemical sclerotherapy of the pleural space may be used in the management of recurrent malignant pleural effusions. Pleural effusions are a cause of chest pain, cough, and dyspnea, which can all be relieved by aspiration of the fluid. However, as many as 97% of malignant effusions will recur within 1 month of drainage. Sclerotherapy is performed by injection of tetracycline, bleomycin, or other chemical agents into the pleural space to irritate the pleura and incite a fibrous response. Tetracycline and bleomycin have both proven effective in preventing recurrence of malignant pleural effusions, with success rates of 62% to 72% reported (19, 20). Other agents, including radioisotopes and nitrogen mustard, are less effective.

Ultrasound guidance may be used to insure accurate catheter placement, especially when loculated effusions are present or when sclerotherapy without guidance has been unsuccessful. The pleural fluid is localized and drained completely using the techniques described previously. The sclerosing agent is then injected through the catheter into the pleural space. Tetracycline is generally given at a dose of 500 mg in 50 ml of saline (19). Bleomycin is given at a dose of 60 mg in 100 ml of saline. Doses of bleomycin larger than 60 mg have no added benefit but are associated with a higher incidence of toxic effects. Following injection, the catheter is removed and the patient is rotated several times to spread the agent throughout the pleural space. Pain and transient fever are reported in 5% of patients following intrapleural installations. Since 45% of the dose installed into the pleural space is absorbed systemically (20), all toxic reactions associated with intravenous use of these agents are a possibility.

Pleural Biopsy

Pleural biopsy has traditionally been performed blindly because pleural lesions often could not be visualized fluoroscopically. Ultrasound guidance of pleural biopsy offers the advantage of directing the biopsy needle to pleural masses or to small loculated pleural effusions, increasing not only the yield but the safety of the procedure (4, 6). Biopsy of large pleural masses can be performed using standard biopsy needles (16- to 22-gauge; Fig. 7.11). Ultrasound is used to localize the mass and select a puncture site. Aspiration cytology or core biopsy specimens are obtained using standard techniques as described in Chapter 1.

Pleural biopsy is performed with the Cope reversed bevel biopsy needle (Randall Fachney, Avon, Mass) An excellent description of the technique of pleural biopsy using this needle is provided by Mueller and co-workers (6). The Cope needle assembly consists of four components: a) a short open-ended outer cannula, b) a longer open-ended trocar with an angled tip, c) a

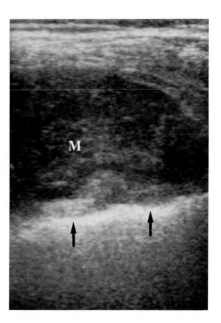

Figure 7.11. Malignant Mesothelioma. Scan in an intercostal space demonstrates a mesothelioma (*M*) as a hypoechoic mass in the pleural space. *Arrows* indicate the interface of the visceral pleura and aerated lung.

solid stylet that fits into the trocar, and d) the Cope needle. The cannula, trocar, and stylet fit together as a three-piece unit approximately 13 gauge in size. Preliminary fine-needle aspiration is performed to confirm the presence of pleural effusion. The three-piece Cope unit is then introduced into the pleural space at the site previously selected by ultrasound localization (Fig. 7.12). The unit is inserted just above the edge of the underlying rib. When puncture of the pleural space is suggested by a sensation of decreased resistance, the stylet is removed and a syringe is attached to the aspirate pleural fluid. If pleural fluid cannot be aspirated, the stylet is replaced and the unit is repositioned. Once within the pleural space, the trocar and stylet are both removed, leaving the outer cannula in place. The operator's thumb is placed over the open cannula to prevent introduction of air. The Cope needle is longer than the cannula, and when passed through the cannula, the

cutting edge protrudes into the pleural space. The needle and cannula are rotated, using the rib as a fulcrum, until the unit is parallel to the chest wall. The whole unit is slowly withdrawn until the reverse bevel of the needle hooks the pleura. The cannula is then rotated and advanced over the needle to biopsy the captured pleura. The biopsy needle containing the specimen is withdrawn, leaving the cannula in place to allow additional needle passes. Mueller and colleagues (6) found this technique to be effective, with an accurate diagnosis in 20 out of 23 patients reported. Significant pneumothorax requiring treatment occurred in only two patients.

COMPLICATIONS

A wide variety of complications is possible as a result of percutaneous interventional procedures in the pleural space, including lung laceration, air embolism, hemothorax, infection, chest wall hematoma,

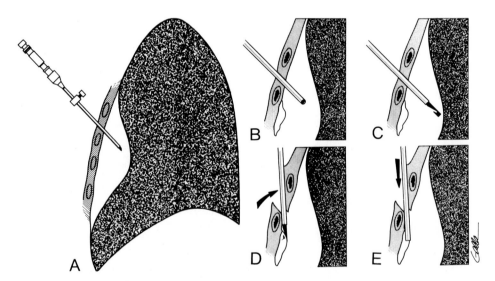

Figure 7.12. Technique for pleural biopsy. Drawings show step-by-step technique for biopsy with the Cope needle assembly. First, the three-piece unit is inserted into a small pleural effusion (shown as a white space) (**A**). The stylet and trocar are removed, leaving the outer cannula within the pleural effusion (**B**). The Cope needle is inserted (**C**). The needle is longer than the outer cannula so that the cutting edge protrudes beyond the end. The outer cannula and needle are angled, with the rib used as fulcrum (**D**). The whole unit is then slowly withdrawn until the hook ''catches'' the pleura (curved arrow). The outer cannula is advanced (straight arrow) with a rotary motion over the needle to capture a piece of pleura (**E**). (Reproduced by permission from Mueller PR, Saini S, Simeone JF et al.: Image-guided pleural biopsies: Indications, technique, and results in 23 patients. *Radiology* 169:1–4, 1988.)

subcutaneous emphysema, and injury to liver, spleen, and stomach. However, the only major complication reported with significant frequency is pneumothorax, usually due to perforation of the lung by needle or catheter. Published series relate pneumothorax as a complication in 0% to 9% of patients undergoing interventional procedures in the thorax. Small pneumothoraces that produce few or no symptoms will resolve without treatment. Larger pneumothoraces can be treated effectively by placement of a catheter into the pleural space and attaching the catheter to a Heimlich valve (Bard-Parker, Rutherford, NJ). A pneumothorax treatment set is available from Cook that includes a 9 F trocar catheter set, a Heimlich valve, and a connecting tube (Fig. 7.13). The catheter is introduced into the pleural space through the second or third anterior intercostal space in the midclavicular line. The catheter is then advanced over the cannula to the apex of the thorax and is attached to the Heimlich valve by the connecting tubing. The Heimlich valve is a one-way valve that allows air and fluid from the pleural space to escape but prevents air or fluid from passing back through the catheter into the pleural space. The valve can be connected to a vented drainage bag or to a trap bottle and regulated suction system.

Lung Parenchyma

Percutaneous transthoracic aspiration biopsy of pulmonary nodules using fluoroscopic guidance is a well established methodology of proven clinical utility (21). However, problems with fluoroscopic visualization of the lesion may be encountered when the lesion is pleural based, near the mediastinum or diaphragm, or in the lung apex (21–25). When a lesion abuts the chest wall or diaphragm, it becomes an acoustic window and can be visualized and biopsied with ultrasound. Aerated lung surrounding a soft tissue nodule causes strong reverberating echoes that make the nodule stand out in strong relief. Linear-array transducers used within the intercostal space provide the best visualization of pleural based nodules because of their wide near-field view. Sonography offers a number of advantages over fluoroscopy and computed tomography in guiding the biopsy of pleural based nodules, including: a) safety, b) accuracy, c) ease of use, and d) speed (23). The incidence of pneumothorax with ultrasound guidance of lesions touching the chest wall is 2% compared to 11% for fluoroscopic guidance (25). Sonography accurately defines the pleural contact point and depth of needle placement of peripheral pulmonary lesions,

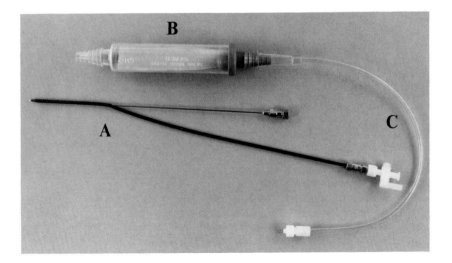

Figure 7.13. Heimlich valve. **A**, Trocar catheter for one-step insertion into the pleural space. **B**, One-way Heimlich valve. **C**, Connecting tubing.

while fluoroscopy may allow passage of the needle through the back of the lesion into lung, or through aerated lung interposed between the lesion and the chest wall (23). The needle position can be continuously monitored with ultrasound but not with computed tomography. Localization of lesions by computed tomography is markedly influenced by small variations in respiration, making it easy to miss the lesion and puncture aerated lung. Sonography involves no radiation exposure to either the patient or the radiologist. Ultrasound compares favorably (22–28) with the 90 to 95% sensitivity reported (21) for the diagnosis of lung cancer by fluoroscopically guided percutaneous needle biopsy. Ultrasound can be performed in a lighted room and at the patient's bedside. Identification of peripheral lesions and the route of access for biopsy is rapid and easy to perform. Ultrasound will also identify peripheral parenchymal nodules that are obscured by pleural effusions.

TECHNIQUE

Peripheral lesions abutting the chest wall are identified by scanning in the intercostal space. The exact location, size, and depth of the lesion is determined. Biopsy can then be performed under continuous ultrasound observations using a biopsy guide if the lesion is small or in a difficult location. If the lesion is large, the needle puncture site, angle, and depth is carefully determined by ultrasound, then the biopsy can be performed without direct observation by using the established landmarks. The patient is asked to suspend respiration momentarily while the needle is placed into the lesion in a single smooth stroke. The patient can then breathe shallow respirations while the needle is allowed to swing freely. The patient is again asked to suspend respiration. A syringe is attached, suction applied, and the biopsy taken. Specimens may be obtained for cytology, histology, Gram stain, or culture.

A wide variety of needles may be effectively used to sample lung lesions. Most authors prefer using 21 or 22-gauge needles to obtain specimens for cytologic diagnosis (21, 23, 25) Needles larger than 19 gauge are reported to be associated with significant and occasionally fatal bleeding problems (21). There is some evidence that small nodules may be easier to biopsy with small needles than with large needles (21). The Rotex screw biopsy needle (Meadox Surgimed, Oakland, NJ) can be used effectively to obtain cytologic specimens in the lung even though it may be suboptimal for use in the abdomen (29, 30). An advantage of the Rotex needle is its excellent visualization characteristics when used with ultrasound guidance. Aspiration specimens examined by cytologic techniques have excellent sensitivity for the diagnosis of malignancy and are all that is needed for most cases. However, some benign conditions and cell type determination of carcinoma require tissue cores for histologic diagnosis. These have been obtained by using large cutting needles such as the 14-gauge Trucut (Travenol, Deerfield, IL) or 15 to 16-gauge Surecut (Meadox Surgimed, Oakland, NJ) needles(28). However, these large needles are associated with a risk of significant and even fatal hemorrhage into the pleural space. Most authors recommend abandoning use of these large needles (21). Specially designed fine needles used in the lung to obtain tissue cores include the 22 to 23 gauge circumferentially bevelled DGBS needle (Cook) and the 21-gauge dual cutting edge PercuCut needle (E-Z-EM, Westbury, NY; 31, 32).

COMPLICATIONS

The most common complications of percutaneous biopsy of lung lesions are pneumothorax and minor bleeding. The incidence of pneumothorax for lesions abutting the chest wall is 2% for ultrasound guidance and 11% for fluoroscopic guidance compared to 10% to 35% overall rate for fluoroscopic guidance of all lung lesions (21). With optimal technique, pleural lesions can be biopsied without passing through aerated lung. Most pneumothoraces encountered are self-limiting and require no treatment. A larger or symptom producing pneumothorax can usually be effectively treated with a small catheter and the Heimlich valve system.

Mediastinum

Although the reported experience of ultrasound guided interventional and biopsy procedures in the mediastinum is limited (24, 25, 28), newer techniques of ultrasound examination of the mediastinum indicate great possibilities (33–36). The potential of percutaneous guided procedures in the mediastinum has been demonstrated by the use of fluoroscopy and computed tomography (37–42). However, the ability of ultrasound to provide continuous real-time imaging of needle and catheter placement offers great advantage over computed tomography and fluoroscopy, particularly in the mediastinum, which is so rich with vital structures.

ULTRASOUND DIAGNOSIS

Using a suprasternal approach, abnormalities in the supraaortic, paratracheal, and aorticopulmonary window areas can be visualized and are amenable to biopsy (33) Patients are examined supine with a cushion placed beneath the shoulders and neck extended. The transducer is placed at the base of the neck just above the manubrium and is angled downward into the mediastinum. Scanning is performed in angled sagittal and coronal planes. Large arteries and veins are identified by their anatomic position, course, and if necessary, by their Doppler flow characteristics. Abnormal masses as small as 1.5 cm can be identified and their relationships to great vessels determined. Masses immediately behind the sternum, posterior to the trachea, and in the pulmonary hila are generally not seen by this approach.

Parasternal scanning with the patient in a lateral decubitus position can provide excellent visualization of the anterior mediastinum and subcarinal regions (34, 35). Wernicke reported sonographic visualization of 95% of tumors in the anterior mediastinum and subcarinal region using a parasternal approach (34). Placing the patient in a right lateral decubitus position results in a gravity-caused mediastinal swing toward the right and creates a right parasternal sonographic window. Scanning of the mediastinum can then be performed in the right anterior intercostal spaces in transverse and parasagittal planes. The ascending aorta, anterior mediastinum, and subcarinal region can be examined in most cases. The left parasternal approach, with the patient in a left lateral decubitus position, allows sonographic access to the pulmonary trunk, anterior mediastinum, and in many cases to the subcarinal region.

Large mediastinal masses often displace paramediastinal lung and create their own sonographic windows (35). Doppler is useful in the diagnosis of vascular masses in the mediastinum (35), and in vessel identification and confirmation of blood flow.

TECHNIQUE

Diagnostic ultrasound is performed to determine the feasibility of ultrasound-guided biopsy, the puncture site, and the needle path. Anterior mediastinal masses are usually biopsied using an anterior parasternal approach. Masses in the posterior mediastinum and middle mediastinum posterior to the superior vena cava are biopsied using a posterior paravertebral approach. The aorticopulmonary window can be reached from the left anterior parasternal region (21). Patients can be placed in the lateral decubitus position to aid visualization and biopsy access. Because of the numerous vital structures present, 22-gauge needles are preferred for initial aspiration biopsy attempts. If the sample is inadequate after several passes, the biopsy can be repeated with a 20-gauge needle. While no large series using ultrasound guidance of mediastinal masses have been reported, 80% to 96% of biopsies performed by fluoroscopic and CT guidance yielded diagnostic material (37–41).

COMPLICATIONS

Hemoptysis and pneumothorax are the most common complications reported with mediastinal biopsies (37–41). Hemoptysis is usually slight and inconsequential. Pneumothorax is reported in 16% to 25% of cases with catheter or chest tube drainage required in about one-fourth.

REFERENCES

1. McGahan JP: Aspiration and drainage procedures in the intensive care unit: Percutaneous sonographic guidance. *Radiology* 154:531–532, 1985.
2. McGahan JP, Anderson MW, Walter JP: Portable real-time sonographic and needle guidance systems for aspiration and drainage. *AJR* 147:1241–1246, 1986.
3. vanSonnenberg E, Nakamoto SK, Mueller PR et al.: CT and ultrasound guided catheter drainage of empyemas after chest-tube failure. *Radiology* 151:349–353, 1984.
4. O'Moore PV, Mueller PR, Simeone JF, et al.: Sonographic guidance in the diagnostic and therapeutic interventions in the pleural space. *AJR* 149:1–5, 1987.
5. Silverman SG, Mueller PR, Saini S, et al.: Thoracic empyema: Management with image-guided catheter drainage. *Radiology* 169:5–9, 1988.
6. Mueller PR, Saini S, Simeone JF, et al.: Image-guided pleural biopsies: Indications, technique, and results in 23 patients. *Radiology* 169:1–4, 1988.
7. Gardner FJ, Clark RN, Kozlowski R: A model of a hepatic mirror-image artifact. *Med Ultrasound* 4:19–21, 1980.
8. Simeone JF, Mueller PR, vanSonnenberg E: The uses of diagnostic ultrasound in the thorax. *Clin Chest Med* 5:281–290, 1984.
9. Lewandowski BJ, Winsberg F: Echographic appearance of the right hemidiaphragm. *J Ultrasound Med* 2:243–249, 1983.
10. Laing FC, Filly RA: Problems in the application of ultrasonography for the evaluation of pleural opacities. *Radiology* 126:211–214, 1978.
11. Marks WM, Filly RA, Callen PW: Real-time evaluation of pleural lesions: New observations regarding the probability of obtaining free fluid. *Radiology* 142:163–164, 1982.
12. Weinberg B, Diakoumakis EE, Kass EG, Seife B, Zvi ZB: The air bronchogram: *Sonographic demonstration. AJR* 147:593–595, 1986.
13. Dorne HL: Differentiation of pulmonary parenchymal consolidation from pleural disease using the sonographic fluid bronchogram. *Radiology* 158:41–42, 1986.
14. Hirsch JH, Rogers JV, Mack LA: Real-time sonography of pleural opacities. *AJR* 136:297–301, 1981.
15. Rosenberg ER: Ultrasound in the assessment of pleural densities. *Chest* 84:283–285, 1983.
16. Light RW: Parapneumonic effusions and empyema. *Clin Chest Med* 6:55–61, 1985.
17. Westcott JL: Percutaneous catheter drainage of pleural effusion and empyema. *AJR* 144:1189–1193, 1985.
18. Merriam MA, Cronan JJ, Dorfman GS, Lambiase RE, Haas RA: Radiographically guided percutaneous catheter drainage of pleural fluid collections. *AJR* 151:1113–1116, 1988.
19. Zaloznik AJ, Oswald SG, Langin M: Intrapleural tetracycline in malignant pleural effusions: A randomized study. *Cancer* 51:752–755, 1983.
20. Ostrowski MJ, Halsall GM: Intracavitary bleomycin in the management of malignant pleural effusions: A multicenter study. *Cancer Treat Rep* 66:1903–1907, 1982.
21. Westcott JL: Percutaneous transthoracic needle biopsy. *Radiology* 169:593–601, 1988.
22. Yang P-C, Luh K-T, Sheu J-C, Kuo S-H, Yang S-P: Peripheral pulmonary lesions: Ultrasonography and ultrasonically guided aspiration biopsy. *Radiology* 155:451–456, 1985.
23. Cinti D, Hawkins HB: Aspiration biopsy of peripheral pulmonary masses using real-time sonographic guidance. *AJR* 142:1115–1116, 1984.
24. Ikezoe J, Sone S, Higashihara T, Morimoto S, Arisawa J, Kuriyama K: Sonographically guided needle biopsy for diagnosis of thoracic lesions. *AJR* 143:229–234, 1984.
25. Pedersen OM, Aasen TB, Gulsvik A: Fine needle aspiration biopsy of mediastinal and peripheral pulmonary masses guided by real-time sonography. *Chest* 89:504–508, 1986.
26. Izumi S. Tamki S, Natori H, Kira S: Ultrasonically guided aspiration needle biopsy in disease of the chest. *Am Rev Respir Dis* 125:460–464, 1982.
27. Afschrift M, Nachtegaele P, Voet D, Noens L, Van Hove W, Van Der Straeten M, Verdonk G: Puncture of thoracic lesions under sonographic guidance. *Thorax* 37:503–506, 1982.
28. Pang JA, Tsang V, Hom BL, Metreweli C: Ultrasound-guided tissue-core biopsy of thoracic lesions with Trucut and Surecut needles. *Chest* 91:823–827, 1987.
29. Nahman BJ, Van Aman ME, McLemore WE, O'Toole RV: Use of Rotex needle in percutaneous biopsy of pulmonary malignancy. *AJR* 145:97–99, 1985.
30. Andriole JG, Haaga JR, Adams RB, Nunez C: Biopsy needle characteristics assessed in the laboratory. *Radiology* 148:659–662, 1983.
31. Greene R, Szyfelbein WM, Isler RJ, Stark P, Jantsch H: Supplementary tissue-core histology from fine-needle transthoracic aspiration biopsy. *AJR* 144:787–792, 1985.
32. Weisbrod GL, Herman SJ, Liang-Che T: Preliminary experience with a dual cutting edge needle in thoracic percutaneous fine-needle aspiration biopsy. *Radiology* 163:75–78, 1987.
33. Wernecke K, Peters PE, Galanski M: Mediastinal tumors: Evaluation with suprasternal sonography. *Radiology* 159:405–409, 1986.
34. Wernecke K, Potter R, Peters PE, Koch P: Parasternal mediastinal sonography: Sensitivity in the detection of anterior mediastinal and subcarinal tumors. *AJR* 150:1021–1026, 1988.
35. Ikezoe J, Morimoto S, Arisawa J et al.: Ultrasonography of mediastinal teratoma. *J Clin Ultrasound* 14:513–520, 1986.
36. O'Laughlin MP, Huhta JC, Murphy DJ: Ultrasound examination of extracardiac chest masses in children: Doppler diagnosis of a vascular etiology. *J Ultrasound Med* 6:151–157, 1987.
37. Linder J, Olsen GA, Johnston WW: Fine-needle aspiration biopsy of the mediastinum. *Am J Med* 81:1005–1008, 1986.
38. Weisbrod GL, Lyons DJ, Tao LC, Chamberlain DW: Percutaneous fine-needle aspiration biopsy of mediastinal lesions. *AJR* 143:525–529, 1984.

39. Moinuddin SM, Lee LH, Montgomery JH: Mediastinal needle biopsy. *AJR* 143:531–532, 1984.

40. Gobien RP, Skucas J, Paris BS: CT-assisted fluoroscopically guided aspiration biopsy of central hilar and mediastinal masses. *Radiology* 141:443–447, 1981.

41. Adler OB, Rosenberger A, Peleg H: Fine-needle aspiration biopsy of mediastinal masses: Evaluation of 136 experiences. *AJR* 140:893–896, 1983.

42. Kuhlman JE, Fishman EK, Wang KP, Zerhouni EA, Siegelman SS: Mediastinal cysts: Diagnosis by CT and needle aspiration. *AJR* 150:75–78, 1988.

8 Interventional Echocardiography

DAVID S. RUSSELL
WILLIAM BOMMER

Introduction

Well established as a tool in the diagnosis of cardiac abnormalities, echocardiography is also valuable in guiding cardiac interventions and in evaluating results. Safe, easily performed at the bedside or in special-procedure environments, and accurate for structure and flow imaging, echocardiography has direct applications in many interventional procedures. These include pericardiocentesis, myocardial biopsy, atrial septostomy, electrophysiologic mapping and ablation, percutaneous translumenal coronary angioplasty, and, with the addition of Doppler flow imaging, percutaneous valvuloplasty.

Intraoperative echocardiography, by both transesophageal and direct epicardial approaches, has evolved to a useful adjunct in coronary artery bypass surgery, valve repair and replacement surgery, and in congenital malformation repair and palliative surgery. It has also proved useful in monitoring cardiac function in high-risk, noncardiac surgical patients.

Pericardiocentesis

DETECTION OF PERICARDIAL EFFUSION AND PERICARDIAL CLOT

Examination of the heart for the diagnosis of pericardial effusion was an early benefit of ultrasound imaging to the practice of cardiology. The one-dimensional (M-mode) echocardiographic finding of an echo-free space between the chest wall and anterior heart wall or between the posterior heart wall and pleural space was described as diagnostic of the presence of fluid within the pericardium (1, 2).

Two-dimensional imaging enhanced the usefulness of echocardiography for evaluating pericardial effusion by improving anatomical orientation in multiple tomographic planes (3). Because of its relatively high sensitivity and specificity for fluid detection in comparison to other testing modalities, echocardiography is the technique of choice for diagnosing pericardial effusions.

Anatomical characteristics

The heart is surrounded by the two layers of the *visceral* and *parietal* pericardium, which are anchored to the outer surfaces of the great vessels as they arise from the heart. The inner visceral layer is adherent to the epicardial surface of the heart, and the outer parietal layer borders the pleural and thoracic structures. The parietal pericardial layer is attached to various supporting ligaments that anchor the entire cardiac structure to the sternum, the thoracic vertebrae, and the diaphragm (4). Between the two layers, a small quantity of clear fluid (approximately 15 ml) lubricates the heart and pericardial sac during the cardiac cycle. Increased amounts of fluid within the pericardium cause the layers to separate by stretching the outer layer to accommodate the increased fluid volume or by compressing the heart.

101

Imaging Techniques

Recognition of pericardial effusion by ultrasound imaging requires identification of the myocardial surfaces, the fluid-containing space within the pericardium, and the surrounding pericardium. Care must be taken to assess the distribution of pericardial fluid as well as to estimate its quantity by examining the heart from multiple echocardiographic windows and tomographic spaces. The customary views for this purpose are the long- and short-axis planes from the left parasternal, apical, and subcostal windows. The heart should be examined routinely from the subcostal approach when evaluating a pericardial effusion, since the fluid may preferentially locate inferiorly and posteriorly. Figure 8.1 shows a large pericardial effusion that is globally distributed around the heart (imaged from orthogonal apical and left parasternal views). The injection of echo contrast agents into a peripheral vein can be helpful to improve definition of the right heart borders and to identify a loculated fluid collection in technically difficult patients.

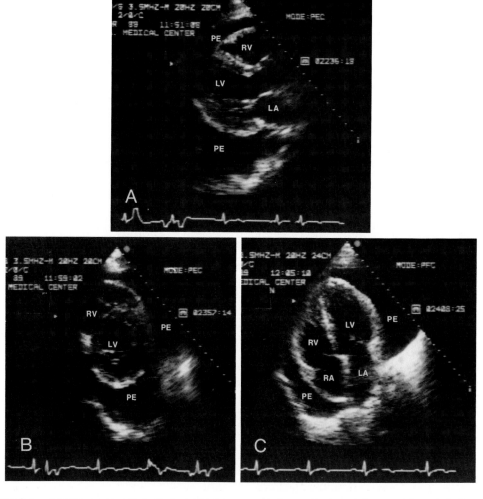

Figure 8.1. A large pericardial effusion which surrounds the entire heart, imaged from **A**, left parasternal long-axis, **B**, short-axis, and **C**, apical 4-chamber views. (*PE* = pericardial fluid; *LV* = left ventricle; *RV* = right ventricle; *LA* = left atrium; *RA* = right atrium.)

Pericardial fluid is usually homogeneous in character; however, fibrinous strands and debris can be recognized within the fluid-filled pericardial space in many diseases, including infectious and malignant effusions. The echocardiographic finding of coarse, irregular reflections within the pericardial space suggests, but is not diagnostic of, pericardial clot. The distinguishing feature of pericardial clot is the nonmobility of these reflections, which can have either a linear or variegated appearance.

Differentiation of Pericardial from Plueral Effusion

Fluid collection in the pleural space can also be encountered in the echocardiographic examination, and differentiation between pleural and pericardial effusions is an important task of the echocardiographer. Pleural effusions can have various patterns of presentation (see Chapter 7) and can occur both in the presence of pericardial effusions and alone. The differences between the ultrasound images of pericardial effusion and of pleural effusion can be related to the position of the echo-free spaces relative to certain anatomical landmarks.

The fairly secure attachment of the parietal pericardium at the base of the heart usually prevents pericardial fluid from extending more superiorly than the atrioventricular groove. In contrast, pleural fluid can extend past the basal structures of the heart.

The best anatomical landmarks for differentiating pleural from pericardial effusion are the thoracic aorta and the pericardium. Normally, the thoracic aorta courses behind the left atrium and lies close to the outer layer of pericardium. Pericardial effusions that extend to this level then lie between the aorta and the atrial wall. Pleural effusions do not usually separate the aorta from the posterior heart wall. Thus, a retrocardiac echo-free space that does not separate the aorta from the posterior heart wall is likely to represent a pleural effusion.

The most important landmark is the pericardial tissue layer itself. With pericardial effusions, the separation between the heart wall and pericardium usually decreases toward the cardiac base and produces a tapering of the echo-free space. The pericardium is clearly recognizable as a strong ultrasound reflector and can be readily distinguished from myocardial surfaces. Reflections from the pericardium can be traced along the fluid compartment border to the point where the pericardium joins the heart wall, usually slightly superior to the level of the mitral valve annulus—except in the setting of an extremely large pericardial effusion (see the section on cardiac tamponade, below). When pericardial and pleural fluid occur together, the pericardium can usually be identified as a thin separation layer between the two regions of fluid collection. Figure 8.2 shows a large pleural effusion and a small pericardial effusion with the pericardial separation layer clearly imaged between them.

In evaluating echo-free spaces around the heart, it is important to recognize potential artifacts that can be confused with pericardial or pleural effusions. These include reflections from fibrotic, echo-dense mitral annulus, which can obliterate the epipericardial images, giving a false impression of posterior fluid; and gross ascites, which can masquerade as anterior or inferior fluid (5). Cystic masses adjacent to the pericardium could also be confused with loculated pericardial effusions, as could fatty tissue deposits along the epicardial surface of the heart (6). It is conceivable that a ventricular pseudoaneurysm could also be taken for a loculated pericardial effusion. Identification of the aneurysmal neck, pulsatile behavior of the aneurysmal sac, and evidence of flow from the true ventricle into the false chamber would be the keys to recognizing this imposter.

DETECTION OF CARDIAC TAMPONADE

Physiologic Considerations

Cardiac tamponade is a clinical emergency caused by restricted filling of the heart. It is caused by increasing pericardial fluid pressure and associated with a reduced cardiac output and elevated systemic venous pressure. The parietal pericardial layer

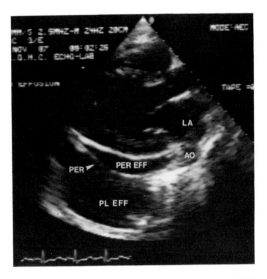

Figure 8.2. Coexistent large pleural (*PL EFF*) and small pericardial (*PER EFF*) effusions, separated by the parietal pericardial layer (*arrow; PER*). Note the position of the thoracic aorta (*AO*) adjacent to the posterior wall of the left atrium (*LA*).

is capable of elastic expansion to accommodate slowly increasing fluid volume in the pericardial space. Rapid accumulation is not well tolerated and leads to cardiac tamponade. The heart's normal compensatory mechanisms of tachycardia, increased vascular tone, and myocardial contractility are rapidly undermined by restricted filling. Rising ventricular and venous diastolic pressures and falling cardiac output and blood pressure complete the clinical picture. Signs of dynamic left ventricular outflow obstruction, mimicking those of hypertrophic obstructive cardiomyopathy (IHSS), have been observed in the setting of cardiac tamponade (7).

Criteria for Evaluation

The echocardiographic features of cardiac tamponade include a marked decrease of right ventricular cavity size with exaggerated respiratory variation of internal dimensions (8), diastolic collapse of the right ventricular cavity (9), diastolic involution of the right atrial wall (10), and altered ventric-

ular inflow patterns by Doppler flow imaging (11).

The body of the right ventricle is best imaged from the apical and subcostal approaches. Respiratory changes in right ventricular dimensions can be appreciated especially well from the subcostal four-chamber view. When intrapericardial pressure has increased to the point of compressing the right ventricle during diastole, the right ventricular anterior and inferior (free) walls move toward the interventricular septum and give the appearance of cavity obliteration. Abnormalities of motion of the interventricular septum are frequent in larger pericardial effusions and may confound measurements of right ventricular size. In cardiac tamponade, the echocardiogram will show an increase of the right ventricular diastolic dimension during inspiration and a corresponding marked decrease in RV dimension with expiration. The sensitivity of the finding of right ventricular compression may be reduced in patients with right ventricular hypertrophy or pericardial adhesions.

Another finding in cardiac tamponade is the involution of the right atrial free wall during diastole. This inward motion of the atrial wall can be best appreciated from the apical four-chamber view, but also from the subcostal four-chamber and parasternal basal views. An incursion of the atrial wall lasting more than one-third of the cardiac cycle is consistent with hemodynamic compromise. Atrial collapse may occasionally occur with large pericardial effusions without clinical signs of cardiac tamponade. Therefore, this echo finding usually requires clinical correlation. Localized tamponade has been described secondary to a loculated intrapericardial clot associated with right atrial compression (12).

Although Doppler flow analysis is not essential to the diagnosis of cardiac tamponade, when the findings described above are present, diastolic flow abnormalities can usually be demonstrated with tamponade. As ventricular inflow patterns reflect diastolic pressure and volume events, wide respiratory variation in the flow velocity occurs with cardiac tamponade. Findings include inspiratory blunting of the spectral envelopes of tricuspid and mitral flow with reduced diastolic flow velocities, marked increases in isovolumic relaxation times, and reduced ventricular ejection times (13).

PERICARDIOCENTESIS GUIDED BY ECHOCARDIOGRAPHY

Pericardiocentesis may be life saving in the patient with cardiac tamponade and of valuable diagnostic help in patients with effusions. However needle aspiration does carry a small but significant morbidity and mortality rate. To minimize these risks a number of precautions can be taken, including careful clinical examination, adequate preparation, and monitoring with fluoroscopy and ECG during the procedure. Additional information and guidance can be provided by echocardiography. The guidelines below can help in the performance of echo guided pericardiocentesis.

Information Needed prior to Pericardiocentesis

1. The spatial distribution of pericardial fluid. (loculated or global)
2. An appreciation of the compartmentalization of the pericardial and any coexisting pleural fluid.
3. An estimate (semiquantitative) of the fluid volume.
4. Cardiac chamber dimensions and wall motion.

This information will help in the selection of the optimal procedure site.

Equipment Needed for Pericardiocentesis

1. Echocardiographic imaging and recording system.
2. Intravenous infusion system with (optional) right heart pressure monitoring catheter.
3. Local anesthetic.
4. Centesis needle, or catheter-over-needle set, connected to closed-system drainage.
5. Syringe for fluid aspiration and for convenient specimen handling.
6. (Optional) Multiport stopcock connected to infusion system.
7. (Optional) Side-hole drainage catheter with introducing sheath, dilator, and guidewire.

Technique

Successful pericardiocentesis permits collection of fluid for chemical, cytologic, and bacteriologic analysis and provides immediate relief of hemodynamic consequences of cardiac tamponade (15, 16). A patient suspected of having cardiac tamponade must be evaluated urgently for a definitive diagnosis. While technical forces are being marshalled for imaging and intervention, appropriate life-support measures should be initiated if required, most importantly to augment cardiac output until hemodynamic relief can be obtained.

Customarily, echocardiographic examinations are performed with the patient in left lateral decubitus position and, for subcostal and various other views, supine. If the patient is orthopneic, optimal position may be impossible. From a combination of parasternal, apical, and subcostal echocardiographic views, the location and distribution of pericardial fluid should be ascertained. Elevation of the upper body during pericardiocentesis often pools fluid inferiorly for better access. Possible puncture sites should be selected for optimal access to the fluid space, potential placement of an indwelling drainage catheter, or other factors dictated by the clinical situation. The site usually preferred is the subcostal region; however, any precordial location that provides clear, unobstructed access to the fluid-filled pericardial sac can be used. Figure 8.3 shows, schematically, the subcostal (four-chamber and short-axis) and apical (two- and four-chamber) transducer positions that provide effective images for monitoring pericardiocentesis. The intended puncture site is marked on the skin surface, then prepared aseptically and draped to form a sterile field. Infiltration with an anesthetic agent should be sufficient to block sensation in the deeper intercostal muscle and parietal pericardial tissues.

A short-bevel, 18-gauge (or larger) needle or flexible catheter over a trochar, long enough to reach the pericardial space from the puncture site and attached to a syringe or a closed-system drainage apparatus, is inserted and directed towards the pericardial sac. An infusion system connected to the

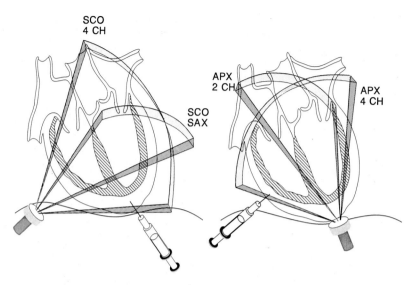

Figure 8.3. Schematic representations of apical (*APX*) and subcostal (*SCO*) transducer positions useful in guiding pericardiocentesis. Optimal tomographic orientations may vary from the standard views shown (*SAX* = short axis; *4 CH* = 4 chamber; *2 CH* = 2 chamber).

needle by means of a stopcock or flow manifold permits flushing of the needle lumen, if necessary, and later connection of an indwelling catheter (Fig. 8.4). The course of the needle should be directed to avoid the neurovascular bundles that lie at the inferior aspect of the ribs. If a flexible catheter and trochar are used, the trochar can be withdrawn and the catheter manipulated under echocardiographic guidance to optimize position for drainage or aspiration.

Echocardiographic guidance of the centesis needle requires selection of a transducer position that will not interfere with penetration of the chest wall and not contaminate the sterile field. A sterile transducer sheath permits closer positioning near the puncture wound, if necessary. The ideal transducer position will permit direct imaging of the needle tip, identification of the surface of the pericardial tissue, the site of needle entry into the pericardial space, and the opposing epicardial surface of the heart (17). When the puncture is performed subcostally, an apical or midprecordial transducer position in various tomographic planes usually allows perpendicular beam orientation to the needle and definition of the heart wall and the apex. Subcostal transducer position is

useful for monitoring changes in the fluid space but poor for resolving a lateral centesis needle entry.

It is important to ensure precise imaging of the tip of the centesis needle by orienting the transducer plane to show its maximum length. Position of the needle tip within the pericardial space can be verified by infusion of a small quantity of saline as a contrast agent while imaging the heart. Contrast effect only within the pericardial space indicates proper needle position. Contrast effect within the heart (right or left ventricle) indicates penetration of the heart wall. In this case the needle should be withdrawn and another contrast test performed to verify placement outside the heart.

Figure 8.5 demonstrates changes pre- and postpericardiocentesis, catheter placement within the pericardial sac, and the saline contrast injection that verified proper position. Approximately 700 ml of bloody fluid was drained during the procedure, with a recognizable change in echocardiographic images of fluid space. Irregular reflections within the pericardial fluid are characteristic of organized thrombotic material and fibrinous strands attached to both epicardial and outer pericardial surfaces. This patient also

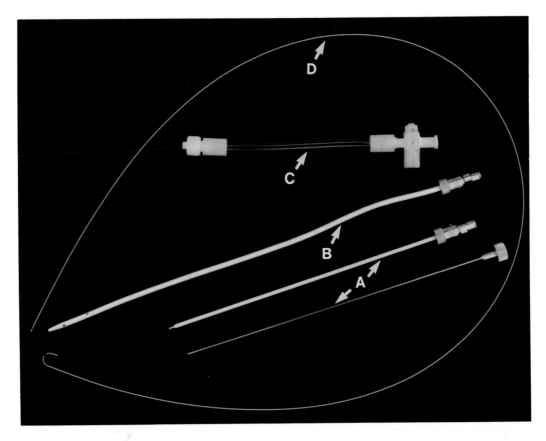

Figure 8.4. Pericardiocentesis needle and catheter system. **A**, 18-gauge introducer needle with sheath, **B**, Side-hole drainage catheter, **C**, connector tube with stopcock, **D**, curved-tip guide wire.

had a pleural effusion. A prosthetic mitral valve caused the dense reflections superimposed on images of the mitral annulus and left atrial cavity. Because of the posterolateral location of the pericardial fluid compartment, a puncture site in a high intercostal space, lateral to the anterior axillary line, was necessary. Echocardiographic imaging and guidance of needle placement was best from mid- and left-precordial transducer positions.

Prior to the availability of echocardiography for guidance, needle placement was performed under fluoroscopic guidance or "blind" with an electrocardiographic lead attached to the needle hilt for recognition of contact with the heart surface (18). The disadvantage of fluoroscopy, in addition to the consequences of radiation exposure, is the difficulty in appreciating the myocardial surface within the fluid-filled pericardial space. Electrocardiographic monitoring for ST segment changes is also disadvantageous, as it provides no visual reference, only evidence of the unwanted encounter of needle tip with myocardium. Echocardiographic imaging is clearly more desirable than either and, when imaging conditions are satisfactory, overcomes these objections. Some operators use fluoroscopy or electrocardiograms as back-up or for verification if ultrasound imaging resolution is suboptimal. A pulmonary artery catheter is useful for documentation of intracardiac pressure changes with relief of tamponade, but otherwise cannot aid in needle placement.

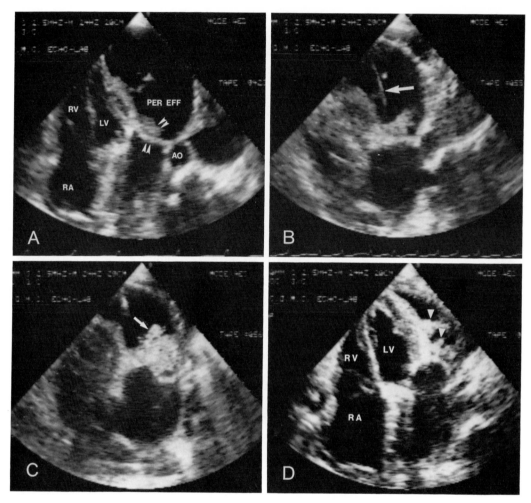

Figure 8.5. Posterolateral pericardial fluid. **A,** Left precordial transducer position prepericardi-ocentesis. **B,** More medial transducer position with the centesis catheter (*arrow*) within fluid space. **C,** Saline injection for verification of catheter position by contrast cloud (*arrow*). **D,** Left precordial transducer position post-pericardiocentesis. Note in *A* and *D,* fibrinous bands and thrombotic mate-rial (*arrowheads*). (*PER EFF* = pericardial effusion, *AO* = descending thoracic aorta, *LV* = left ventri-cle, *RV* is right ventricle, *RA* = right atrium, *LA* = left atrium).

Post pericardiocentesis Evaluation

Changes to be documented echocardi-ographically after successful drainage of pericardial fluid include:

1. Reduction in pericardial fluid volume.
2. Relief of hemodynamic compromise and car-diac tamponade, demonstrated by reversal of abnormal right ventricular and right atrial wall motion, and normalization of Doppler in-flow velocities, ejection times, and isovolumic relaxation times.
3. Proper position of the flow ports of an in-

dwelling catheter placed for continuous drain-age or infusion of medications.

Monitoring for recurrence of pericardial effusion and signs of hemodynamic com-promise should be performed following per-icardiocentesis. Further evaluation should be dictated by progress of the patient's clinical condition. Removal of an indwelling catheter should include echocardiographic evaluation, in order to show adequate de-compression of the pericardial space and to identify any cause of difficulty in removing the catheter, such as adhesion or clot formation.

Complications

Possible complications of pericardiocentesis include arrhythmia, infection, ventricular puncture, myocardial infarction, hemopericardium and cardiac tamponade, vasovagal reactions with hypotensive response, cardiac bradyarrhythmia and arrest, and death (15, 16). The results of pericardiocentesis should be evaluated by an experienced cardiologist-echocardiographer at the time of examination, so that further intervention can be started immediately in the case of complications.

PERCUTANEOUS INTRACARDIAC INTERVENTIONS

Myocardial Biopsy

In addition to pericardiocentesis, certain intracardiac procedures such as myocardial biopsy can be performed under echocardiographic guidance. Echocardiography permits bioptome tip identification and biopsy site location during percutaneous endomyocardial biopsy and enhances the information available from fluoroscopy. Biopsy of heart muscle tissue is a valuable aid in the diagnosis and evaluation of heart muscle abnormalities, such as inflammatory myocarditis, infiltrative cardiomyopathy, and tissue rejection after heart transplantation (19, 20).

A sheathed bioptome is introduced into the right internal jugular vein or femoral vein for right heart access and into a femoral artery for left heart access and advanced. Entrance of the bioptome into the heart is readily recognized echocardiographically because of the highly reflective metal tip. Direct observation of the course of the bioptome and position of the cutting tip aids in preventing inadvertent puncture of the free right ventricular wall or damage to atrioventricular valve structures.

In the case of a right ventricular biopsy, the position of the bioptome cutting tip should be on the interventricular septum near the apex of the heart, well away from septal attachments of the tricuspid valve and from the right ventricular free wall. Left ventricular biopsy requires retrograde passage of the bioptome well into the body of the left ventricle, with care to avoid the papillary muscles, mitral valve support apparatus, and left ventricular free wall. With fluoroscopy, the landmarks of the cardiac silhouette and a characteristic curve of the bioptome towards the plane of the interventricular septum are the only available clues to proper position. Echocardiographic imaging from the apical, parasternal, or subcostal approach allows more confident placement of the bioptome. The capability of imaging from various tomographic planes in many instances permits demonstration of the entire length of the biopsy catheter with respect to intracavitary structures. Figure 8.6 shows a bioptome within the right heart, imaged from the subcostal four-chamber view, and positioned in an arc directed away from the right ventricular free wall to a point along the distal segment of the septum. By direct observation of catheter position in this manner and meticulous selection of biopsy sites, multiple specimens can be obtained from recognizably different myocardial segments.

Potential complications of myocardial biopsy include perforation of the heart wall, pneumothorax, hemopericardium and cardiac tamponade, systemic and pulmonary embolism, arrhythmia, myocardial infarction, and acute mitral or tricuspid valve insufficiency. The procedure should be performed by a skilled, experienced operator and in a setting where appropriate emergency support measures are available, including surgical intervention if necessary.

Interventions in Congenital Heart Disease

Echocardiographic guidance of palliative treatments of congenital heart defects has significant potential as an effective alternative or adjunct to cardiac catheterization (21, 22, 23). Benefits of echocardiographic guidance include avoidance or minimizing of exposure to ionizing radiation and radiographic contrast media as well as the pre-

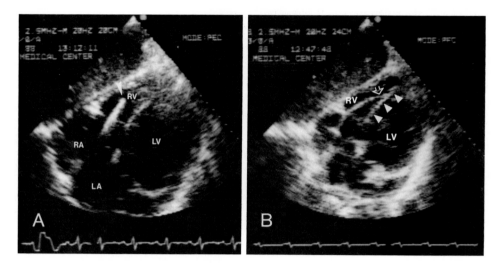

Figure 8.6. Percutaneous myocardial biopsy, subcostal four-chamber view. **A,** Bioptome cutting tip (*arrow*) visible in the right ventricle near the tricuspid valve; **B,** Bioptome tip (*arrow*) in contact with distal interventricular septum in an arc directed away from the right ventricular free wall. (*LV* = left ventricle, *RV* = right ventricle, *LA* = left atrium, *RA* = right atrium)

viously mentioned capabilities for internal structure identification. Atrial septostomy by balloon, blade, or laser can be readily directed under echocardiographic control.

The balloon septostomy catheter, introduced via a transvenous route into the right atrium, can be identified from multiple echocardiographic views, and its position at the right side of the foramen ovale verified. Once advanced across the foramen and with the balloon inflated in the left atrium, the ideal position prior to withdrawal (left to right) can be demonstrated, and safe deflation of the balloon and identification of the resultant atrial septal defect achieved. Analogous utilization of echocardiographic guidance can be applied to blade atrial septostomy (24) and laser atrial septostomy (25). Doppler color flow imaging and spectral flow analysis are also useful techniques for verification of atrial septal defects and interatrial blood flow.

Additional interventions that can be monitored by Doppler echocardiography include transcatheter closure of patent ductus arteriosis (26); and balloon dilatation of aortic coarctation (27), pulmonic valvular stenosis (28), discrete peripheral pulmonic stenosis, and hypoplastic pulmonary arteries (29).

Figure 8.7 demonstrates excellent visualization of cardiac structures by echocardiography used for direct observation of catheter placement from the right atrium into the right ventricle and the pulmonary artery.

Electrophysiologic Evaluation and Myocardial Ablation

Because of the multiple tomographic planes possible for evaluation of the heart, echocardiographic guidance of catheters for intracardiac pacing and electrophysiologic studies has been described as advantageous (30), and utilized clinically in transseptal cardiac catheterization (31). The additional advantage in electrophysiologic mapping is the recognition of catheter tip location within a specific segment of the ventricular endocardial surface. Resolution errors and reverberation artifacts can be overcome by a catheter tip ultrasonic transponder system developed recently for ventricular endocardial mapping (31). The ultrasonic transponder signal can be precisely located with reference to intracardiac anatomical landmarks and yields a reproducible mapping system for interventional electrophysiology.

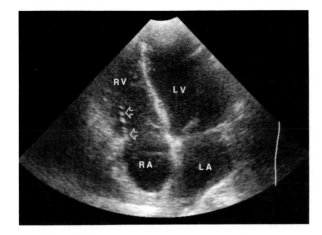

Figure 8.7. Catheter (*arrows*) placed under direct echocardiographic guidance from right atrium (*RA*) into right ventricle (*RV*) and into the pulmonary artery. (*LA* = left atrium, *LV* = left ventricle)

Echocardiography may also play a role in tissue characterization in myocardial ablation procedures. It may be possible to determine the extent of ablation from the echo image.

Valvuloplasty

Echocardiography also has a role in percutaneous valvuloplasty in acquired heart disease. Balloon dilatation by transatrial septum approach for the mitral valve, by retrograde aortic approach for the aortic valve, and by antegrade approach for the tricuspid and pulmonic valves can be directed by echocardiography in combination with fluoroscopy. Echocardiographic recognition of valve orifices and associated structures permits direct observation of catheter placement (Fig. 8.8). Since balloon inflations must be done in stages, the progress of serial dilatations can be monitored by Doppler flow analysis for both residual stenosis and developing regurgitation. Immediate post-valvuloplasty results can be utilized as a baseline for long-term follow-up of patients and provide an accurate indicator for ultimate benefit from the procedure.

Angioplasty and Thrombolysis Therapy

The value of echocardiography in routine percutaneous translumenal coronary angio-plasty and thrombolysis therapy is its ability to image in real-time ventricular wall motion changes. Wall motion patterns and overall ventricular systolic function can be assessed before, during, and after infusion of thrombolytic agents. Balloon angioplasty procedures also can be monitored and show marked wall motion abnormalities during balloon-induced ischemia in a number of patients.

INTRAOPERATIVE APPLICATIONS

Intraoperative utilization of Doppler echocardiography is a more recent expansion of the technique's interventional role. Both transesophageal and direct epicardial approaches are important adjuncts for evaluation of results in various types of open heart surgery.

Aortocoronary Grafting

Echocardiography is particularly useful for assessment of ventricular wall motion immediately after reversal of cardioplegia and discontinuance of artificial circulatory bypass. The technique also permits assessment of myocardial function immediately after aortocoronary grafts are placed. Demonstration of an unanticipated abnormally moving ventricular wall segment calls for reevaluation of the anastomoses and graft vessels and, if necessary, immediate intervention. The echocardiographic transducer,

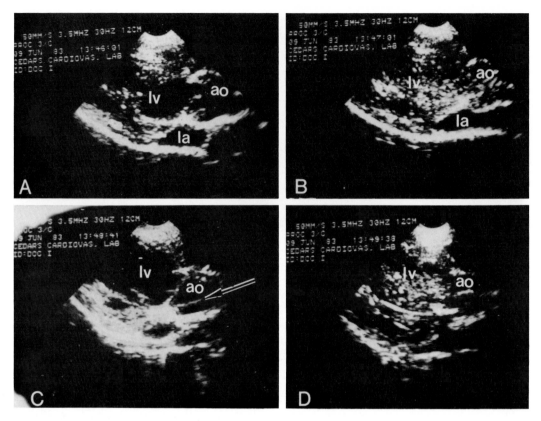

Figure 8.8. Aortic valvuloplasty using argon laser. (**A, C**) The laser catheter (*arrow*) can be seen adjacent to the aortic valve in these parasternal long-axis views. When the laser is fired, (**B and D**) contrast echoes appear in the aorta (*ao*) and left ventricle (*lv*) as white dots representing the vapor trail of the laser (*la* = left atrium).

within a sterile sheath, can be placed directly on the epicardial surface of the heart. Images are usually of high quality because of the absence of intervening reflectors and use of high-resolution, high-frequency transducers.

Doppler color-flow imaging also is useful in assessing graft patency by direct imaging of graft and anastomosis flow. Direct epicardial transducer placement on graft vessels and distal coronary arteries, using multiple orientations of the imaging plane, can verify flow patency and identify flow irregularities. Postoperatively, grafts imaged from the chest surface are more difficult to resolve; however, reliable documentation of patency intraoperatively contributes to the clinical information in following postsurgical patients.

Valve Repair and Replacement

Doppler echocardiography can demonstrate the adequacy of sewing ring attachment, relief of stenosis in valve repair, proper positioning of mitral prosthesis stents relative to the left ventricular outflow tract, and adequacy of repair of insufficient mitral and tricuspid valves.

Structural Revision and Palliative Procedures

Similar perioperative, direct epicardial imaging of structural repairs and palliative procedures for congenital heart defects, such as shunt placement, atrial and ventricular septal defect patch placement, and venoatrial reanastomosis allows immediate assessment of surgical results.

Assessment of Cardiac Function

Transesophageal echocardiography is frequently useful for intraoperative monitoring of ventricular function in noncardiac surgical patients. Transducer position within the esophagus permits high-resolution imaging of the heart and yields continuous, real-time assessment of ventricular volumes, overall systolic function, and regional wall motion. In these patients, Doppler flow analysis also provides information for assessment of valvular function and changes during surgery.

EXPANDING ROLE OF ECHOCARDIOGRAPHY

Although routine echocardiographic procedures provide valuable information during the standard cardiologic interventions discussed in this chapter, it is likely that echocardiography will play a much larger role in the future. With improvements in transducers, high-frequency, high-resolution images will provide pictures with a resolution of 100 um or better. Ultrasound images will soon surpass those of the best x-ray systems. Echo contrast agents will soon be released which will provide real-time perfusion scanning for myocardial ischemia. Three-dimensional pictures will be available, and already available are echo transducers smaller than 1 mm in diameter that can provide detailed images from within the coronary arteries along with Doppler flow information. These catheters can be coupled with laser or mechanical atherectomy catheters to provide a truly unique approach to the atherosclerotic vessel. Indeed, clinicians may soon be making an incredible journey through the vascular system. Lesions will be routinely identified by ultrasound and removed from inside, leaving clear vessels and minimal scarring.

ACKNOWLEDGEMENTS

The contributions of technologists Tom Jackson and Michael Skeels, RN, RDMS are gratefully acknowledged.

REFERENCES

1. Edler I: Diagnostic use of ultrasound in heart disease. *Acta Med Scand*, 308:32, 1955.
2. Feigenbaum H Waldhausen JA, Hyde LP: Ultra-sound Diagnosis of pericardial effusion. *JAMA* 191:107, 1965.
3. Tajik AJ: Echocardiography in pericardial effusion. *Am J Med* 63:29, 1977.
4. Holt JP: The normal pericardium. *Am J Cardiol* 26:455, 1970.
5. D'Cruz IA: Echocardiographic simulation of pericardial effusion by ascites. *Chest* 85:93, 1984.
6. Isner JM et al.: Subepicardial adipose tissue producing echocardiographic appearance of pericardial effusion. *Am J Cardiol* 51:565, 1983.
7. Pandi AS and Kronik G: Pseudoidiopathic hypertrophic subaortic stenosis in a patient with cardiac tamponade. *Chest* 91:631, 1987.
8. D'Cruz IA et al.: Diagnosis of cardiac tamponade by echocardiography: Changes in mitral valve motion and ventricular dimensions, with special reference to paradoxical pulse. *Circ* 52:460, 1975.
9. Armstrong WF et al.: Diastolic collapse of the right ventricle with tamponade: An echocardiographic study. *Circ* 65:1491, 1982.
10. Gillam LD et al.: Hydrodynamic compression of the right atrium: A new echocardiographic sign of cardiac tamponade. *Circ* 68:294, 1983.
11. Bommer WJ Everhart, R Smith, D et al.: Is Doppler echocardiography better than 2D echo in the detection of pericardial tamponade? *Clin Res* 35(I):101, 1987.
12. Dreyfus G et al.: Hemopericarde compressif de l'oreillette droite apres chirurgie cardiaque. *Arch Mal Coeur* 79:499, 1986.
13. Appleton CP et al.: Cardiac tamponade and pericardial effusion: Respiratory variation in transvalvular flow velocities studied by Doppler echocardiography. *J Am Coll Cardiol* 11(5):1020, 1988.
14. King SW, Pandian NG, Gordian JM: Doppler echocardiographic findings in pericardial tamponade and constriction. *Echocardiography* 5:361, 1988.
15. Callahan JA et al.: Diagnosis and treatment of pericardial effusion using ultrasonic guidance. In van-Sonnenberg E (ed): *Interventional Ultrasound*, vol 21 of *Clinics in Diagnostic Ultrasound*. New York, Churchill Livingstone, 1987, p 189.
16. Krikorian JG, Hancock EW: Pericardiocentesis. *Am J Med* 65:808, 1978.
17. Berger BC: Pericardiocentesis using echocardiography. In Schroeder JS (ed): *Invasive Cardiology*, vol 15, no 1 of *Cardiovascular Clinics*. Philadelphia, Davis, 1985, p 269.
18. Bishop LH et al.: The electrocardiogram as a safeguard in pericardiocentesis. *JAMA* 162:264, 1956.
19. Mason JW: Myocardial biopsy. In Yu PN, Goodwin JF (ed): *Progress in Cardiology*, vol 9. Philadelphia, Lea & Febiger, 1980, p 113.
20. French JW, Popp RL, and Pitlick PT: Cardiac localization of transvascular bioptome using 2-dimensional echocardiography. *Am J Cardiol* 51:219.
21. Rashkind WJ: Interventional cardiac catheterization in congenital heart disease. In Schroeder JS (ed): *Invasive Cardiology*, vol 15, no 1 of *Cardiovascular Clinics*. Philadelphia, Davis, 1985, p 303.
22. Allan LD, Ranjut L, Wainwright R et al.: Balloon atrial septostomy under two-dimensional echocardiographic control. *Br Heart J* 47:41, 1982.
23. Perry LW, Ruckman RN, Galioto FM, Jr et al.: Echo-

cardiographically assisted balloon atrial septostomy. *Pediatrics* 70:403, 1982.

24. Park SC, Neches WH, Zuberbuehler JR, et al.: Clinical use of base atrial septostomy. *Circ* (Suppl III):172, 1977.

25. Bommer WJ, Lee G, Riemenschneider TA et al.: Laser atrial septostomy. *Am Heart J* 106:1152–156, 1983.

26. Portsmann W, Wierny L, and Warnke H. Closure of persistent ductus arteriosus without thoracotomy. *Thoraxchirurgie* 15:199, 1967.

27. Lock JE, Niemi T, Burke BA et al.: Transcutaneous angioplasty of experimental aortic coarctation. *Circ* 66:1280, 1982.

28. Kan JS, White RI, Mitchell SE et al.: Transluminal balloon valvuloplasty for the treatment of congenital pulmonary valve stenosis. *J Am Coll Cardiol* 2: 588, 1983.

29. Lock JE, Castaneda-Zuniga WF, Fuhrman BP et al.: Balloon dilatation angioplasty of hypoplastic and stenotic pulmonary arteries. *J Am Coll Cardiol* 2: 588, 1983.

30. Drinkovic N: Subcostal echocardiography to determine right ventricular pacing catheter position and control advancement of electrode catheters in intracardiac electrophysiologic studies: M-mode and two-dimensional studies. *Am J Cardiol* 47:1260, 1981.

31. Kronzon I, Glassman E et al.: Use of two-dimensional echocardiography during trans-septal cardiac catheterization. *J Am Coll Cardiol* 4:425, 1984.

32. Langberg JJ, Frankclin JO, Landzberg JS et al.: The echo-transponder electrode catheter: A new method for mapping the left ventricle. *J Am Coll Cardiol* 12:218, 1988.

9 Intraoperative Abdomen

JUNJI MACHI
BERNARD SIGEL

Intraoperative ultrasonography plays a significant role in abdominal surgery where it has been widely used during liver, biliary tract, and pancreatic operations (1–4). During operative management of abdominal abscesses, gastrointestinal tumors, and other abdominal tumors, intraoperative ultrasonography may also be used. This chapter will describe the instrumentation, technique, indications, and the clinical results of intraoperative abdominal ultrasonography.

Instrumentation

During surgery, the most appropriate ultrasound instrument is a high-frequency, real-time B-mode system. High-resolution images can be obtained using transducer frequencies ranging from 5 to 10 MHz during abdominal operations. With instruments in this frequency range, a sound penetration depth of from 5 to 10 cm can be achieved, and this is usually sufficient for intraoperative abdominal scanning. Several American, Japanese, and European companies produce the 7.5-MHz instruments that are most frequently employed during abdominal surgery. It is even possible to scan the entire liver, the largest solid organ, with a 7.5-MHz instrument; however, a 5-MHz transducer may be required to penetrate the severely cirrhotic or markedly enlarged liver. On the other hand, the extrahepatic biliary tract or normal-sized pancreas can be scanned with a 10-MHz instrument.

Important features of the intraoperative instrumentation are the size and the shape of the ultrasound probe, and the type of probe selected for scanning is determined by the anatomic structure to be examined. In the abdominal cavity, a small probe with a flexible, easily manipulated cable is most appropriate. A thin cylindrical pencil-like probe and a flat linear-array probe are the two main types of intraoperative probes. When scanning the extrahepatic biliary tree, which is occasionally located deep in the operative field at the hepatoduodenal ligament, or for other abdominal organs, such as the pancreas, the pencil-like probe is utilized. For examining the liver, a flat "T" or "I"-shaped linear-array tranducer is essential (Fig. 9.1). This side-viewing probe has a 3- to 6-cm footprint and a wide image is obtained from a near field. In addition to the liver, other portions of the abdominal cavity may also be scanned with the flat probe.

Either an electronic or mechanical transducer is employed for B-mode real-time scanning. Also, color Doppler imaging systems have recently been introduced.

Techniques

Before the probes are introduced into the surgical field, they are either sterilized with cold gas or placed in a sterile plastic covering. Probe preparation is described in Chapter 4.

Contact and probe-standoff are the two principal scanning techniques used during intraoperative ultrasonography. In contact

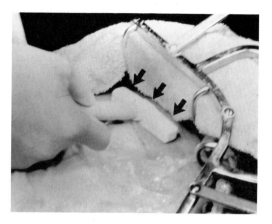

Figure 9.1. Intraoperative contact scanning of the liver using a T-shaped probe (*arrows*). (Reproduced with permission from Machi J: *Operative Ultrasonography—Fundamentals and Clinical Applications*. Tokyo, Life Science, 1987.)

scanning, the probe is placed directly on the tissue; in the probe-standoff technique, the probe is positioned 1 to 2 cm away from the surface of the structures. To obtain acoustic coupling between the probe and tissue during standoff scanning, saline solution is poured into the abdominal cavity. The distance between the probe and the target organ or the area of interest determines which method is chosen. For example, contact scanning is chosen to examine the interior of the liver (Fig. 9.1), and standoff scanning is used to examine the extrahepatic bile duct (Fig. 9.2) because it permits clear visualization of the surface of tissue. To image the deep portion of the pancreas, contact scanning can be used, whereas to image the pancreatic surface or superficial area of 0.5 to 1.0 cm in depth, standoff scanning is required.

It is important to scan the area of interest thoroughly from various positions and directions. Utilizing lateral, rotational, and angular movements of the probe, the examiner should obtain longitudinal and transverse views, and sometimes oblique views, of the organ or the lesions. This is particularly essential when screening or localizing small lesions in the solid organ. Systematic examinations using both longitudinal and transverse sections of the liver, for example, are

required in order to detect small or occult tumors in the liver.

For scanning of the extrahepatic bile duct, the supraduodenal portion is first visualized in a longitudinal plane (Fig. 9.2). The probe is moved from the hepatic hilum to the duodenum along the course of the duct. The intrapancreatic portion of the bile duct is imaged through the duodenum. Air in the duodenum, when present, is displaced by gently compressing the duodenum with the probe. Following scanning of the retroduodenal portion of the common duct, the supraduodenal portion of the duct is again surveyed to the level of the hilum of the liver. This survey should include visualization of the junction of the cystic and common hepatic ducts and the confluence of the right and left hepatic ducts. Whenever calculi are detected in an extrahepatic biliary system or intrahepatic calculi are suspected, the intrahepatic ducts are examined by scanning through the substance of the liver.

The pancreas is situated more deeply within the abdominal cavity and is obscured by the stomach, duodenum, colon, and the

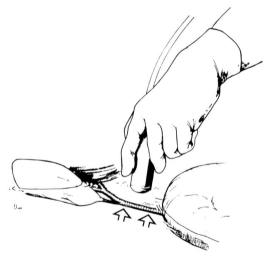

Figure 9.2. Standoff scanning of the extrahepatic bile duct using a pencil-like probe. The duct (*arrows*) and the head of probe are immersed in saline solution, and the longitudinal section of the duct is imaged. (Reproduced with permission from Machi J: *Operative Ultrasonography—Fundamentals and Clinical Applications*. Tokyo, Life Science, 1987.)

peritoneal membrane between these organs. Although the pancreas can be imaged through these structures, imaging is best achieved after surgical exposure. Surgical exposure of the pancreas for intraoperative ultrasonography is usually accompanied by transection of the gastrocolic ligament and entry into the lesser omental sac. Once the surface of the pancreas is exposed, ultrasound scanning is usually performed in longitudinal and transverse planes along the course of the gland, moving from the pancreatic head to the pancreatic tail (Fig. 9.3).

When intraoperative needle placement is needed for liver or pancreatic biopsy or other purposes, it is performed under ultrasound guidance. A probe-adaptor for needle guidance or a biopsy probe is commercially available; however, in the majority of instances, intraoperative ultrasound-guided needle placement can be performed in a freehand fashion. This method is described in detail in Chapter 1.

Depending on the purpose of the study, scanning may be performed at any time during abdominal surgery. Intraoperative ultrasonography can reveal information that is not evident during preoperative studies or during surgical explorations before tissue dissection. To obtain this new information, intraoperative ultrasonography may be used immediately after laparotomy, but prior to intraabdominal tissue dissection. Ultrasound scanning may also be used during the main surgical procedures. During hepatectomy, for example, intraopertive ultrasonography is used to guide resection of the liver parenchyma. Following surgical procedures, extirpation of tumors or extraction of biliary stones may be verified by ultrasound examination. Intraoperative ultrasonography is safe and noninvasive, and thus can be repeated as often as necessary during an operation.

Indications and Clinical Results

Liver

During liver surgery, intraoperative ultrasonography is used primarily to detect and evaluate primary malignant tumors, metastatic liver tumors, and benign lesions, and to guide hepatic surgical procedures.

The use of intraoperative ultrasonography for primary tumors developed initially in Japan (2, 3, 5–8), where there was a problem localizing hepatocellular carcinoma in the posthepatitic cirrhotic liver. Approximately 80% of hepatocellular carcinomas are associated with cirrhosis of the liver. Because approximately 50% of all carcinomas and 65% of carcinomas less than 5 cm in the cirrhotic liver are nonpalpable and invisible during surgery, it was crucial to find an intraoperative imaging method capable of detecting or localizing these tumors (8). Intraoperative ultrasonography appears to be more sensitive in detecting hepatocellular carcinomas than preoperative imaging stud-

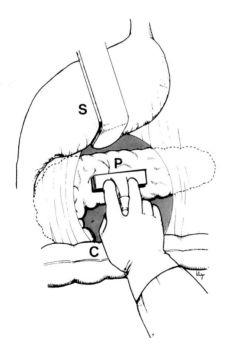

Figure 9.3. Scanning of the exposed pancreas using a T-shaped probe, which may be placed directly on the pancreas, after the gastrocolic ligament is transected. (S = Stomach, P = Pancreas, C = Transverse colon.) (Reproduced with permission from Machi J: *Operative Ultrasonography—Fundamentals and Clinical Applications.* Tokyo, Life Science, 1987.)

ies or surgical inspection and palpation. Makuuchi and colleagues reported that in a study of 203 hepatocellular carcinomas less than 5 cm in size, the sensitivity of intraoperative ultrasonography (99%) was significantly superior to that of preoperative ultrasonography (89.3%), angiography (84.1%), and computed tomography (89.6%) (8). The hepatocellular carcinoma in the cirrhotic liver demonstrated in Figure 9.4 was precisely localized by intraoperative scanning even though it was not palpable or visible.

During examinations to detect the intrahepatic spread of hepatocellular carcinoma, intraoperative ultrasonography has also played an important role in localizing previously undetected secondary lesions such as daughter (accessory) tumors, intrahepatic metastases, and intravascular tumor throbi, particularly in the tumor-bearing portal vein. Makuuchi and coworker reported that the sensitivity of intraoperative ultrasonography (41.7%) in detecting daughter tumors was significantly better than preoperative ultrasonography (12.5%), angiography (14.0%), and computed tomography (22.4%) (8). It was also reported that intraoperative ultrasonography (70%) had a markedly higher sensitivity in detecting intravascular tumor thrombi than preoperative ultrasonography (21%) and angiography (21%). These findings are the result of a study involving 152 patients in which surgically resected specimens were compared to the results of various imaging methods used to evaluate secondary lesions. A small daughter tumor from hepatocellular carcinoma, which was unrecognized during preoperative studies, is also shown in Figure 9.4. In order to determine the resectability of a tumor and decide on the type of hepatic operation to be performed, accurate evaluation of the extent of hepatocellular carcinoma in the liver is essential, and intraoperative examination with ultrasonography has become a valuable source of information for this purpose.

During laparotomy for the treatment of other abdominal malignancies, including gastrointestinal cancer, pancreatic cancer, and retroperitoneal tumors, intraoperative

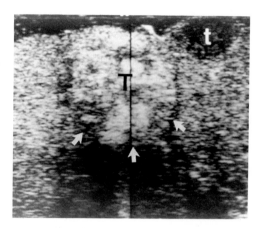

Figure 9.4. A hepatocellular carcinoma and its daughter tumor at the anterior-superior segment of the right lobe. The main tumor (T) was hyperechoic, 4 cm in diameter, and located near the liver surface; however, it was nonpalpable and invisible because of the severely cirrhotic liver. The daughter tumor (t) was hypoechoic and 17 x 12 mm. It was unknown preoperatively and was initially detected by intraoperative ultrasonography. (Reproduced with permission from Machi J: *Operative Ultrasonography—Fundamentals and Clinical Applications.* Tokyo, Life Science, 1987.)

ultrasonography may be used to examine the liver for metastasis, probably with higher accuracy than with preoperative studies (3, 9–11). Intraoperative ultrasonography is particularly helpful in screening for liver metastasis during operations for cancer with a high liver metastatic rate, such as colorectal cancer.

While screening for liver metastasis during 120 colorectal cancer operations, we have performed intraoperative ultrasonography on a routine basis. (3, 9). These screenings were performed regardless of the presence or absence of metastasis during preoperative studies or surgical exploration. In 88 of the 120 operations, none of the diagnostic methods revealed any metastases. A total of 69 metastatic tumors were detected in the remaining 32 operations. In 14 operations (11.7% of the total operations) 18 tumors were detected for the first time by intraoperative ultrasonography even though these same tumors were unrecognized during preoperative screening studies and surgical inspection and palpation. These 18 nonpalpable metastatic tumors were located 5 cm in depth from the liver surface and ranged in size from 4 x 4 mm to 13 x 18 mm. A small, nonpalpable metastatic tumor that was unidentified before operation is demonstrated in Figure 9.5. The comparative accuracy of various screening methods for liver metastases in 120 colorectal operations is summarized in Table 9.1. When compared to preoperative ultrasonography, computed tomography, and surgical exploration, the sensitivity, predictability of a negative test, and overall accuracy of intraoperative ultrasonography were significantly higher. A sensitivity and specificity rating greater than 95% indicates that intraoperative ultrasonography can become a valuable screening procedure during colorectal cancer surgery.

In addition to evaluating malignant tumors, intraoperative ultrasonography can also be used during hepatic operations for various benign lesions (1–3). Intrahepatic stones and cystic lesions are two types of benign hepatic lesions that require surgical intervention. From the liver surface, intrahepatic stones are almost always nonpalpable; however, because intraoperative ultrasonography is highly sensitive to biliary calculi and can locate intrahepatic stones precisely, it is a valuable imaging modality

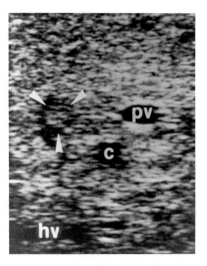

Figure 9.5. A metastic tumor from rectal cancer at the anterior-inferior segment of the right lobe. The tumor (*arrowheads*) was 7 mm in size, located 2.5 cm in depth, and thus was nonpalpable. *pv* = portal vein branch; *c* = small cyst; *hv* =right hepatic vein branch. (Reproduced with permission from Machi J: *Operative Ultrasonography—Fundamentals and Clinical Applications.* Tokyo, Life Science, 1987.)

during surgical procedures such as hepatectomy or hepatolithotomy. Surgery is not usually required for nonparasitic liver cysts, but when an operation is performed for liver cysts due to enlarged size or parasitic origin, intraoperative ultrasonography aids in at-

Table 9.1
Comparative Accuracy of Intraoperative Ultrasonography and other Methods in Diagnosing Liver Metastases from Colorectal Cancers

	Preoperative Ultrasound	Preoperative Computed Tomography	Surgical Exploration	Intraoperative Ultrasonography
Sensitivity	43.5%	46.4%	65.2%	95.7%*
Specificity	96.8%	94.7%	87.4%	95.8%
Predictability of negative test	70.2%	70.9%	77.6%	96.8%*
Predictability of positive test	90.9%	86.5%	78.9%	94.3%
Overall Accuracy	74.4%	74.4%	78.0%	95.7%

*p <0.01

Reprinted from Machi J: *Operative Ultrasonography—Fundamentals and Clinical Applications.* Tokyo, Life Science, 1987.

taining accurate localization. Intraoperative ultrasonography during liver abscess operations assists in achieving adequate drainage, thereby preventing the recurrence of symptoms (3, 12).

During imaging studies, it is clinically important to differentiate benign liver abnormalities (such as hemangioma, hyperplastic and regenerative nodules of liver cirrhosis, adenoma, adenomatous hyperplasia, localized fatty deposition, localized fibrosis, and calcification) from primary or metastatic malignant tumors. Intraoperative ultrasonography is generally sensitive in detecting lesions, but distinguishing benign lesions from malignancy is sometimes difficult; for example, a hyperplastic nodule or adenoma cannot be easily distinguished from a small hepatocellular carcinoma or daughter tumor. An intraoperative biopsy should be performed in such instances.

Intraoperative hepatic ultrasonography has become a popular imaging modality because it is useful not only in diagnosing various lesions accurately, but in guiding various hepatic surgical procedures (1–3, 5–8, 13–16). Needle placement into the liver and hepatic resection are the two main pro-

cedures that are facilitated by intraoperative ultrasound guidance. During surgery, needle placement is frequently performed to obtain tumor biopsies and to aspirate cystic lesions. In the case of a deep lesion that is not palpable, blind insertion of a needle is usually not successful. Blind needle placement may result in complications even when the lesion is visible or palpable. On the other hand, intraoperative ultrasonography guides the needle and places it precisely at the site of a lesion as shown in Figure 9.6. This biopsy was performed using the freehand method described in detail in Chapter 1. Use of ultrasound guidance for needle placement can prevent inadvertent insertion of a needle into the major vessels or the bile duct. Intraoperative ultrasound guidance may also assist in injecting agents, such as a dye or a drug, into the selected portal vein branch.

Intraoperative ultrasonography plays an extremely important role in hepatic resection, particularly in anatomically oriented hepatectomy. To perform hepatectomy appropriately, it is important to have an understanding of the anatomic relationships of the intrahepatic vessels (such as the portal

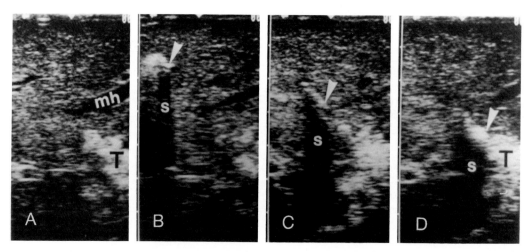

Figure 9.6. Intraoperative ultrasound guidance of needle placement for biopsy. **A,** A tumor (*T*) was detected at the posterior-inferior segment of the right lobe; (*mh* = middle hepatic vein). **B** through **D,** A biopsy needle (*arrowhead*) was introduced into the liver and advanced toward the tumor; *s* = the shadow of the needle. The tumor was a metastasis from rectal cancer. (Reproduced with permission from Machi J: *Operative Ultrasonography—Fundamentals and Clinical Applications.* Tokyo, Life Science, 1987.)

system and the hepatic veins) to a target lesion, and this can be achieved with intraoperative ultrasonography. By providing images of the spatial orientation of intrahepatic vessels, intraoperative ultrasonography helps to demarcate each segment or even subsegment of the right and left lobe and define the exact location and extent of lesions. This anatomic information enables the surgeon to establish the resection line for hepatectomy and perform various types of hepatic resections, including lobectomy, segmentectomy, extended segmentectomy, and subsegmentectomy. Systematic subsegmentectomy and inferior right hepatic-vein-preserving hepatectomy are two operations that have developed as a result of intraoperative ultrasound guidance, and hepatic surgeons recognize the importance of these new procedures in the treatment of hepatocellular carcinoma (2, 5, 8, 13). Ultrasonography can be used repeatedly during resection procedures to evaluate and control the direction of the resection plane. The use of intraoperative ultrasonography during a hepatic resection is demonstrated in Figure 9.7. On the ultrasound images, the resection plane is discernible as a hyperechoic line, and thus the extent and direction of resection and its relationship to the tumor can be recognized readily.

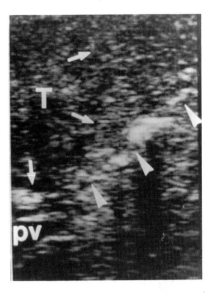

Figure 9.7. Intraoperative ultrasound guidance of hepatic resection. A tumor (*T* and *arrows*), metastasis from colon cancer, was located at the anterior-inferior segment of the right lobe. A right portal vein branch (*pv*) was seen behind the tumor. The hepatic resection plane exhibited a hyperechoic line (*arrowheads*). It confirmed that the resection was proceeding appropriately toward the portion between the tumor and the vein. (Reproduced with permission from Machi J: *Operative Ultrasonography—Fundamentals and Clinical Applications.* Tokyo, Life Science, 1987.)

Biliary Tract

Intraoperative ultrasonography is indicated during biliary tract operations for the detection of gallstones, the screening of common bile duct stones, the evaluation of biliary tumors, and the localization of the obscured extrahepatic biliary duct.

Gallstones are usually diagnosed without difficulty by preoperative imaging studies. Intraoperative ultrasonography, however, is a valuable tool for diagnosing or excluding gallstones when preoperative gallbladder examination has not been performed or when the examination findings are indeterminate. The extreme sensitivity of high-resolution intraoperative ultrasonography to biliary calculi enables stones as small as 1 mm to be detected readily.

Screening for common bile duct stones at the time of cholecystectomy for gallstones is the most common indication for using intraoperative ultrasonography during biliary surgery (1–3, 17–21). Intraoperative radiographic cholangiography, the established procedure for this screening purpose, has certain disadvantages in terms of its limited accuracy, adverse effects, and complications. In our experimental and clinical studies, we compared the results of intraoperative ultrasonography and intraoperative cholangiography (1, 3, 17–19, 22). In 580 operations, intraoperative ultrasonography was performed to screen for common duct stones, and in 368 of these operations, operative cholangiography was performed simultaneously (3, 17). The comparison of both methods is presented in Table 9.2. The sensitivity, specificity, predictability of a negative test, and the overall accuracy of

Table 9.2
Comparative Accuracy of Intraoperative Ultrasonography and Cholangiography in Diagnosing Common Bile Duct Stones

	Intraoperative Ultrasonography	Intraoperative Cholangiography
Sensitivity	92.8%	85.4%
Specificity	99.2%	95.4%
Predictability of a negative test	99.0%	98.0%
Predictability of a positive test	94.1%	71.4%*
Overall Accuracy	98.4%	94.2%

*p <0.005

Reprinted from *Operative Ultrasonography—Fundamentals and Clinical Applications* (1987) with the permission of Junji Machi, MD, PhD, and Life Science Co, Ltd, Tokyo, Japan

each screening method were at high and comparable values. The predictability of a positive test with intraoperative ultrasonography, however, was significantly superior to that with cholangiography. In the case of common duct stones, predictability of a positive test reflects how often the stones are present when the test is positive; that is, a low score for predictability of a positive test will lead to a higher rate of negative common duct explorations. Our clinical results suggest that negative common duct explorations can be reduced by using intraoperative ultrasonography. A small common duct stone that was detected only with intraoperative ultrasonography is demonstrated in Figure 9.8..

Intraoperative ultrasonography possesses several advantages besides accuracy over intraoperative cholangiography. First, because various directions and multiple planes can be imaged with intraoperative ultrasonography and because it provides real-time two-dimensional images, more information is obtained. Second, it enhances the surgeon's anatomic understanding of the relationship of the biliary system to the liver, pancreas, and vessels, including the hepatic artery and the portal vein. Third, unlike intraoperative cholangiography, it does not expose the patient to the risks associated with cannulation of the duct, injection of contrast material, or irradiation. Therefore, intraoperative ultrasonography is safer and less invasive. Finally, it can be performed more quickly than intraoperative cholangiography; for example, intraoperative scanning of the extrahepatic biliary duct can usually be achieved within 5 minutes.

The possibility of replacing intraoperative cholangiography with intraoperative ultrasonography in the screening of common duct stones is an important issue. Based on its accuracy and advantages, we believe that intraoperative ultrasonography can be the first choice diagnostic procedure for this use. However, both intraoperative ultrasonography and cholangiography should be used simultaneously until the examiner gains confidence in the scanning technique and image interpretation of intraoperative ultrasonography. After this experience and knowledge have been acquired, the physician can utilize intraoperative ultrasonography routinely during gallstone operations. When the results of intraoperative ultrasonography are equivocal or inconclusive or when additional information regarding biliary tract abnormalities (e.g., strictures) is

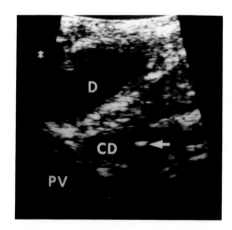

Figure 9.8. A 2-mm biliary stone (*arrow*) in the common bile duct (*CD*) detected by intraoperative ultrasonography and not demonstrated with intraoperative cholangiography; *PV* = portal vein; *D* = duodenum. (Reproduced with permission from Sigel B: Biliary tract surgery. In Sigel B (ed): *Operative Ultrasonography*, ed 2. New York, Raven Press, 1988, p 107.)

necessary, intraoperative cholangiography can be performed. The use of intraoperative ultrasonography on a routine basis and intraoperative cholangiography on a selective basis reduces the number of radiographic studies and may be more cost-effective than the routine use of cholangiography during biliary stone operations.

Intraoperative ultrasonography provides valuable imaging information during biliary tumor examination. Small preoperatively unrecognized gallbladder polyps are at times discovered. During examinations to assess the extent of biliary tumor, including primary gallbladder and bile duct cancer, intraoperative ultrasonography assists in deciding whether or not the tumor is resectable and in determining the type of operation to be performed. In particular, when compared to preoperative studies, intraoperative ultrasonography provides a more precise evaluation of direct invasion of the biliary tumor to the liver parenchyma and to vessels such as the portal vein. The metastatic spread of cancer to the liver and regional lymph nodes may also be investigated with this modality.

During biliary operations in which the anatomy around the biliary system is distorted, localization of the extrahepatic bile duct may become a difficult problem, although this is a rare occurrence. Tissue adhesion resulting from previous surgery, inflammation caused by cholecystitis, cholangitis, pancreatitis, biliary and pancreatic fistula, and biliary or other malignancies are the most common causes of an obscured biliary duct. In such situations, locating the biliary duct requires prolonged tissue dissection, most likely with blind needle puncture, which presents the risks of duct injury and longer operating time. These risks may be avoided and operating time may be reduced by the use of intraoperative ultrasonography to localize the duct.

Pancreas

During pancreatic operations, intraoperative ultrasonography is indicated for the diagnosis or definition of the complications of pancreatitis, pancreatic cancer evaluation, and islet cell tumor localization.

Chronic pancreatitis is associated with various complications such as dilatation of the pancreatic duct, pancreatic pseudocyst, stenosis of the common bile duct, and splenic or portal vein thrombosis, and intraoperative ultrasonography has been used to diagnose, exclude, or localize these lesions (1, 3, 18, 19, 23–26). Intraoperative ultrasonography also provides anatomic information about the area around the pancreas. Preoperative imaging studies are the usual means of making primary diagnoses of dilated pancreatic ducts or pseudocysts. When intraoperative ultrasonography is applied, however, previously unidentified lesions may be detected. New lesions are detected most often in the presence of secondary lesions. During an operation for a large pseudocyst or a dilated duct, for example, a small pseudocyst may be detected for the first time by intraoperative ultrasonography. Intraoperative ultrasonography is also useful in excluding abnormalities suspected during preoperative studies or surgical exploration. Pancreatic tissue swelling due to pancreatitis, in particular, occasionally suggests the presence of a pseudocyst. With intraoperative ultrasonography, pancreatic enlargement would be imaged as a solid mass, and thus the suspicion of pseudocyst would be ruled out.

A particularly valuable role of intraoperative ultrasonography is localization of preoperatively diagnosed lesions. Because of dense inflammation, even an extremely dilated pancreatic duct or a large pseudocyst may frequently be nonpalpable during an operation. The precise location of such lesions is easily demonstrated with intraoperative ultrasonography, and it assists in guiding exploratory needle placement into these lesions. Intraoperative ultrasound guidance also facilitates the procedure of pancreatic incision for drainage of the duct or the cyst. A dilated but nonpalpable pancreatic duct localized by intraoperative ultrasonography is demonstrated in Figure 9.9..

In treating pancreatic cancer, intraoperative ultrasonography is indicated for both establishing the diagnosis and stage of the cancer (1, 3, 18, 19, 24, 27). In the absence of

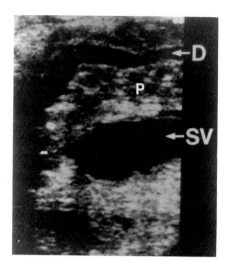

Figure 9.9. A high-resolution scan through the pancreas demonstrated a dilated main pancreatic duct (*D*) caused by chronic pancreatitis. The duct was not palpable during operation and was localized by intraoperative ultrasonography; *SV* = splenic vein behind the pancreas (*P*). (Reproduced with permission from Machi J: *Operative Ultrasonography—Fundamentals and Clinical Applications.* Tokyo, Life Science, 1987.)

vides images of the relationship of a tumor to vessels or the biliary duct. In particular, when tumor encasement of the vein is visualized, as demonstrated in Figure 9.10, cancer invasion to the portal system may be a strong suspicion. Pancreatic cancer metastasis to the liver and regional lymph nodes is also determined using intraoperative ultrasonography. These ultrasound findings help the surgeon to decide soon after laparotomy whether a radical resection or a palliative operation should be performed, thereby reducing operating time and unnecessary massive tissue dissection.

Surgical management is significantly affected by the ability of intraoperative ultrasonography to detect and localize small islet cell tumors (1, 3, 24, 28–30). During ultrasound imaging, islet cell tumors, including insulinoma and gastrinoma, exhibit a characteristic hypoechogenicity that enables their distinction from normal pancreatic tissue. Functioning islet cell tumors are usually small and are occasionally nonpalpable during surgery. Tumors that are unidentified by preoperative studies and surgical explora-

a preoperative histologic diagnosis of pancreatic cancer, an intraoperative biopsy is usually performed. Even when a tumor is visible or palpable, a blind biopsy entails the risks of intraoperative bleeding or postoperative infection and fistula resulting from inadvertent puncture of blood vessels or of the pancreatic duct. Through the use of intraoperative ultrasonography, the risks associated with the blind procedure can be avoided. Under direct needle visualization, a biopsy can be performed and the specimen can be obtained at the exact site of interest. In determining the resectability of a tumor, evaluating an advanced stage of pancreatic cancer is very important because pancreatic tumor resection is a major abdominal operation associated with relatively high mortality and morbidity. Surgical exploration by inspection and palpation for this staging evaluation often necessitates extensive tissue dissection. However, an evaluation prior to tissue dissection may be obtained using intraoperative ultrasonography, which pro-

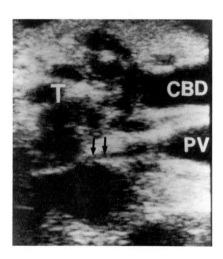

Figure 9.10. Portal vein invasion of a pancreatic head cancer. The tumor (*T*) encased and partially occluded (*arrows*) the portal vein (*PV*). The common bile duct (*CBD*) was involved in the tumor and completely obstructed. (Reproduced with permission from Machi J: *Operative Ultrasonography—Fundamentals and Clinical Applications.* Tokyo, Life Science, 1987.)

tion can be detected and precisely localized with intraoperative ultrasonography. Islet cell tumors as small as 3 or 4 mm are delineated with high-resolution intraoperative ultrasound instruments (Fig. 9.11). Intraoperative ultrasonography can also be used to confirm or exclude that a palpable pancreatic nodule is a tumor. Because islet cell tumors sometimes occur multiply, this is of value when multiple nodules are discovered by palpation. If indicated, intraoperative ultrasonography is used after localization to guide tumor enucleation.

In a total of 122 pancreatic operations, we employed intraoperative ultrasonography during 90 operations for the complications of pancreatitis, 27 operations for pancreatic cancer and 5 operations for islet cell tumors (24). The uses of intraoperative ultrasonography were categorized as beneficial if diagnosis or definition of lesions was provided. Diagnosis was defined as new detection of previously unrecognized conditions and exclusion of suspected conditions. Definition included localization of lesions, spatial assessment of lesions and the surrounding anatomy, and tissue feature distinction. The results indicated that intraoperative ultra-

sonography was useful in 69% of the operations for the complications of pancreatitis and in 66% of the operations for pancreatic tumors, including cancers and islet cell tumors (Table 9.3).

Other Abdominal Surgery

During abdominal operations for lesions other than hepato-biliary-pancreatic diseases, intraoperative ultrasonography can be used. For intraabdominal, retroperitoneal, and solid organ abscesses (for example, liver, pancreatic, or splenic abscess), the first choice procedure currently in use is percutaneous drainage under ultrasound or computed tomographic guidance. Surgical drainage is performed when percutaneous methods are unsuccessful because a safe access drainage route is unavailable or because there are multiple abscesses. Surgical exploration for abscesses is, however, often tedious and time-consuming because of severe inflammatory conditions. During surgical drainage of abdominal abscesses, intraoperative ultrasonography assists by precisely localizing all abscesses before extensive tissue dissection and by guiding needle placement for aspiration (3, 12). Ultrasound imaging may reduce the complications caused by difficult tissue dissection

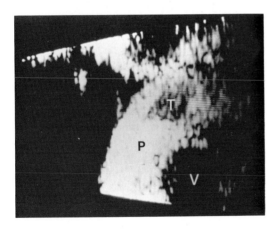

Figure 9.11. A 4-mm gastrinoma (*T*) localized by intraoperative ultrasonography in the tail of the pancreas. It was markedly hypoechoic as compared to the pancreatic parenchyma (*P*); V = splenic vein. (Reproduced with permission from Sigel B, et al.: The role of imaging ultrasound during pancreatic surgery. *Ann Surg*, 100(4):1984, p 491, © JB Lippincott.

Table 9.3
Value of Intraoperative Ultrasonography during Pancreatic Operations

Benefits	Complications of Pancreatitis	Pancreatic Tumors
Diagnosis		
Detection	8%	6%
Exclusion	24%	19%
Definition		
Localization	20%	6%
Spatial Assessment	17%	19%
Tissue Feature	0%	16%
Subtotal Useful	69%	66%
Not Useful	31%	34%
Total	100%	100%

Reprinted by permission from Sigel B, Machi J, Ramos JR, Duarte B, Donahue PE: The role of imaging ultrasound during pancreatic surgery. *Ann Surg* 200:486, 1984, © JB Lippincott.

and may reduce the recurrence of infection resulting from incomplete drainage of all abscesses.

Intraoperative ultrasonography can be used during operations for abdominal malignancies, including gastrointestinal cancer, retroperitoneal tumor, or ovarian cancer, for the same purpose as in hepato-biliary-pancreatic cancer: to determine the extension of local invasion of tumor and the existence of lymph nodes or liver metastases. The choice of type of operation can be made on the basis of intraoperative ultrasound findings.

Of particular interest in imaging diagnosis is the layered appearance of the gastrointestinal wall on the ultrasound images (3, 31). A five-layer wall is visualized using high-resolution intraoperative instruments, and these layers correspond to the stomach wall layer structure obtained during histologic examination as follows: the innermost hyperechoic layer corresponds to the mucosal surface boundary; the second hypoechoic layer to the mucosa and the muscularis mucosa; the third hyperechoic layer to the submucosa; the fourth hypoechoic layer to the muscularis propria; and the outermost hyperechoic layer to the subserosa and the serosa. Intraoperative ultrasound imaging can reveal the distortion or destruction of the normal five-layer appearance that occurs as a result of cancer; and therefore the depth of tumor invasion and intramural lateral tumor extension can be determined. This intraoperative ultrasound information assists in drawing a resection line of the stomach during gastric cancer surgery. Intraoperative ultrasonography can also localize a nonpalpable early gastric cancer, as in Figure 9.12. This figure also demonstrates the normal five-layer stomach wall.

Summary

Intraoperative abdominal ultrasonography is a relatively new imaging technique with a number of advantages compared to intraoperative radiography. First, it provides unique information that is otherwise unavailable. Second, it assists in guiding surgical manipulations. Third, it is noninvasive. As a result, intraoperative ultrasonography has had a significant impact on the management of abdominal surgery. Because detection and localization of benign and malignant lesions are possible, intraoperative ultrasound reduces operative time and facilitates appropriate operative decision making and surgical tissue dissection. The use of intraoperative ultrasonography has reduced the need for intraoperative radiographic studies, such as cholangiography. In the liver or pancreas or at anatomically distorted structures, intraoperative ultrasound guidance can achieve safe and expedient needle aspiration of cystic lesions or biopsies of deep-seated tumors. Intraoperative ultrasonography has also led to refinements in surgical procedures. New abdominal procedures such as anatomically oriented subsegmentectomy have been developed.

Because of the remarkable benefits of this modality, we urge that practitioners attain the skill and experience required for its use

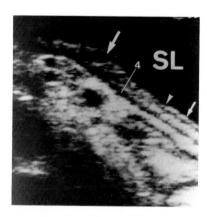

Figure 9.12. An early gastric cancer (*large arrow*) with invasion to the submucosa. A *small arrow* indicates the portion of normal stomach wall, exhibiting normal five-layer appearance. At the cancer, layers 1 to 3 (the mucosal and submucosal layers) were distorted, while layer 4 (the muscle layer) was intact. An arrowhead points out the lateral extension of the tumor. *SL* = stomach lumen. (Reproduced with permission from Machi J, Takeda J, Kakegawa T, Sigel B: Normal stomach wall and gastric cancer: Evaluation with high-resolution operative US. *Radiology* 159(1): 85–87, 1986 © Radiological Society of North America.)

and thereby expand the utilization of intraoperative ultrasonography for the surgical management of hepatic, biliary, pancreatic, and other abdominal diseases.

REFERENCES

1. Sigel B (ed): Biliary tract surgery. In *Operative Ultrasonography,* ed 2. New York, Raven Press, 1988.
2. Makuuchi M: *Abdominal Intraoperative Ultrasonography.* Tokyo, Igaku-Shoin, 1987.
3. Machi J: *Operative Ultrasonography: Fundamentals and Clinical Applications.* Tokyo, Life Science, 1987.
4. Sigel B, (ed): Progress symposium: Advances in intraoperative ultrasound. *World J Surg* 11:557–671, 1987.
5. Mukuuchi M, Hasegawa H, Yamazaki S: Intraoperative ultrasonic examination for hepatectomy. *Jpn J Clin Oncol* 11:367–390, 1981.
6. Nagasue N, Suehiro S, Yukaya H: Intraoperative ultrasonography in the surgical treatment of hepatic tumors. *Acta Chir Scand* 1984; 150:311–316.
7. Igawa S, Sakai K, Kinoshita H, Hirohashi K: Intraoperative sonography: Clinical usefulness in liver surgery. *Radiology* 1985; 156:473–478.
8. Makuuchi M, Hasegawa H, Yamazaki S, Takayasu K, Moriyama N: The use of operative ultrasound as an aid to liver resection in patients with hepatocellular carcinoma. *World J Surg* 1987; 11:615–621.
9. Machi J, Isomoto H, Yamashita Y, Kurohiji T, Shirouzu K, Kakegawa T. Ultrasonography in screening of liver metastases from colorectal cancer: Comparative accuracy with traditional procedures. *Surgery* 1987; 101:678–684.
10. Boldrini G, Gaetano AM, Giovannini I, Castagneto M, Colagrande C, Castiglioni G: The systematic use of operative ultrasound for detection of liver metastasis during colorectal surgery. *World J Surg* 11: 622–627, 1987.
11. Angelini L, Bezzi M, Tucci G, et al.: Intraoperative high-resolution hepatosonography in the detection of occult metastases in colorectal carcinoma. *Ital J Surg Sci* 13:203–208, 1983.
12. Machi J, Sigel B, Beitler JC, Nyhus LM, Donahue PE: Ultrasonic examination during surgery for abdominal abscess. *World J Surg* 7:409–415, 1983.
13. Makuuchi M, Hasegawa H, Yamazaki S: Ultrasonically guided subsegmentectomy. *Surg Gynecol Obstet* 1985;161;346–350.
14. Gozzetti G, Mazziotti A, Bolondi L, et al.: Intraoperative ultrasonography in surgery for liver tumors. *Surgery* 1986;99:523–530.
15. Sheu JC, Lee CS, Sung JL, Chen DS, Yang PM, Lin TY: Intraoperative hepatic ultrasonography. An indispensable procedure in resection of small hepatocellular carcinomas. *Surgery* 1985;97: 97–103.
16. Bismuth H, Castaing D, Garden OJ: The use of operative ultrasound in surgery of primary liver tumors. *World J Surg* 1987;11:610–614.
17. Sigel B, Machi J, Beitler JC, et al.: Comparative accuracy of operative ultrasound and cholangiography in detecting common duct calculi. *Surgery* 1983;94:715–720.
18. Sigel B, Coelho JCU, Machi J, et al.: The application of real-time ultrasound imaging during surgical procedures. *Surg Gynecol Obstet* 157:33–37, 1983.
19. Sigel B, Machi J, Anderson KN, et al.: Operative sonography of the biliary tree and pancreas. *Sem Ultrasound CT MR,* 6:2–14, 1985.
20. Lane RJ, Coupland GAE: Ultrasonic indication to explore the common bile duct. *Surgery* 1982;91: 268–274.
21. Jakimowicz JJ, Rutten H, Jurgens PJ, Carol EJ: Comparison of operative ultrasonography and radiography in screening of common bile duct for calculi. *World J Surg* 1987;11:628–634.
22. Machi J, Sigel B, Spigos DG, Beitler JC, Justin JR: Experimental assessment of imaging variables associated with operative ultrasonic and radiographic cholangiography. *J Ultrasound Med* 1983;2: 535–538.
23. Sigel B, Coelho JCU, Donahue PE, et al.: Ultrasonic assistance during surgery for pancreatic inflammatory disease. *Arch Surg* 1982; 117:712–716.
24. Sigel B, Machi J, Ramos JR, Duarte B, Donahue PE: The role of imaging ultrasound during pancreatic surgery. *Ann Surg* 1984;200:486–493.
25. Smith, SJ, Vogelzang RL, Donavan J, Atlas SW, Gore RM, Nieman, HL: Intraoperative sonography of the pancreas. *AJR* 1985;144:557–562.
26. Hernigou A, Plainfosse MC, Chapuis Y, et al.: Operative ultrasound of the pancreas: A review of 53 cases. *J Belge Radiol* 169:37, 1986.
27. Sigel B, Coelho JCU, Nyhus LM, et al.: Detection of pancreatic tumors by ultrasonography during surgery. *Arc Surg* 117:1058–1061, 1982.
28. Lane RJ, Coupland GAE: Operative ultrasound features of insulinomas. *Am J Surg* 1982; 144:585–587.
29. Norton JA, Sigel B, Baker AR, et al.: Localization of an occult insulinoma by intraoperative ultrasound. *Surgery* 1985;97:381–384.
30. Charboneau WJ, James EM, Van Heerden JA, et al.: Intraoperative real-time ultrasonographic localization of pancreatic insulinoma: Initial experience. *J Ultrasound Med* 2:251–254, 1983.
31. Machi J, Takeda J, Kakegawa T, Sigel B: Normal stomach wall and gastric cancer: Evaluation with high-resolution operative ultrasound. *Radiology* 159:85–87, 1986.

10 Abdominal Abscesses: The Role of CT and Sonography

R. BROOKE JEFFREY, JR.

Introduction

Percutaneous catheter drainage of abdominal abscesses developed as a combination of cross-sectional imaging with computed tomography (CT) and sonography and modified angiographic techniques (1). It has proven to be a safe and effective alternative to operative drainage that avoids the morbidity and expense of general anesthesia and surgical dissection. Percutaneous abscess drainage is one of the most successful and gratifying of all intraabdominal interventional procedures. It has gained wide acceptance in the surgical community and is now the technique of choice in draining the majority of abdominal abscesses. This chapter will focus on the role of CT and sonography in guiding percutaneous catheter drainage and managing intraabdominal abscesses.

Diagnosis of Abdominal Abscess

Clinical Features

The epidemiology of abdominal abscesses has changed significantly in the past few decades. Previously, gastrointestinal perforation from lesions such as appendicitis, diverticulitis, or duodenal ulcer disease was the most common cause of intraabdominal abscesses (2). At present, however, postoperative complications are the single most common etiologic factor in the development of abdominal abscesses (3). The clinical signs and symptoms of abdominal abscesses have similarly changed to reflect different trends in patient presentation. The increasing number of immunocompromised and immunodeficient patients has made the early diagnosis of abdominal abscesses even more clinically challenging.

Although the majority of patients with intra-abdominal abscesses present with localized pain, fever, and leukocytosis, this is not invariably the case. There are a growing number of patients with clinically occult or silent abdominal abscesses that may pose significant problems in diagnosis (4). Not infrequently, these are elderly patients with chronic walled off gastrointestinal perforations or patients with some degree of immunocompromise. In addition, patients may be receiving corticosteroids or prolonged antibiotic therapy for other clinical indications that may mask systemic signs of infection (4). Focal abdominal pain should always be considered as a symptom of a possible abdominal abscess even in the absence of system signs of sepsis.

The clinical presentation as well as the CT and sonographic findings of an abdominal abscess may be nonspecific. Therefore, a high index of suspicion, as well as an aggressive approach to guided diagnostic needle aspiration is essential for precise diagnosis of abdominal abscesses. In a previous CT series of nine patients with abnormal fluid collections and clinically silent abscesses (i.e., no fever or leukocytosis), the diagnosis of an abscess was not made prior to laparotomy in four patients (4). Abscess was not considered due to the "benign" clinical presentation and the failure to perform a guided aspiration (4).

Imaging with CT and Sonography

The CT and sonographic features of abdominal abscesses are variable and can be mimicked by other fluid collections such as seromas, pancreatic pseudocysts, bilomas, or loculated ascites (5–15). The most characteristic finding of an abdominal abscess demonstrated is a complex fluid collection with mass effect. Noninfected fluid collections are passive, and rarely displace adjacent bowel loops or solid viscera. The presence of gas bubbles with a fluid collection with mass effect is highly suggestive of an abdominal abscess. It should be noted, however, that gas is detected in only one-third of abdominal abscesses on CT (5). Thus, guided needle aspiration is essential for precise diagnosis of all abnormal intraabdominal fluid collections.

The sonographic appearance of abdominal abscesses depends on the viscocity of the abscess fluid, the degree of internal septations and the presence or absence of microbubbles or gas (12–15). Although the majority of abscesses on sonography are hypoechoic lesions (Fig. 10.1), there are numerous examples of both isoechoic and hyperechoic abscesses. (Figs. 10.2 and 10.3) Isoechoic abscesses with little enhanced sound transmission may mimic solid lesions (Fig. 10.2) (15). The degree of enhanced-through-sound transmission produced by abdominal abscesses is similarly variable and depends on the extent of sound attenuation or scattering by the debris within the abscess (Fig. 10.4). It should be noted that, on occasion, solid lesions may, in fact, mimic complex fluid collections sonographically by demonstrating internal septations and enhanced through sound transmission (Fig. 10.5).

One of the main disadvantages of sonography in evaluating intraperitoneal inflammatory masses is the difficulty in distinguishing a liquified abscess from a phlegmon. Phlegmons are nonliquified areas of indurated soft tissue inflammation that are not appropriate for percutaneous or surgical drainage. Contrast-enhanced CT is clearly superior in identifying the low-density areas of liquified pus versus phlegmon.

The majority of abdominal abscesses on CT are low-density lesions with attenuation values slightly greater than simple fluid (15–25 HU) (5–11). Phlegmons are of soft density (25–40 HU). Areas of adjacent edema often result in soft tissue infiltration of adjacent fat planes. Inflammation of the omentum or mesentery can be readily appreciated

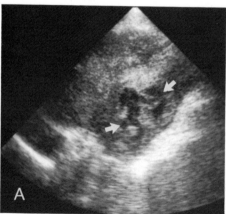
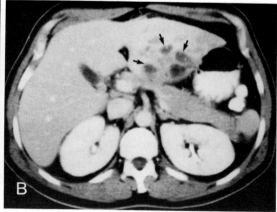

Figure 10.1. Sonographic (**A**) and CT (**B**) appearance of hepatic abscess. A Transverse scan of the left lobe of the liver demonstrating coalescing hypoechoic microabscesses in the lateral segment (*arrows*). Corresponding CT demonstrates well-defined hypodense lesion in the lateral segment of the left lobe. Bacteroides microabscesses were confirmed via ultrasound-guided needle aspiration.

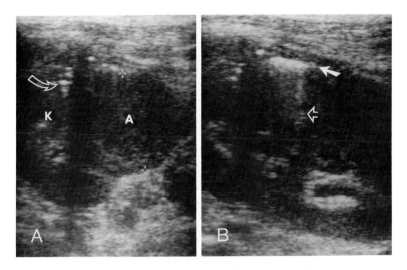

Figure 10.2. Isoechoic renal abscess with gas forming subcapsular extension. **A,** sagittal sonogram of the left kidney demonstrates an isoechoic renal abscess (*A*) between cursors. *K* = kidney. Linear high-amplitude echoes are noted (*curved arrow*) representing gas in the subcapsular and perinephric space. **B,** Sagittal sonogram in same patient demonstrating the high-amplitude echoes in the subcapsular region (*arrow*) representing gas. Note ring down artifact from the gas (*open arrow*). (Reproduced with permission from Jeffrey RB Jr: *CT and Sonography of the Acute Abdomen.* New York, Raven Press, 1989.)

by CT as the density of the normal fat (−80 to −10 HU) is elevated to near water density −10 to +10 HU). In addition, CT can clearly identify adjacent fascial thickening that is rarely, if ever, appreciated sonographically.

Gas bubbles within abdominal abscesses on occasion may be difficult to identify with sonography, but are readily identified with CT. Prominent air-fluid levels present in abscesses with enteric fistulas may entirely pre-

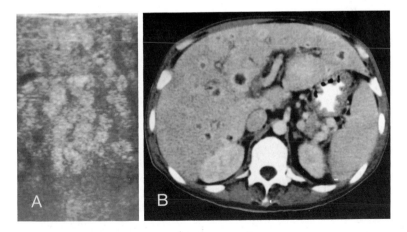

Figure 10.3. Hyperechoic hepatic cryptococcal abscesses. **A,** transverse sonogram of the left lobe of the liver demonstrating innumerable rounded echogenic foci representing cryptococcal microabscesses. Corresponding CT (**B**), demonstrates relatively few of the lesions, which appear as focal low-density areas with enhancing rims. Patient had AIDS and cryptococcal hepatic microabscesses. (Reproduced with permission from Jeffrey RB Jr: *CT and Sonography of the Acute Abdomen,* New York, Raven Press, 1989.)

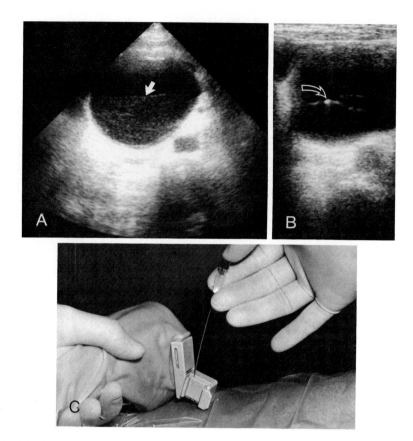

Figure 10.4. Infected pancreatic pseudocyst diagnosed by sonographically guided needle aspiration. **A,** Transverse sonogram of head of the pancreas demonstrating a large pseudocyst containing a fluid debris level (*arrow*). **B,** Using sonographic guidance, a fine-needle aspiration was performed (*arrow = needle tip*). Notice that in order to sample the viscous debris within the abscess, the needle must be inserted at least to the fluid debris interface. **C,** Simulated ultrasound fine-needle aspiration. The needle is placed through a sidearm attachment that permits constant sonographic monitoring of the needle insertion. (Reproduced with permission from Jeffrey RB Jr: *CT and Sonography of the Acute Abdomen,* New York, Raven Press, 1989.)

clude sonographic imaging of the abscess (Fig. 10.6).

Choice of Imaging Modality

Plain chest and abdominal radiographs should be performed in the initial evaluation of all patients with clinically suspected abdominal abscesses. Abdominal radiographs may show obvious ectopic gas, abnormal calcifications such as an appendicolith, or other compelling findings that may greatly expedite the clinical evaluation. In many patients with abscesses, however, plain abdominal radiographs are nonspecific and provide insufficient information for precise abscess localization or guided drainage.

CT and sonography are the imaging methods of choice for diagnosis and guided drainage of the vast majority of abdominal abscesses. The choice between these two modalities varies from institution to institution depending upon availability, expertise, and clinical philosophy. In general, suspected right upper quadrant or pelvic abscesses can readily be demonstrated by sonography. CT is clearly superior in demonstrating extraperitoneal abscesses such as pancreatic, renal, and psoas abscesses. Ab-

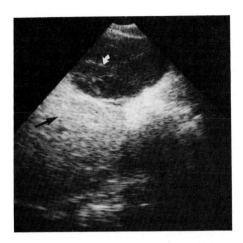

Figure 10.5. Solid mass mimicking complex fluid collection. Patient presented with fever and right upper quadrant pain. Sagittal sonogram of the liver demonstrates a well-defined hypoechoic lesion with internal septations (*curved arrow*) and enhanced through sound transmission (*black arrow*). Diagnostic needle aspiration revealed hepatic lymphoma.

Accuracy of Diagnosis

Although statistics vary from institution to institution, in general, CT is slightly more accurate for detection of intraabdominal abscesses than sonography, largely because of the poor sensitivity of sonography in detecting abscesses in the gastrointestinal tract and the retroperitoneum. The greatest accuracy of imaging is only achieved with an aggressive approach to diagnostic needle aspiration. CT can detect approximately 90% to 95% of all abdominal abscesses when combined with diagnostic needle aspiration (8–10).

PERCUTANEOUS ABSCESS DRAINAGE

Patient Selection

The majority of abdominal abscesses are appropriate for percutaneous drainage

scesses related to gastrointestinal perforations such as periappendiceal, diverticular, or perirectal abscesses are similarly best imaged with CT (Fig. 10.6).

One of the main advantages of sonography is that both real-time imaging and guided percutaneous drainage can be performed at the bedside of critically ill patients (16). In general, these are patients in the intensive care unit with relatively large and superficial abscesses that have no intervening bowel or vascular structures to preclude catheter insertion.

Intravenous contrast enhancement is essential for accurate abscess detection with CT. Sonography, on the other hand, requires no potentially nephrotoxic contrast media and can be readily performed in patients with renal insufficiency or frank renal failure. Postoperative patients, however, with open wounds and surgical drains are often best imaged with CT. This is particularly true if there are no localizing signs of an abscess in the right upper quadrant pelvis. Open wounds and surgical drains may limit transducer skin contact with and preclude a complete sonographic examination.

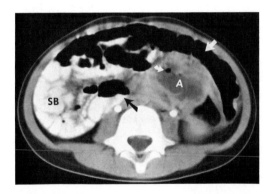

Figure 10.6. False-negative sonogram for diagnosis of left-sided periappendiceal abscess readily demonstrated by CT. Abdominal sonography (not shown) failed to identify an abdominal abscess. Contrast CT demonstrates a well-defined low-density abscess (*A*) with a gas bubble (*curved white arrow*). Note overlying transverse colon (*white arrow*) that precluded sonographic imaging. There was nonrotation of the small bowel (*SB*) with a midline cecum (*black arrow*). Left lower quadrant abscess was secondary to appendiceal perforation. (Reproduced with permission from Barakos JA, Jeffrey RB Jr., Federle MP, Wing VW, Laing FC:. CT in the management of periappendiceal abscess. *AJR* 146:1161–1164, 1986, © American Rutgers Ray Society.)

(17–19). Even when percutaneous drainage fails, it is often a useful temporizing measure to improve the patient's overall clinical condition prior to semielective surgical drainage (20). Criteria for patient selection vary, but in general there are four major contraindications to percutaneous drainage: 1) lack of a safe access route for catheter insertion due to overlying bowel, adjacent vascular structures, or pleural space; 2) poorly defined and extensive abscesses with multicompartmental involvement; 3) infected pancreatic necrosis with predominantly necrotic solid tissue; and 4) major bleeding diasthesis or coagulopathy (19, 20). With few exceptions, amebic abscesses are treated with antibiotics and not referred for percutaneous drainage.

CT is often critical in determining a safe access route for catheter insertion. This is particularly true of intraperitoneal or interloop abscesses surrounded by bowel. (Fig. 10.7) Sonography is often unreliable in depicting the exact anatomic relationship of these abscesses to the gastrointestinal tract. In selected patients, contrast CT may also define to better advantage major vascular structures to be avoided by catheter insertion. Duplex sonography, particularly with color flow, may greatly enhance sonographic visualization of adjacent vasculature.

Extensive, poorly defined abscesses that involve multiple anatomic compartments are often best treated surgically. The only exception to this is in patients who are poor operative candidates. There are a growing number of reports of successful percutaneous drainage of infected pancreatic pseudocysts and fluid collections (21). However, patients with infected pancreatic necrosis, in general, are best treated with aggressive surgical debridement. The necrotic tissue and pancreatic debris that accompany such abscesses can often not be drained via a cathe-

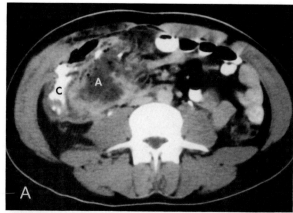

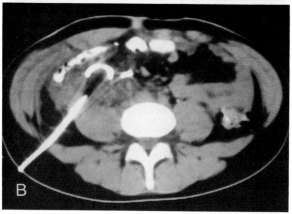

Figure 10.7. CT guidance for periappendiceal abscess adjacent to bowel. **A,** Contrast-enhanced scan demonstrating a periappendiceal abscess (*A*) with adjacent cecum (*C*). Using CT guidance, a safe access for catheter insertion was identified in a position posterior and lateral to the abscess. **B,** Following catheter insertion the abscess has been completely evacuated.

ter. The overall morbidity and mortality of infected pancreatic necrosis, however, has been reduced by an aggressive approach with CT-guided needle aspiration for early detection of pancreatic infection. (22).

The decision to perform percutaneous abscess drainage must always be made in close consultation with the referring physician, the surgeon, the interventional radiologist, and the patient. The potential risks and possible complications must be understood by all involved. The responsibility for catheter management and clinical follow-up must be clearly defined and the potential benefits of percutaneous drainage should be carefully outlined to the patient.

Patient Preparation

An abdominal abscess detected by CT or sonography is first confirmed by diagnostic needle aspiration and immediate Gram stain. Based on the anatomic site and the imaging characteristics, the abscess is analyzed with respect to safety of catheter insertion and likelihood of success. If the abscess appears appropriate for percutaneous drainage, then the referring clinician, surgical service, and the patient are consulted with regard to the feasibility of this technique. If percutaneous drainage is to be performed, specific complications such as bacteremia and hemorrhage are discussed and informed consent is obtained. The patient is then given appropriate broad-spectrum intravenous antibiotics. Antibiotics should always be administered prior to catheter insertion or any manipulation of the abscess cavity in order to minimize bacteremia.

Although it would be ideal to have recent coagulation studies confirming normal clotting factors and platelets, in the majority of patients undergoing percutaneous drainage this is not mandatory unless there is a clinical suspicion of a coagulopathy or a known bleeding diasthesis during prior surgery.

Techniques with CT and Sonography

A variety of techniques may be utilized for guided percutaneous drainage. In patients in the intensive care unit, the procedure may be performed entirely with portable real-time sonographic guidance (Fig. 10.8 and 10.9). In other patients, percutaneous abscess drainage can be performed solely under CT guidance using digital scout radiographs to guide tract dilation and catheter insertion (Fig. 10.10). And in some patients, a combined approach with imaging and fluoroscopy is frequently useful. The abscess is first identified with sonography or CT and then confirmed with fine-needle aspiration. The abscess cavity is then punctured and a guidewire is coiled in the abscess. Initial CT puncture will require patient transfer. However, using ultrasound in the interventional suite, tract dilation and catheter insertion may be monitored fluoroscopically. Immediately following abscess evacuation, real-time portable sonography is used to determine any residual collections of pus necessitating insertion of a second catheter (23). (Fig. 10–11).

No single method of percutaneous drainage is appropriate for all abscesses. Of the last 152 abdominal abscesses drained percutaneously at San Francisco General Hospital, 112 were drained entirely under CT guidance. Twenty-four were performed with a combination of imaging and fluoroscopy and six patients underwent drainage with portable sonography in the intensive care unit. Many experienced observers advocate direct trocar catheter insertion under CT guidance for relatively superficial abscesses. Alternatively, a Seldinger technique can be utilized that involves a guidewire exchange method. With this technique, the abscess cavity is punctured with a needle or a sheath needle and then an angiographic guidewire (.035 or .038 inch) is coiled within the abscess cavity. It is essential to use a floppy tipped J-shaped wire in order to avoid perforation of the abscess cavity. When slight resistance is encountered on insertion of the guidewire, fluoroscopy is used to determine catheter position. A PA and/or lateral digital scout radiograph can be performed to confirm coiling of the guidewire within the abscess cavity. If there is any question of the guidewire's location, a single axial CT scan can be obtained. When the distance from the abdominal wall to the abscess cavity has been precisely calculated,

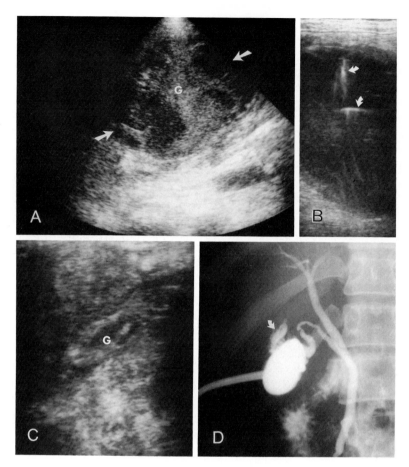

Figure 10.8. Sonographically guided percutaneous drainage of staphylococcal empyema of the gallbladder. Because of sepsis and hypotension, the procedure was performed at the patient's bedside. **A,** Sagittal sonogram of a markedly distended gallbladder (G) containing mixed hyper- and hypoechoic pus (*arrows*). **B,** Under sonographic guidance, the gallbladder was punctured with an 18-gauge needle and a guidewire was coiled in the gallbladder (*arrows*). A 12-F sump catheter was then inserted into the gallbladder and the pus was evacuated. **C,** Immediately following the aspiration, the gallbladder has been completely decompressed; G = gallbladder. **D,** 5 days later, a cholangiogram was performed that demonstrates contrast extravasation (*arrow*) from the gall-bladder from a perforation. The patient made an uneventful recovery following successful percutaneous drainage.

the tract can then be dilated over the guidewire and an appropriate drainage catheter inserted.

One of the main advantages of total CT guidance of percutaneous drainage is that after evacuation of the abscess, scans can be performed to quickly ascertain whether the entire contents of the abscess have been evacuated. In many patients with apparent multiseptated abscesses, a single catheter will suffice to drain all the various locules of the abscess (Fig. 10.12). This is because the

locules actually intercommunicate, though this may not be readily apparent on cross-sectional imaging with CT or ultrasound.

One of the chief disadvantages of exclusive use of CT in guiding percutaneous drainages is that the tract dilatation and catheter insertion are relatively blind. In some instances, buckling of the guidewire by fascial dilators or actual abscess cavity perforation may not be readily appreciated. However, with experience, total CT drainage offers a number of important advan-

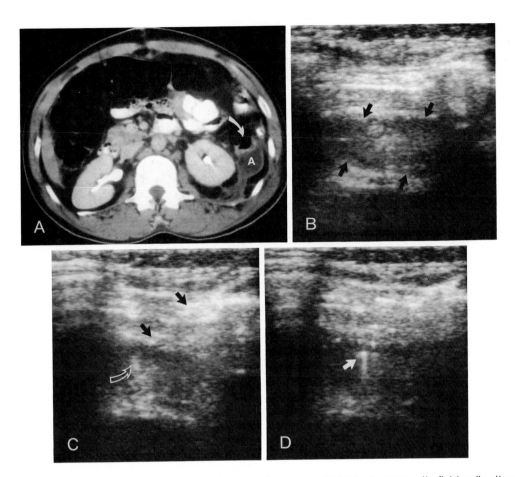

Figure 10.9. Sonographic guided percutaneous drainage of infected pancreatic fluid collections at the bedside. Patient was septic and had adult respiratory distress syndrome. **A,** Preliminary CT done 2 days previously demonstrates a possible left anterior pararenal space abscess (**A**) posterior to the left descending colon (*curved arrow*). Because of the patient's respiratory status, it was decided to undergo percutaneous drainage at the bedside. **B,** Coronal sonogram of the left anterior pararenal space demonstrates a hypoechoic abscess (arrows). **C,** Under real-time sonographic monitoring, an 18-gauge needle was inserted into the abscess cavity. (*Closed arrows* = Needle shaft, *curved arrow* = needle tip). **D,** A guidewire was then inserted into the abscess cavity (*arrow*). The abscess resolved with percutaneous drainage alone.

tages in critically ill patients. Perhaps the chief value is that patients with multiple life-support systems do not need to be transported to the interventional suite for catheter insertion and then back to CT for repeat scans to determine the adequacy of abscess evacuation.

Sonography may be utilized alone to guide percutaneous drainage at the bedside in critically ill patients or combined with fluoroscopy in the interventional suite. McGahan reported successful sonographically

guided abscess aspiration or catheter drainage at the bedside in 12 patients (16). Although the exact spatial relationship of the catheter and guidewire may be difficult to appreciate, the specular reflection from both catheter and guidewire can be visualized within the abscess cavity with sonography. (Figs. 10.8 and 10.9). Immediately after evacuation of the abscess cavity, real-time sonography should be performed to assess the adequacy of the drainage. Using real-time sonography to monitor percutaneous

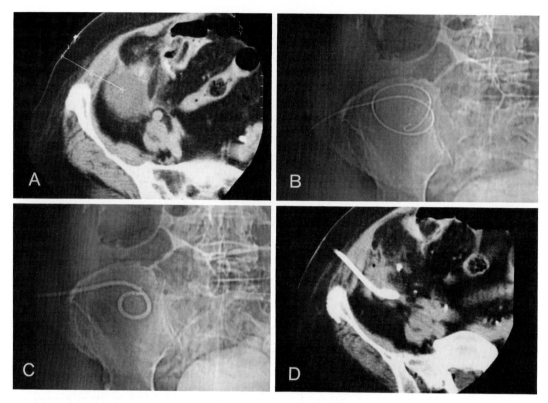

Figure 10.10. Digital scout radiograph monitoring a CT-guided abscess drainage. **A,** CT precisely identifies the appropriate site of catheter insertion and measures the distance required for diagnostic needle aspiration. **B,** Following puncture of the abscess cavity and insertion of a guidewire, a digital scout radiograph confirms that the wire is coiled within the abscess cavity. **C,** Digital radiograph identifying the final catheter position. **D,** Axial scan obtained immediately after evacuation of the abscess cavity demonstrating no residual pus.

drainage in 50 patients, Jeffrey and co-workers noted residual pus in five patients, requiring insertion of a second catheter (23).

Catheter Selection

To date there have been no randomized prospective studies that clearly identify the superiority of one type of percutaneous drainage catheter to any other. The most frequently used percutaneous catheters range in size from 8 to 16 French (Fig. 10.13). Although double lumen sump catheters have been advocated by some authorities as being highly effective for percutaneous drainage, this has not been proven to have any specific advantages over single lumen drainage catheters such as a nephrostomy pigtail catheter.

The choice of catheter selection for percutaneous drainage should be based on the size of the abscess, the viscocity of the fluid, and the presence of continuous drainage or fistula to the abscess cavity. In general, small abscesses (3–5 cm in maximal diameter) are readily drained via nephrostomy or angiographic pigtail catheters. Larger abscesses with viscous fluid are often best evacuated with double lumen sump catheters, particularly if there is extensive debris or a likely enteric fistula. These include periappendiceal or peridiverticular abscesses or infected pancreatic fluid collections that frequently have communications to the main pancreatic duct.

Retention loop devices are often of considerable value in securing the catheter within the abscess cavity. They are particu-

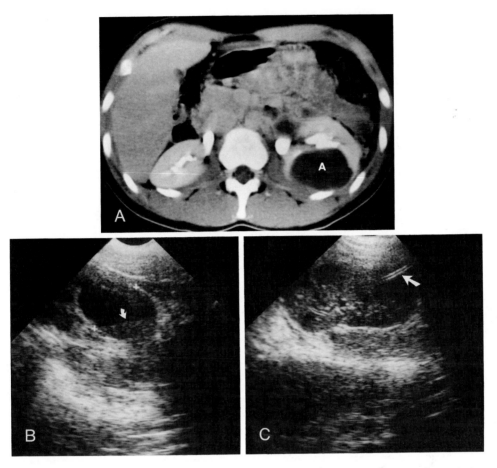

Figure 10.11. Real-time sonographic monitoring of renal abscess drainage. **A,** Left renal abscess (*A*) was identified on contrast CT. The patient was then transferred to the interventional suite. **B,** Sagittal sonogram of the left kidney demonstrates the abscess with a fluid debris level (*curved arrow*). **C,** Following catheter insertion and evacuation of the pus, real-time sonography demonstrates no residual evidence of the abscess; *arrow* = percutaneous drainage catheter.

larly helpful if patients are to be discharged with a draining catheter in place to return for outpatient sinography of the abscess cavity.

Success of Guided Percutaneous Drainage of Abdominal Abscesses

In the largest clinical series to date, van Sonnenberg reported a success rate of 209 in 250 patients (83.6%) undergoing percutaneous drainage (18). A lower success rate is encountered in pancreatic and splenic abscesses as well as in extensive multilocular abscesses. In analyzing the reasons for failure of percutaneous drainage, Lang and colleagues emphasized technical errors (premature catheter withdrawal and inappropriate approach to the abscess) as common causes of difficulty (24). Because of the lower morbidity and expense compared to surgery, percutaneous abscess drainage should be attempted first in all abdominal abscesses unless there is a major contraindication.

CT and Sonography in Follow-up

Success of percutaneous catheter drainage is determined by both clinical and laboratory response. There is often decreased pain and normalization of temperature and blood cell count. In patients successfully treated with

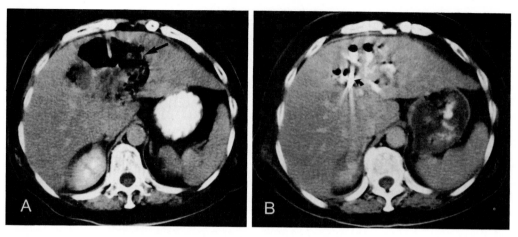

Figure 10.12. Multiseptated appearing abscess (*arrow*) drained with a single catheter under CT guidance. **A**, CT demonstrates a gas-forming abscess in the left lobe of the liver. The abscess has a complex, multiseptated appearance. **B**, 3 days following percutaneous drainage, a CT abscessogram was performed by injecting dilute water-soluble contrast into the abscess drainage catheter (*curved arrow*). Note that all the locules of the abscess intercommunicate. The abscess resolved with percutaneous drainage alone. (Reproduced with permission from Jeffrey RB Jr: *CT and Sonography of the Acute Abdomen,* New York, Raven Press, In Press.)

percutaneous techniques, it is often not necessary to perform a repeat CT or sonogram after the initial procedure merely to document resolution of the abscess cavity. This is often best performed with fluoroscopically controlled abscess sinography. Abscess sinography is useful not only in positioning the drainage catheter optimally within the abscess cavity but in demonstrating any fistulous communications (25, 26). In patients

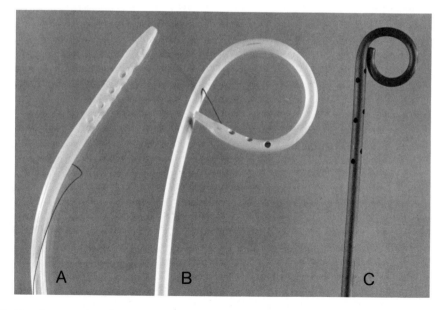

Figure 10.13. Commonly utilized percutaneous drainage catheters. **A**, 12-F double lumen sump catheter (retention loop is optional). **B**, 10-F nephrostomy pigtail catheter with retention loop. **C**, 8-F angiographic pigtail catheter.

with pancreatic, enteric or biliary fistulas, often the nature and volume of the drainage fluid changes 48 to 72 hours after percutaneous drainage. In some patients, occult fistulas may not be demonstrable until 1 or 2 weeks after the drainage catheter has been in place. The demonstration of a fistula is important not only for subsequent catheter management but to clarify the etiology of the underlying abscess.

In general, low-output fistulas pose no problems in clinical management and will often close with a combination of percutaneous drainage and antibiotic therapy alone (26). Jeffrey and colleagues reported a 45% incidence of fistulas to the appendiceal stump or cecum following percutaneous drainage of periappendiceal abscesses. All fistulas closed within 2 weeks of percutaneous drainage. Patients were discharged with a draining catheter in place following adequate, clinical and laboratory response, acute percutaneous drainage and antibiotics (27). Similar low-output fistulas to the colon and small bowel may also be successfully treated if the underlying bowel is normal. Pancreatic fistulas and fistulas in patients with Crohn disease are notoriously difficult to manage and may require weeks to months for the fistula to close spontaneously. Abscess sinography is essential in documenting the anatomic site of fistulous communication, so catheter sideholes can be positioned in close proximity to the fistula for optimal drainage. Tomographic techniques such as CT and sonography have little value in demonstrating fistulous communication.

The main value of CT and sonography following percutaneous drainage is in patients who demonstrate an initial poor clinical response. These patients are often persistently febrile 72 hours after percutaneous drainage and have continued leukocytosis. CT or sonography may demonstrate significant undrained locules of pus not appreciated at the initial procedure or unsuspected complications due to gastrointestinal perforation or hemorrhage. It is essential to perform repeat imaging as well as an abscessogram in patients who fail to respond initially to percutaneous drainage.

Catheter Management and Patient Follow-Up

There have been few scientifically controlled studies attempting to examine critically specific methods of catheter management following percutaneous abscess drainage. To date, much of the experience in this area has largely been derived through anecdotal trial and error attempting to emulate prior time-tested surgical procedures. However, the technique of percutaneous drainage of abdominal abscess differs in several important respects from open surgical drainage. With a percutaneous approach, dependent drainage is not mandatory, nor is the preference of an extraperitoneal approach to intraperitoneal abscesses. (19). Thus, it is hazardous merely to extrapolate from prior surgical experience with open drainage when formulating techniques for catheter management. Important considerations in catheter management include: 1) immediate and subsequent catheter irrigation; 2) the role of abscess sinography; 3) the parameters that determine the success or failure of percutaneous drainage; 4) management of the abscess-fistula complex; and 5) the timing of catheter withdrawal.

Many respected interventional radiologists have advocated careful, yet copious irrigation of the abscess cavity immediately after catheter insertion, based largely on their surgical experience with operative abscess drainage (19). Following evacuation of pus, the abscess cavity is irrigated with small aliquots of sterile saline until the aspirated return is clear and all the internal debris has been evacuated. To date, there has not been a controlled study demonstrating any clear advantage of immediate catheter irrigation. Indeed, there is a potential theoretical disadvantage of immediate catheter irrigation in that, unlike open surgical drainage, irrigation occurs within a closed space and can induce bacteremia. This may be of particular concern for the patient who has received only a single bolus of intravenous antibiotics prior to percutaneous abscess drainage of a visceral abscess such as a liver abscess immediately adjacent to parenchymal vascular structures. Again, there are no scientific data to substantiate or refute the claim that immediate irrigation of the abscess cavity is of any clinical benefit. My own bias is not to perform vigorous irrigation immediately after catheter insertion. After aspiration of all the pus, the catheter is simply placed in a reasonably dependent position within the abscess cavity. The abscess cavity is immediately imaged with repeat CT or portable real-time sonography to determine if all the pus has been drained. If there are significant undrained locules of pus, a second catheter is immediately inserted. If significant debris is noted within the abscess cavity at 48 to 72 hours, a larger catheter may be required as well as gentle saline irrigation. By this time, however, the patient has tissue levels of appropriate antibiotics, thus reducing the risk of bacteremia.

Immediately after percutaneous drainage, the patient's vital signs should be monitored carefully with specific orders to identify any episode of hypotension, tachycardia, or spiking fevers. In approximately 2% to 3% of patients undergoing percutaneous abscess drainage, significant bacteremia and/ or septicemia may occur immediately after the drainage procedure (18). The initial management of bacteremia and/or septicemia includes: 1) intravenous bolus of broad-spectrum antibiotics that are appropriate for the Gram stain of the abscess fluid or the presumed etiology of the abscess, and 2) rapid infusion of intravenous fluids. As with all invasive procedures, patient monitoring by nurses in the radiology department is of considerable clinical value in the early identification of problems and in their subsequent management. The clinical team must be consulted as soon as possible to monitor the patient carefully on the ward or, if appropriate, in the intensive care unit.

Optimal catheter management includes careful daily follow-up by the interventional radiologist. The patency of the catheter should be established by flushing the catheter on the ward once or twice a day to ensure patency. In my experience, if management of the catheter is left solely to nonradiologic colleagues or nursing staff who are not experienced in the management of such catheters, problems frequently arise. There is no substitute for the direct interview with the patient about symptoms and for personal management of the catheter at the bedside to assure that the drainage system is adequate or that the catheter is patent. For simple drainage catheters, a small volume (5–10 cc) is often sufficient to determine catheter patency. With typical sump catheters, it is very useful to do a simultaneous injection of the sideport while aspirating through the suction lumen of the catheter. Stopcocks on percutaneous catheters should be avoided as they are often inadvertently turned off by well-meaning but misinformed ancillary personnel.

Although many patients demonstrate a prompt response to percutaneous drainage, it is important to emphasize to other clinical colleagues that it may take up to 72 hours for some patients to demonstrate a significant clinical response. Unless there is clinical deterioration (hypotension, profound septicemia), surgery should not be performed in stable patients until adequate time has elapsed in order to ascertain the success of percutaneous drainage. In patients who are persistently febrile 72 hours after percutaneous drainage, repeat imaging of the abscess cavity is mandatory with CT or sonography to exclude an undrained locule of pus. In addition, a fluroscopically controlled abscess sinogram is essential to determine the adequacy of catheter position within the abscess cavity or to identify an unsuspected fistula tract. At 72 hours, the patient should have an improved sense of well-being with decreased abdominal pain, decreased fever and leukocytosis. However, percutaneous drainage should not be abandoned if at this point the patient is still mildly febrile. Often the situation can be remedied by inserting a second percutaneous catheter or simply repositioning the existing catheter.

Management of abscesses with underlying enteric or pancreatic fistulas is significantly more complex than that of other abdominal abscesses. Abscesses with fistulas often require prolonged drainage and multiple catheter exchanges. In general, the prognosis depends on the volume of the output and the etiology of the fistula. Most low-output enteric fistulas (less than 50 ml/day) will generally resolve with a combination of percutaneous drainage and antibiotic therapy alone. A typical example is percutaneous drainage of a periappendiceal abscess. Cecal fistulas are noted in approximately 45% of patients undergoing percutaneous drainage for periappendiceal abscess (27). However, the fistulas are nearly always low-output and resolve within a 2-week period (27). Patients with a fistula can be discharged with a draining catheter in place following normalization of temperature and white count and can be followed on an outpatient basis with repeat abscess sinography. Again, the catheter should not be withdrawn until sinography demonstrates that the fistula has closed.

Perhaps the most difficult of all fistulas to manage are those to the pancreatic duct. These are often high in output (over 200 ml/day) and may not close if there is proximal obstruction to the duct. Management of the fistula-abscess cavity relationship is best controlled with abscess sinography. In general, with high-output pancreatic fistulas, larger (12–14 F) sump catheters are preferred. The sideholes of the catheter should be positioned in close proximity to the site of the fistula. Hyperalimentation is extremely useful to decrease the volume of pancreatic secretions and maintain nutrition. Some pancreatic fistulas will not close despite adequate percutaneous catheter positioning and can only be cured by distal pancreatectomy and resection of the perforated portion of the duct.

In patients with fistulas, withdrawal of the percutaneous catheter is determined by a combination of both clinical and laboratory response as well as of imaging findings. The catheter should not be withdrawn as long as the patient is febrile, demonstrates leukocytosis, or has a significant residual abscess cavity identified on sinography. The catheter should be slowly withdrawn when the abscess cavity has been obliterated on sinography and no underlying fistula is present.

REFERENCES

1. Gronwall S, Gammelgaard J, Haubek A, Holm HH: Drainage of abdominal abscesses guided by sonography. *AJR* 138: 527–529, 1982.

2. Altemeier WA, Culbertson WR, Fullen WP, Shook CD: Intraabdominal abscess. *Am J Surg* 125:70–79, 1973.

3. Fry DE, Garrison RN, Heitsch RC, Calhoun K, Polk HC: Determinants of death in patients with intraabdominal abscesses. *Surgery* 1980; 88:507–523.

4. Jeffrey RB Jr, Federle MP, Laing FC: Computed tomography of silent abdominal abscesses. *J Comput Assist Tomogr* 1984; 8:67–70.

5. Callen PW: Computer tomographic evaluation of abdominal and pelvic abscesses. *Radiology* 1978; 131:171–175.

6. Koehler PR, Moss AA: Diagnosis of intraabdominal and pelvic abscesses by computerized tomography. *JAMA* 1980; 244:49–52.

7. Wolverson MK, Jagannadharao B, Sundaram M et al.: CT as a primary diagnostic method in evaluating intraabdominal abscess. *AJR* 133:1089–1096, 1979.

8. Korobkin M, Callen PW, Filly RA et al.: Comparison of computer tomography, ultrasonography and gallium-67 scanning in the evaluation of suspected abdominal abscesses. *Radiology* 1978; 129: 89–93.

9. Haaga JR, Alfidi RJ, Havrella TR et al.: CT detection and aspiration of abdominal abscesses. *AJR* 128: 465– ,1977.

10. Aronberg DJ, Stanley RJ, Levitt et al.: Evaluation of abdominal abscess with computed tomography. *J Comput Assist Tomogr.* 2:384–387, 1978.

11. Chiu LC, Shapiro RL, Yiu VS: Abdominal abscess. Computed tomographic appearance, differential diagnosis and pitfalls in diagnosis. *J Comput Assist Tomogr* 1978; 2:195–209.

12. Newlin N, Silver TM, Stuck KJ, Sandler MA: Ultrasonic features of pyogenic liver abscesses. *Radiology* 1981; 139:155–159.

13. Kressel HY, Filly RA: Ultrasonographic appearance of gas-containing abscesses in the abdomen. *AJR* 130:71–73, 1978.

14. Kuligowska E, Conners SK, Shapiro JH: Liver abscess: Sonography in diagnosis and treatment. *AJR* 138:253–257, 1982.

15. Subramanyam BR, Balthazar EJ, Raghavendra BN, Horii SC, Hilton S, Naidich DP: Ultrasound analysis of solid-appearing abscesses. *Radiology* 1983; 146:487–491.

16. McGahan JP: Aspiration and drainage procedures in the intensive care unit: Percutaneous sonographic guidance. *Radiology* 1985; 154:531–532.

17. Van Sonnenberg E, Mueller RP, Ferrucci JT Jr: Percutaneous drainage of abdominal abscesses and fluid collections. Techniques, results and applications. *Radiology* 1982;142:1–10.

18. Van Sonnenberg E, Mueller PR, Ferrucci JT Jr: Percutaneous drainage of 250 abdominal abscesses and fluid collections. Part I: Results, failures and complications. *Radiology* 1984; 151:337–341.

19. Mueller PR, Van Sonnenberg E, Ferrucci JT Jr: Percutaneous drainage of 250 abdominal abscesses and fluid collections. Part II: Current procedural concepts. *Radiology* 151:343–347, 1984.

20. Van Sonnenberg E, Wing VW, Casola G et al.: Serious complications following transgression of the pleural space in drainage procedures. *Radiology* 152:335–341, 1984.

21. Freeny PC, Lewis GP, Traverso LW, Ryan JA: Infected pancreatic fluid collections: percutaneous catheter drainage. *Radiology* 167:435–441, 1988.
22. Jeffrey RB Jr, Grendell JH, Federle MP, et al.: Improved survival with early CT diagnosis of pancreatic abscess. *Gastrointest Radiol* 162:331–336, 1987.
23. Jeffrey RB Jr, Wing VW, Laing FC: Real-time sonographic monitoring of percutaneous abscess drainage. *AJR* 144:469–470, 1985.
24. Lang EK, Springer RM, Glorioso LW III, Cammarata CA: Abdominal abscess drainage under radiologic guidance: Causes of failure. *Radiology* 1986; 159:329–336.
25. Kerlan RK Jr, Pogany AC, Jeffrey RB Jr, et al.: Radiologic management of abdominal abscesses. *AJR* 144:145–149, 1985.
26. Kerlan RK Jr, Jeffrey RB Jr, Pogany AC, Ring EJ: Abdominal abscess with low output fistulae: Successful percutaneous drainage. *Radiology* 1985; 155:73–75.
27. Jeffrey RB Jr, Tolentino CS, Federle MP, Laing FC: Percutaneous drainage of periappendiceal abscesses: Review of 20 patients. *AJR* 149:59–62, 1987.

11 Hepatobiliary Techniques

PETER L. COOPERBERG
ANDOU CORET
SERGIO AJZEN

Introduction

In the clinical evaluation of hepatobiliary disease, the clinician has a limited range of findings to aid in diagnosis of specific abnormalities in the liver and biliary tree. The history and physical examination in this area are relatively crude techniques. Biochemical liver function tests are notoriously nonspecific, and there is considerable overlap between different diagnoses. The newer imaging techniques have made a considerable impact on the diagnosis of both focal and diffuse diseases in the liver and in the evaluation of obstructive versus nonobstructive jaundice as well as on the ability to differentiate the cause of obstructive jaundice. However, it is the ability of these imaging studies to guide needle and catheter placement for cytologic aspiration and therapeutic drainage that has made the most impact in the diagnosis and management of hepatobiliary disease.

In this chapter, we will discuss the use of ultrasound to guide fine-needle aspiration in the liver, both for fluid collection and for obtaining cytologic material from solid lesions. Sonography can be useful to guide core biopsies of the liver, and both cysts and abscesses in the liver can be drained percutaneously under sonographic guidance (1–4). Percutaneous transhepatic cholangiography is not a new technique and does not usually require sonographic guidance. However, sonography can aid in the traditional right-sided approach for PTC as well as guidance for the approach to the left hepatic ducts (5, 12). In addition, ultrasound can be used intraoperatively both to diagnose small lesions within the liver, guide subsegmental hepatic resection and in the identification of common bile duct stones (6–11).

FNAB

All of the newer cross-sectional imaging techniques are useful in evaluating the hepatic parenchyma for the presence of focal abnormalities. Real-time ultrasound is particularly valuable for identifying focal areas of inhomogeneity within the liver parenchyma. Yet, in most cases, the appearance of focal lesions is nonspecific and requires further evaluation to make a definitive diagnosis. It is recognized that cysts can usually be easily differentiated from solid lesions. Once a structure is identified as a cyst, there usually is no benefit in further analysis of the fluid within the cyst. Most cysts are asymptomatic and do not require further investigation. Occasionally, an arteriovenous fistula or malformation will mimic a cyst. If there is a clinical suspicion, Doppler scanning may be helpful. If the patient has clinical findings suggestive of an abscess, it is more important to aspirate the fluid. However, abscesses and hematomas generally have echogenic fluid and are easily differentiated from the echo-free fluid of simple cysts.

Solid lesions in the liver may have a wide range of appearances. They may be echo-poor, echogenic, or isoechoic and identified only by their surrounding halo. They may present with a combination of these appearances. Lesions in the liver may be suspected in the patient with known primary malignancy, by the palpation of a nodule or nodules, or may be unsuspected clinically. In most cases of hepatic metastases, the patient will admit to recent weight loss.

In most situations, where one or more focal solid lesions are identified within the liver, it is difficult to be specific about their nature. Even if the patient has a known primary, this does not mean that the lesion in the liver is a secondary from that primary. It could be a second primary, a secondary from a different primary, or even an incidental hemangioma unrelated to the malignant lesion. It therefore becomes important to make a specific diagnosis by identifying the cells within the lesion. Fortunately, many pathologists have developed great expertise in cytological interpretation and diagnosis of malignancy from the aspirated material. Even when there is a strong clinical suspicion of liver metastases, clinicians still place greater confidence in a pathology report than in a radiology report. With greater confidence in sonographic and computed tomographic diagnoses, this is becoming less so, but usually the clinician wants the "final" pathological diagnosis.

It is important to point out that only malignant lesions can be identified cytologically. There are no identifying features of cells obtained from benign lesions in the liver. Furthermore, if no malignant cells are seen in the aspirate, there is no certitude that the needle tip was within the lesion. And even if the tip of the needle was definitely seen within the lesion, it is possible that the sample was not adequate. Therefore, it is only worthwhile to aspirate the lesions that are more likely malignant. If the lesion has the typical sonographic features of a hemangioma, especially in the asymptomatic patient without weight loss, a fine-needle aspiration biopsy can be a frustrating technique, since no malignant cells can be expected.

Benign Lesions

There are four main benign lesions in the liver: regenerative nodules, focal nodular hyperplasia, hepatoadenoma, and hemangioma. They may be clinically suspected because of a palpable mass, pain caused by hemorrhage, or more commonly are detected at the time of sonographic or CT examination. If these diagnoses are suspected, a fine-needle aspiration biopsy is not worth performing. The aspirate will only contain relatively normal hepatic cells. Furthermore, in the case of hepatoadenoma, there is the possibility of hemorrhage, either spontaneous or caused by the fine-needle aspiration. In special circumstances, there may be a benefit to a fine-needle aspiration to reinforce a strong clinical suspicion of a benign lesion by the lack of malignant cells.

Hemangiomas represent a major problem with the newer imaging techniques. These studies tend to detect hemangiomas with great frequency, especially in the large number of patients who are referred for possible gallbladder disease or other vague upper abdominal problems. Finding a focal lesion within the liver always causes concern. If the lesion is relatively small, very echogenic and well-defined, especially in the asymptomatic person without weight loss, we do not recommend any further procedure. If the lesion is large enough (over 2.5 cm), we recommend a blood pool scan with technetium-99-labeled red blood cells. Dynamic CT scans or magnetic resonance imaging can also be used to confirm the diagnosis of a hemangioma. However, hemangiomas may have an atypical appearance. With experience, we are even able to suggest the appropriate diagnosis in these atypical cases. Again, this is especially true if the patient is asymptomatic without weight loss. Rarely, if the patient has a known primary, or occasionally, with atypically occurring hemangiomas, a fine-needle aspiration may be necessary. If malignant cells are obtained, the diagnosis of hemangioma will be proven wrong. Although the lack of identifying malignant cells, especially if the needle tip is definitely within the lesion, is suggestive, it is not completely diagnostic of a hemangioma. (13) Fears of possible hemorrhage from fine-needle aspiration of hemangiomas have been shown to be unfounded (14).

Malignant Lesions

It is, of course, the malignant lesion in the liver that is most amenable to confirmation and further characterization by fine-needle aspiration. Frequently, there is a known primary with histological material already available from previous surgery. In these situations, it is easy to compare the cytological material with the previous specimen. In other situations, the patient presents with liver lesions and the cytological examination provides the only material available. Usually, the cytological examination identifies the cells as malignant. This identification is easiest if the cells are very poorly differentiated. However, the tissue of origin of the poorly differentiated malignancy cannot usually be determined. Conversely, if the malignancy is well differentiated, it can be easier to determine the tissue of origin and the cell type, but may be more difficult to identify the lesion as malignant.

It is frequently possible to identify and differentiate hepatocellular carcinoma from other malignancies. Pigment granules may be seen within the cells and the malignant cells resemble hepatocytes. Sonographic examination may help define the lesion as primary by noting the invasion of the portal or hepatic veins.

Cholangiocarcinomas, on the other hand, are more difficult to diagnose by fine-needle aspiration cytology. This is due to the desmoplastic reaction with considerable fibrosis and a relatively small number of relatively well-differentiated malignant cells. These lesions are more easily biopsied under fluoroscopic guidance following a transhepatic catheter placement or by transcatheter brushings (15).

Ultrasound Technique

When focal lesions are identified in the liver on an ultrasound examination, the referring physician should be contacted to obtain approval for the fine-needle aspiration biopsy (FNAB) while the patient is still on the examining table. We now have blanket permission from many of our referring clinicians to do a biopsy if we feel it is indicated. The reason for the biopsy, the procedure itself, and the absence of any significant risks are explained to the patient and a signed consent is obtained. We do fine-needle aspirations on outpatients without any special arrangements. We feel fasting is not routinely needed for FNAB. If the patient has no history of bleeding problems and is not on medication that can prolong bleeding, we do not obtain coagulation studies.

We choose the simplest method possible to guide the biopsy, considering the size, depth, and movement of the lesion. The easiest technique is indirect ultrasound guidance as explained in Chapter 1. A skin puncture site is chosen by ultrasound that allows the needle to be inserted vertically, since this is the easiest direction to reproduce. If necessary, it is possible to angle the needle in either the craniocaudal or mediolateral direction. If angulation is required in both planes, it is helpful to have an assistant at the foot of the stretcher to confirm that the appropriate needle angulation is being used. It is important to appreciate the depth of the lesion from the skin surface. However, the transducer compresses the subcutaneous tissue more than the needle does, so that the measured depth may be underestimated by as much as 2 to 4 cm. The motion of the lesion during respiration is noted, especially if it is excessive. The puncture site is marked by applying pressure with a fingernail, a drinking straw, or the hub of a needle. With the memory technique, it is most important for the operator to imagine the lesion in its location relative to the skin and to superficial landmarks. Handing the materials to the operator to avoid a break in concentration is helpful.

If the lesion is small, deep, or moves excessively with respiration, it is preferable to visualize the needle with real-time scanning as it is advanced into the lesion (Figs. 11.1–11.3). This is easily accomplished using the freehand method. To optimize needle visualization, two positions are important. One is for the transducer and the other for the needle entrance site. It is important to visualize the needle entrance site and the lesion in the same plane of section. Thus, the length of the needle will be within the plane of section. Furthermore, it is important that the needle passes approximately perpendicularly to the ultrasound beam in the central vectors of the plane of section (Fig. 11.1). Nonetheless, usually only the tip of the needle can be visualized by its artifact, and only while it moves in and out along its longitudinal axis. It is also easier for the person holding the needle to watch the screen for best hand-eye coordination (Fig. 11.2). It is much more difficult to identify the echo of the needle tip if someone else is moving it. If the needle is seen to enter the lesion, all is well (Fig. 11.3). If the needle is seen in the plane of section, but away from the lesion, it is easiest to direct the needle towards the transducer, or away from the transducer. It is more difficult to change the position of the needle if it is out of the plane of section. In this situation, the plane of section must be moved to find the needle tip, and then back to the lesion again. Then it is easy to determine whether the position of the needle should be shifted cranially or caudally. It is only by the back-and-

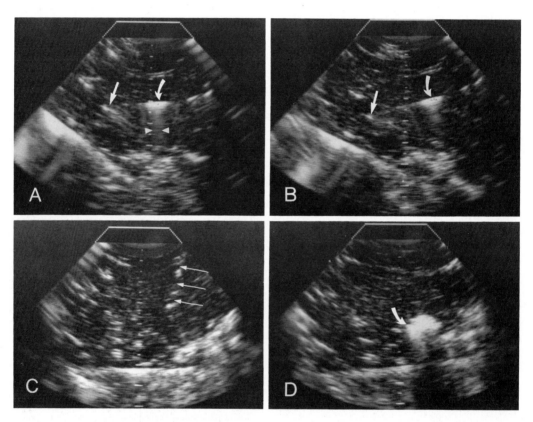

Figure 11.1. Sonographic visualization of the needle in liver specimen. **A,** The needle is horizontal. Note the artifact from the tip of the needle (*arrow*). The portion of the needle perpendicular to the beam is also visible (*curved arrow*). Note the ring down artifact (*arrow heads*) coming from the portion of the shaft of the needle perpendicular to the ultrasound beam. **B,** The same needle is slightly off the perpendicular and oblique. Note the artifacts from the tip of the needle (*arrow*). The visible portion of the needle shaft is now further away from the tip of the needle, but is still perpendicular to the beam (*curved arrow*). **C,** The needle (*arrows*) is almost parallel to the ultrasound beam (as in many practical situations, and in this case, using a biopsy guide). Note that there are only a few isolated echoes from the shaft of the needle and a stronger echo from the tip of the needle. **D,** An echogenic area after gas has been expressed from the tip of the needle in **C** (*curved arrow*).

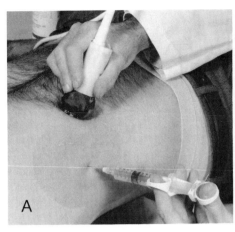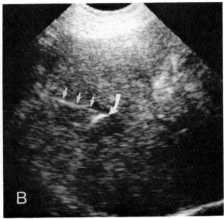

Figure 11.2. **A,** Biopsy of a liver lesion in an ambulatory patient, showing the transducer anteriorly and subcostally in a transverse plane of section with the spinal needle on the control syringe entering the liver from a right lateral lower intercostal approach. **B,** Real-time sonographic visualization of the needle (*arrows*) with its tip (*curved arrow*) in a liver metastasis.

forth motion of the plane of the section that the relative position of the needle to the lesion can be appreciated.

There are numerous other techniques employed for identifying the needle. Some people use a linear-array transducer. However, a large window on the skin surface is needed. Some use the parallel approach with the linear-array transducer whereas others aim the transducer perpendicular to the plane of the needle. Biopsy guides are available to direct the needle appropriately. The use of these biopsy guides is explained in detail in chapter one and elsewhere throughout this text (Figs. 11.4 and 11.5).

Fine-needle aspiration biopsies are treated very much like any routine intramuscular injection. Masks are not worn unless the patient is severely immunosuppressed. The skin is prepped with topical antiseptic but not draped. Usually no local anesthetic is necessary, except if the patient requests it or if the

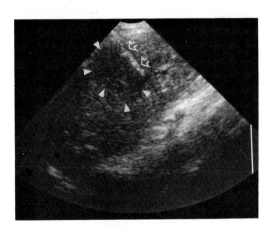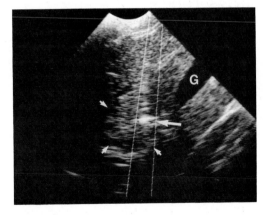

Figure 11.3. Biopsy: freehand method. Hypoechoic lesions (*arrowheads*) in the left lobe of the liver is biopsied using the freehand technique with the entire shaft of the roughened Teflon-coated needle visualized (*open arrows*).

Figure 11.4. Biopsy: needle-guidance system. Using a needle biopsy guidance system, a 22-gauge needle is placed in between the electronic calipers into a focal hepatic mass (*small arrows*). The artifact from the needle tip is well identified (*long arrow*) (G = gallbladder).

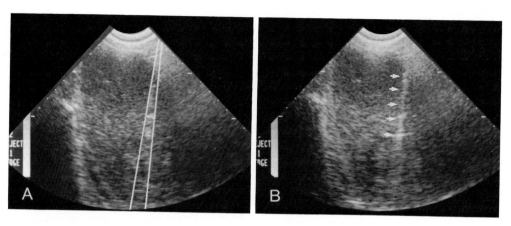

Figure 11.5. Hepatoma-needle guidance system. **A,** Electronic grid lines are used for guidance of a 22-gauge Chiba needle. **B,** After removal of these grid lines, the needle is well identified (*arrows*). Biopsy confirmed hepatoma.

biopsy is likely to be technically difficult. However, in most cases, the injection of local anesthetic is more painful than the single needle pass usually required for a positive FNAB (16, 17).

We usually use a 22-gauge 9-cm length spinal needle. These are stiff enough so that they go in the appropriate direction and can be advanced through the skin even after the stylet has been removed and the needle has been attached to the syringe. If the longer length of a Chiba needle is required, it is more difficult to advance through the skin and one cannot control the direction as easily. Others (18–20) have reported using larger needles to obtain more cytological material. Fortunately, our cytologists do not seem to require the larger needles. When the architecture of the tissue sample is needed, a core biopsy needle is used.

Although any syringe can be used, we prefer the 10-cc Luer Lok control syringe with finger rings that facilitate one-handed aspiration (Fig. 11.2). Alternatively, an ordinary syringe can be fitted into an aspiration gun for a one-handed operation. When the tip of the needle is in the lesion, 5 to 10 cc of suction are applied and the tip of the needle is moved in and out 1 to 3 cm several times. It is important to avoid aspirating blood into the syringe, because this makes the cytological examination more difficult, so the suction is released before needle withdrawal.

The entire needle aspiration should take only a few seconds.

It is preferable to have the cytopathology technician in the room to prepare the slides immediately. These can be fixed and stained for determination of diagnostic adequacy while the patient is still in the department. If necessary, repeat aspirations can be performed. Alternatively, if there is confidence that material will be easily obtained, the aspirate can be expressed into a vial of saline solution for centrifugation so that a cell block can be prepared for subsequent diagnosis.

In our experience, immediate cytological examination after each fine-needle pass limited the number of passes required for positive diagnosis. The diagnosis was made in the first pass in 69% of cases, after two passes in another 18%, and after three passes in 8%. In only 5% of cases were four or more punctures required (16). Ferrucci and co-workers reported similar results (19).

Outpatients are released immediately and inpatients return promptly to the ward. The referring physician is contacted immediately with the preliminary biopsy results for outpatients, and the preliminary results are recorded in the charts of inpatients.

CT Guidance

An alternative imaging guidance procedure is computed tomography. This technique is used widely in many institutions, especially where ultrasound expertise is lacking. Although it does definitively show the needle tip in the lesion, CT demonstrates where the needle has been placed rather than guides one into the lesion. For the most part, CT is a more cumbersome technique than real-time sonographic guidance. Furthermore, there is more demand on CT scanner time. Usually, fine-needle biopsies can be just as successfully obtained by sonographic guidance (21). We use CT whenever the lesion cannot be seen on ultrasound, but size of lesion is not a criterion for using one technique or the other. In fact, we (17) as well as Reading and colleagues (20) have found it preferable to guide FNAB for small lesions with real-time sonographic guidance.

Rarely, MRI may be necessary to guide fine-needle aspiration biopsy if this is the only technique that shows the lesion (22). Occasionally, fluoroscopy can be used to guide needle aspiration biopsy in the biliary tree, but only if there is a catheter in the biliary tree so that it can be delineated with contrast material.

Results

Our previous results on all upper abdominal biopsies show a sensitivity (percentage of patients with malignancy who had positive FNAB) of 87% and specificity (percentage of patients without malignancy who had a negative biopsy) of 100% (17). False-positive diagnosis should be exceedingly rare if ever. Although this can happen in pancreatic lesions, where rarely an inflammatory process can be misdiagnosed as a neuroendocrine tumor, this should not happen in hepatic lesions. The specificity of the technique is therefore a function of the expertise of the cytopathologist.

The sensitivity of the technique depends upon the adequacy of the specimen. A false-negative biopsy can occur under several circumstances. An obvious cause is if the tip of the needle did not pass through the lesion. Occasionally, the tip of the needle is clearly seen within the lesion, but no malignant cells are obtained. This can be a sampling error, but usually means that the tumor is well differentiated or contains considerable fibrosis. In most of our false-negative cases,

the result was predictable. Because of lack of patient cooperation, or technical difficulty in directing the needle through an intercostal space at a particularly high or posterior lesion, we were aware that the tip of the needle was not going into the lesion, but could not accomplish the entry. When the risk of persisting with the procedure outweighs the advantage of the diagnosis, the attempt should be terminated. In fact, these are not really false-negative biopsies, but rather inadequate attempts. On the other hand, with the tip of the needle clearly within the lesion, the false-negative rate for liver lesions is exceedingly low.

Complications

There have been some exaggerated concerns over the potential hazards of fine-needle aspiration. Although elsewhere in the abdomen the needle frequently traverses bowel or spleen, this does not occur in the aspiration of liver lesions.

Livraghi and co-workers reviewed 11,700 FNABs and found only one related death (18). This was in a pancreatic biopsy. In a series of 63,000 patients by Smith, there were three deaths from hemorrhage and one from pancreatitis (23). We have been made aware recently of a death following fine-needle aspiration biopsy of a metastatic carcinoid tumor in which there was profound shock that did not respond to resuscitation (24). The mortality rate previously reported for liver biopsies up to 1950 was as high as 0.12%, but this relates primarily to blind core biopsies with much larger needles (25).

Minor complications that may occur after FNAB are hemorrhage and bile leak. We had one patient who developed severe right upper quadrant pain and shortness of breath following a fine-needle aspiration. There was no evidence of any abnormal fluid collection around the liver or pneumothorax on chest x-ray. Another patient did have a pneumothorax following needle aspiration from the anterior approach towards a more posterosuperiorly situated lesion. Numerous patients have been operated on following fine-needle aspiration biopsy procedures. Rarely, a delayed hemorrhage may occur (26).

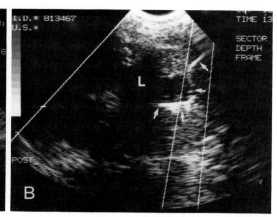

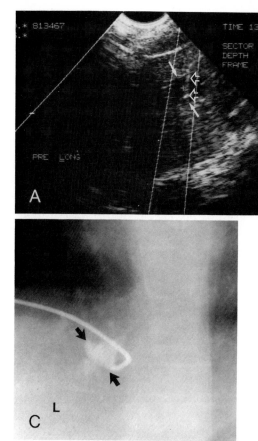

Figure 11.6 Drainage of infected biloma on a 1-year-old child with a liver transplant. A, Sonogram shows a well-circumscribed fluid collection (1 cm in diameter) in left lobe (*arrows*). A roughened Teflon-coated needle (*open arrows*) is placed into infected biloma. B, Sonogram shows a 0.018-inch guidewire (*arrows*) passing through the 22-gauge needle and coiling within the fluid collection (*L* = liver). C, Using a modified Seldinger technique, a 5 French catheter was placed under fluoroscopic control. Injection of contrast material outlines biloma cavity (*arrows*). (Reproduced with permission from McGahan JP, Anderson MW, Walter JP: Portable real-time sonographic and needle guidance systems for aspiration and drainage. *AJR* 147:1241–1246, 1986. ©American Roentgen Ray Society.)

Although there is a theoretical risk of spreading tumor cells around the needle tract (23), disease to the liver already, further tracking should not be a significant problem in those cases. Essentially, 22-gauge needles can be used with impunity.

Contraindication for Fine-Needle Aspiration

There is no absolute contraindication for fine-needle aspiration biopsy of the liver lesion. A known coagulopathy should be corrected before fine-needle aspiration. In a cirrhotic patient with portal hypertension, especially if a coagulopathy is present, the biopsy should be very strongly indicated to justify the risk. Although echinococcal cysts

are considered a contraindication for aspiration because of possible anaphylactic reaction, there are several reports of successful aspiration (42).

CORE BIOPSY

Cutting needles for large-bore core biopsy are still used to diagnose causes of diffuse parenchymal disease of the liver. Real-time sonographic guidance can be helpful, especially if the liver is small, or if there is portal hypertension. Vessels and the gallbladder and porta hepatis can be avoided by guiding cutting needle placement. The recent availability of the Biopty gun with the 18-gauge core needle should make ultrasound guidance the technique of choice, even for diffuse parenchymal disease.

Therapeutic Aspiration of Cysts and Abscesses

Once a cavity has been demonstrated sonographically, and entered with a fine needle it is easy to guide a therapeutic catheter insertion (Figs. 11.6 to 11.8). Either an introduction set with a fine wire through the 22-gauge needle (Fig. 11.6), or, since these fluid collections are fairly large, a one-step procedure with a catheter piggy backed onto a large needle can allow efficient drainage. Although it is clear that pyogenic abscesses require such a drainage (28, 29), there is controversy as to whether an amebic abscess needs drainage or can be treated by antibiotics alone (30). Occasionally, a large hepatic cyst can cause pain, biliary obstruction or respiratory difficulty (31, 32). We have under-

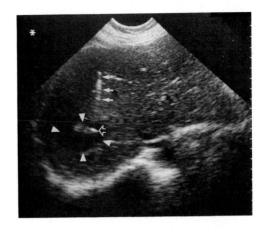

Figure 11.7. Hepatic abscess. Needle (*arrows*) almost parallel to the ultrasound beam with its tip (*open arrow*) in a liver abscess (*arrowheads*). Remainder of the abscess drainage was carried out under fluoroscopic guidance.

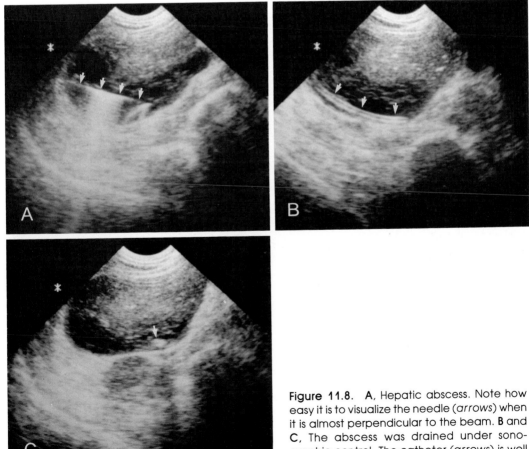

Figure 11.8. **A**, Hepatic abscess. Note how easy it is to visualize the needle (*arrows*) when it is almost perpendicular to the beam. **B** and **C**, The abscess was drained under sonographic control. The catheter (*arrows*) is well visualized in both long (**B**) and short (**C**) axes.

taken therapeutic drainage in a few cases. However, they most commonly recur and eventually require deroofing at surgery.

Percutaneous Transhepatic Cholangiography

Percutaneous transhepatic cholangiography is usually performed under fluoroscopic guidance alone. We have used ultrasound to help plan the procedure, since we find it most useful to know ahead of time whether we can expect dilated or nondilated ducts. It is also helpful to know if the obstruction is high near the bifurcation or lower down, and if there is concomitant ascites, since the catheter can curl in the fluid space between the abdominal wall and the liver. Ultrasound can help assess the level of the needle puncture site above the table top so that it passes horizontally towards the porta hepatis (Fig. 11.9). We have found this particularly valuable in cases with nondilated ducts. We do not actually guide the needle placement with ultrasound during the cholangiogram. Once the planning is completed, the remainder of the technique is performed under fluoroscopic guidance alone.

On the other hand, there are occasional indications for directed transhepatic cholangiograms into specific ducts. Sometimes it is preferable to use the left hepatic duct for

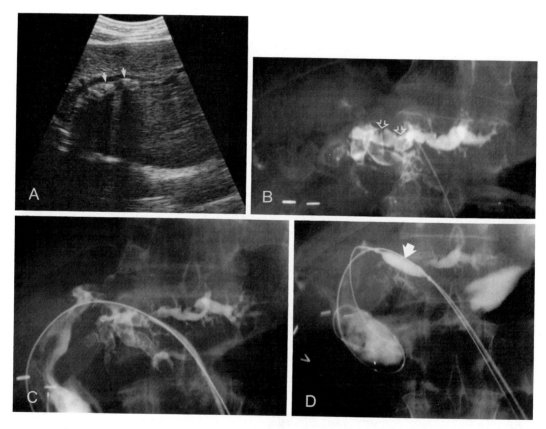

Figure 11.9. Sonographically guided left percutaneous transhepatic cholangiography, drainage and stricture dilatation. **A,** Transverse real-time scan showing several calculi in a left hepatic duct (*arrows*) posterior to a left portal vein. **B,** Radiograph after sonographically guided needle placement into a left hepatic duct containing calculi (*arrows*). **C,** Radiograph showing guide wire through the stone-filled ducts, stenotic portion, and common bile duct. **D,** Balloon catheter (*arrow*) dilating strictured portion in proximal left hepatic duct.

a drainage procedure (5). In this situation, ultrasound is necessary to guide the needle toward the dilated duct. Also, if there are segmentally obstructed ducts, especially those containing calculi, as in recurrent pyogenic cholangitis, it is important to do a directed cholangiogram into the appropriate ducts (Fig. 11.9). A routine nondirected cholangiogram may opacify the noninvolved ducts and miss the diagnosis and opportunity for percutaneous therapy (3, 4). After the appropriate duct has been entered and contrast can be administered, the remainder of the procedure is done most efficiently under fluoroscopic guidance alone. Opacification of the gallbladder can be performed in a similar manner, as explained in Chapter 12 (Fig. 11.10).

Intraoperative Ultrasound: Future Applications

Some recent developments include a report by Makuuchi, of intraoperative ultrasound used not only to identify hepatic lesions, but also to guide injection of the feeding portal vein with a blue dye to indicate on the surface of the liver the limits of the subsegment to be resected (35). Infiltration of the dye around the portal vein also indicated the apex of the segment.

A recent paper has discussed the use of a new device for cryotherapy of hepatic lesions under sonographic guidance. The cryoprobe (36), at present, is too large to be used percutaneously and must be used at operation. Livraghi and colleagues (7–9) and Shiina (40) have described the percutaneous injection of ethanol for the treatment of hepatic neoplasms. They claim these techniques are potentially valuable in the treatment of selected small neoplastic lesions in poor-risk patients. Thus ultrasound guidance may be used for selective therapeutic applications using the percutaneous route for focal application of hepatic neoplasms. This may be performed on an outpatient basis.

Summary

Although imaging techniques have come a long way to aid in the diagnosis of focal lesions in the liver, a great advance has been the ability to guide fine-needle aspiration biopsies for definitive diagnosis. The tech-

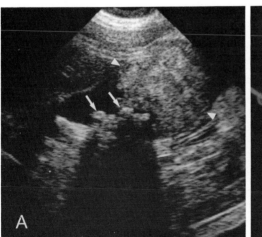
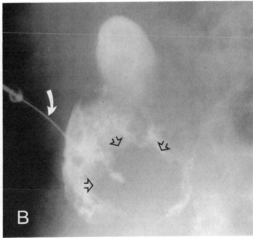

Figure 11.10. Gallbladder carcinoma. **A,** Longitudinal ultrasound demonstrating a large mass (*arrowheads*) within the gallbladder lumen. Note associated cholelithiasis (*arrows*). **B,** Using ultrasound guidance, a biopsy of the mass was performed and then the needle (*curved arrow*) was inserted into the gallbladder lumen with opacification of the gallbladder under fluoroscopic control, demonstrating the mass (*open arrows*) corresponding to carcinoma of the gallbladder.

nique is safe and widely accepted, such that it is almost an integral part of the sonographic examination of the liver. Sonography can also be used in selected situations to help percutaneous transhepatic cholangiography. The possibility of percutaneous therapy of tumors by freezing or alcohol is yet another exciting example of the penetration of interventional ultrasound into the totality of patient care.

REFERENCES

1. Cappell SM: Obstructive jaundice from benign, nonparasitic hepatic cysts: Identification of risk factors and percutaneous aspiration for diagnosis and treatment. *Am J Gastroenterol* 83:93–96, 1988.
2. Yarenchuk MJ, Kane R, Cady B: Ultrasound-guided catheter localization of intrahepatic abscesses—An aid in open surgical drainage. *Surgery* 91(4): 482–484, 1982.
3. Kuligowska, E., Connors, S.K., Shapiro, J.H.: Liver abscess: Sonography in diagnosis and treatment. *AJR*138:253–257,1982.
4. Kimura M, Tsuchiya Y et al.: Ultrasonically guided percutaneous drainage of solitary liver abscess: Successful treatment in four cases. *J Clin Gastroenterol* 3:61–65, 1981.
5. Lameris, JS, Obertop, H, Jeekel J: Biliary drainage by ultrasound-guided puncture of the left hepatic duct. *Clin Radiol* 36, 269–274, 1985.
6. Castaing D, Emond J, et al: Utility of operative ultrasound in the surgical management of liver tumors. *Ann Surg* 204 (5): 600-605, 1986.
7. Bowerman RA, McCracken S et al.: Abdominal and miscellaneous applications of intraoperative ultrasound. *Radiol Clin North Am* 23(1): 107–119, 1985.
8. Chardavoyne R, Kumari-Subhaya S: Comparison of intraoperative ultrasonography and cholangiography in detection of small common bile duct stones. *Ann Surg* 206(1): 53–55, 1987.
9. Rifkin MD, Rosat F, et al.: Intraoperative Ultrasound of the liver, an important adjunctive tool for decision making in the operating room. *Ann Surg* 205(5): 466–472, 1987.
10. Machi J, Isomoto H et al.: Intraoperative ultrasonography in screening for liver metastases from colorectal cancer. Comparative accuracy with traditional procedures. *Surgery*101(6):678–684, 1987.
11. Igawa S, Sakai K, et al.: Intraoperative sonography: Clinical usefulness in liver surgery. *Radiology* 156: 473–478, 1985.
12. Makuuchi M, Bandai Y, et al.: Ultrasonographically guided percutaneous transhepatic bile drainage: A single-step procedure without cholangiography, *Radiology* 136:165–169, 1980.
13. Cronan JJ, Esparza AR, et al.: Cavernous hemangioma of the liver: Role of percutaneous biopsy. *Radiology* 166:135–138, 1988.
14. Solbiati L, Livraghi T, et al.: Fine-needle biopsy of hepatic hemangioma with sonographic guidance. *AJR* 144: 471-474, 1985.
15. Kuroda C, Yoshioka H, et al.: Fine-needle aspiration biopsy via percutaneous transhepatic catheter-

16. Lewis GP, Cooperberg PL: Fine-needle abdominal aspiration. In Sigel B (ed): *Diagnostic Patient Studies in Surgery*. Philadelphia Lea & Febiger, pp 401–412, 1986.
17. Rowley VA, Cooperberg PL: Ultrasound guided biopsy. In vanSonnenberg E (ed): *Clinics in Diagnostic Ultrasound, Interventional Ultrasound*. New York, Churchill Livingstone, pp 59–76, 1987.
18. Livraghi T, Damascelli, et al.: Risk in fine needle abdominal biopsy. *J Clin Ultrasound* 11:77, 1983.
19. Ferrucci, JT, Jr., et al.: Diagnosis of abdominal malignancy by radiologic fine needle aspiration biopsy. *AJR* 134:323, 1980.
20. Reading CC, Charboneau JW, et al.: Sonographically guided percutaneous biopsy of small (3 cm or less) masses. *AJR* 151:189–92, 1988.
21. Limberg B, Hopker WW, Kommerell B: Histologic differential diagnosis of focal liver lesions by ultrasonically guided fine needle biopsy. *Gut* 28: 237–241, 1987.
22. VanSonnenberg E, Hajek P et al.: A wire-sheath system for MR-guided biopsy and drainage: Laboratory studies and experience in 10 patients. *AJR* 151(4):815–817, 1988.
23. Smith EH: The hazards of fine-needle aspiration biopsy. *Ultrasound Med Biol* 10:628–634, 1984.
24. Gibney RG: Vancouver, B.C., personal communication.
25. Terry R: Risks of needle biopsy of the liver. *Br Med J*1:1102–1105, 1952.
26. Yankaskas BC, Stabb EV et al.: Delayed complications from fine-needle biopsies of solid masses of the abdomen. *Invest Radiol* 21:325–328, 1986.
27. Mueller PR, Dawson SL: Hepatic echinococcal cyst: Successful percutaneous drainage. *Radiology* 155: 627–628, 1985.
28. Bernardino ME, Beckman WA, et al.: Percutaneous drainage of multiseptated hepatic abscess. *JCAT* 8(1):38-41, 1984.
29. Johnson RD, Mueller PR, et al.: Percutaneous drainage of pyogenic liver abscesses. *AJR* 144: 463–467, 1985.
30. Berry M., Bazaz R., Bhargava S.: Amebic Liver abscess: Sonographic diagnosis and management. *J Clin Ultrasound* 14:239–242, 1986.
31. Brockman WP, Klapdor R: Palliative punctures in polycystic liver and kidney disease under sonographic monitoring. *Digit Bilddiagn* 5:80–84, 1985.
32. Trinkl W, Sassaris M, Hunter FM: Nonsurgical treatment for symptomatic nonparasitic liver cyst. *Am Gastroenterol* 80(11):907–911, 1988.
33. Gibney RG, Cooperberg PL, Scudamore CH, Nagy AG: Segmental biliary obstruction: False-negative diagnosis with direct cholangiography without US guidance. *Radiology* 164:27–30, 1987.
34. Park JH, Choi BI, et al.: Percutaneous removal of residual intrahepatic stones. *Radiology* 1633: 619–623, 1987.
35. Makuuchi M, Hasegawa H, et al.: Ultrasonically guided subsegmentectomy. *Surg, Gynecol Obstet* 161:346–350, 1985.
36. Ravikumar TS, Kane R, et al.: Hepatic cryosurgery with intraoperative ultrasound monitoring for met-

astatic colon carcinoma. *Arch Surg* 22:403–409, 1987.

37. Livraghi T, Salmi A, et al: Small hepatocellular carcinoma: Percutaneous alcohol injection—results in 23 patients. *Radiology* 168–313–317, 1988.

38. Livraghi T, Sangalli G, Vettori C: Adenomatous hyperplastic nodules in the cirrhotic liver: a therapeutic approach. *Radiology* 170:155–157, 1989.

39. Livraghi T, Festi D, et al.: US-guided percutaneous alcohol injection of small hepatic and abdominal tumors. *Radiology* Nov. 161:309–312, 1986.

40. Shiina S, Yasuda H, et al.: Percutaneous ethanol injection in the treatment of liver neoplasms. *AJR* 149:949–952, Nov. 1987.

41. Buckley J, Scudamore CH, Becker CD, Cooperberg PL: Intraoperative imaging of the biliary tree: Sonography vs. operative cholangiography. *Ultrasound Med* 6(10):589–595, 1987.

42. Buckley J: Vancouver, B.C., personal communication.

12 Gallbladder

JOHN P. McGAHAN

Introduction

Diseases of the gallbladder are a common and disabling problem affecting a large portion of the population of many countries. For instance, in the United States, it is estimated that over one million Americans develop gallstones each year and that upwards of twenty million people have gallbladder disease (1). It is postulated that cholelithiasis occurs in more than 40% of patients over 70 years of age (2). Cholelithiasis may result in acute cholecystitis, gallbladder perforation, choledocholithiasis, and gallstone pancreatitis, and it has been implicated in the development of carcinoma of the gallbladder. Other diseases affecting the gallbladder include acute acalculous cholecystitus, hyperplastic cholecystoses, and metastatic lesions. While many methods have been advocated, cholecystectomy remains the most widely accepted definitive treatment of gallbladder disease. In the United States alone, it is estimated that over one-half million cholecystectomies are performed annually with an estimated cost of well over one billion dollars (3).

Only recently have a number of alternative procedures for treatment of gallbladder disease been developed. Several of these nonsurgical methods use ultrasound guidance. Present methods and future applications of ultrasound-guided invasive gallbladder techniques will be reviewed in this chapter.

GALLBLADDER BIOPSY

The technique for gallbladder biopsy for the diagnosis of malignancy is similar to other percutaneous biopsy procedures. In four cases of gallbladder biopsy presented within the literature, all biopsies were successful for retrieval of tumor cells (4). Primary carcinoma of the gallbladder was diagnosed in three patients and undifferentiated carcinoma was diagnosed in the fourth. Sonography is an excellent method for needle guidance into a gallbladder mass. The lesion is localized by ultrasound. The route is selected, the skin anesthetized, and the needle passed into the gallbladder under sonographic control as in other aspiration-biopsy procedures (Fig. 12.1). Biopsies are performed with a small (20- to 22-gauge) needle, preferably using the transhepatic route with a technique similar to that outlined in Chapter 1. A pathologist is available to check for adequacy of tissue specimen. Cytological staining techniques are as described in Chapter 2. Preoperative knowledge of gallbladder carcinoma may change the surgical management of the patient from a simple cholecystectomy to a cholecystectomy with wedge resection of the liver in an area of possible hepatic invasion (Fig. 12.1).

DIAGNOSTIC CHOLECYSTOGRAPHY

Diagnostic cholecystography for opacification of the biliary system may be performed after failed percutaneous transhepatic cholangiography (PTC), or may be used to better delineate confusing gallbladder or biliary anatomy (Fig. 12.2, 12.3).

Percutaneous ultrasound-guided puncture of the gallbladder has been reported using the transperitoneal route (5). In that

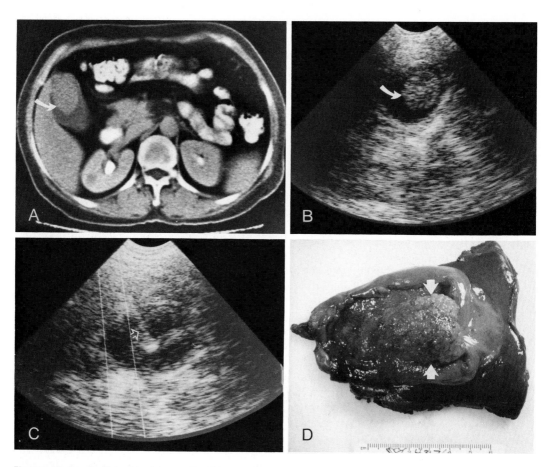

Figure 12.1. Gallbladder biopsy. **A,** CT scan showing well-circumscribed soft tissue mass within the gallbaldder (*curved arrow*). **B,** Ultrasonography demonstrating well-circumscribed echogenic mass originating from the anterior gallbladder wall (*curved arrow*). **C,** Percutaneous biopsy needle (*open arrow*) being passed into the soft tissue mass. Cytology demonstrated carcinoma. **D,** Wedge resection of the liver with opened gallbladder, demonstrating polypoid carcinoma (*arrows*). (Reproduced with permission from McGahan JP, Gerscovich E, Lindfors KK: Gallbladder disease: Perspectives in diagnosis and treatment. *Radiology Report: 171–179, 1989, ©The C.V. Mosby Company.)*

series, five transperitoneal punctures of the gallbladder were performed to opacify the gallbladder and biliary tract immediately prior to surgery. In all five patients, there was mild bile staining of the gallbladder wall and in two patients, there was a bile leakage. The most significant bile leakage occurred in a patient who had obstructive jaundice and in who dilute contrast was injected into the gallbladder. The risk of bile leakage with cholangiography performed through the transperitoneal cholecystic route may be increased in patients with bil-

iary obstruction because of increased biliary ductal pressure. Further risk of bile leakage may increase with use of larger bore needles. If the puncture needle is left in place for long periods of time, there may be considerable movement of the gallbladder with respiratory motion, thus increasing the risk of bile leakage at the puncture site. Therefore, whenever possible, the transhepatic route is selected for any needle placement into the gallbladder. The liver may thus tamponade the gallbladder puncture site to prevent bile leakage. A recent report has

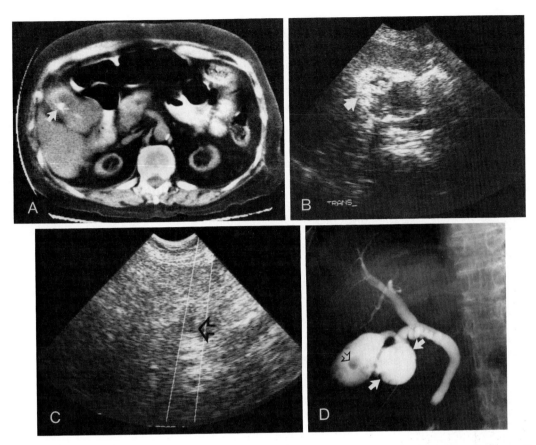

Figure 12.2. Diagnostic cholecystography. **A,** CT scan of the right upper quadrant showing soft tissue mass and calcification in the gallbladder fossa (*arrow*). **B,** Ultrasonography of this region demonstrating gallbladder wall thickening and confusing gallbladder anatomy (*arrow*). **C,** Under ultrasound guidance, a thin needle (*arrow*) was placed transhepatically to the gallbladder fossa. **D,** Injection of contrast under fluoroscopic control demonstrated gallstones (*open arrow*) and a presumed gallbladder diverticula (*arrows*). (Reproduced with permission from McGahan JP, Gerscovich E, Lindfors KK: Gallbladder disease: Perspectives in diagnosis and treatment. *Radiology Report:* 171–179, 1989, © The C.V. Mosby Company.)

demonstrated that in most instances the liver is interposed between the subcutaneous tissue and the gallbladder, making the transhepatic route of access feasible (6). The main risk of gallbladder puncture using the transhepatic route is hepatic hemorrhage. The complication has been reported infrequently and usually only in those with known coagulopathies (7). The risk of hemorrhage is probably minimal using the transhepatic route because only the periphery of the liver is punctured, so only distal and small arteries or veins are potentially traumatized.

Real-time ultrasound combined with fluoroscopy is used for performance of diagnostic cholecystography. The method for ultrasound guided cholecystic cholangiography is similar to other ultrasound-guided aspiration procedures. Fine-needle ultrasound-guided puncture of the gallbladder is performed in the fluoroscopy suite. The gallbladder is opacified under fluoroscopic control to evaluate the gallbladder and/or the bile ducts (Fig. 12.2, 12.3).

When the gallbladder is used as an access, there may be difficulty in opacifying the intrahepatic biliary ducts. As contrast material

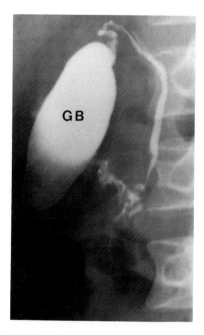

Figure 12.3. Cholangiography performed after gallbladder (*GB*) puncture demonstrates preferential flow of contrast to the common bile duct rather than the intrahepatic ducts in this nonobstructed system. Trendelenburg positioning of the patient may help opacify the intrahepatic ducts.

is injected into the gallbladder, it may flow into the common bile duct rather than the more proximal intrahepatic biliary system (Fig.12.3). Placing the patient in the Trendelenburg position may be of some help in opacifying the intrahepatic bile ducts (4). Fortunately, most ductal obstructions are distal, thus making the procedure adequate for diagnosis. If biliary ductal obstruction is encountered, the puncture needle may be exchanged for a cholecystostomy catheter. This technique will be further explained below.

DIAGNOSTIC ASPIRATION

A recent report has correlated the results of gallbladder bile aspiration and culture with the presence or absence of acute cholecystitis in the hospitalized septic patient (8). The impetus to perform diagnostic aspiration of the gallbladder comes from the difficulty in diagnosing acute cholecystitis,

especially in the hospitalized patient (9). Patients with symptoms of acute cholecystitis are often suffering from pancreatitis, gastroenteritis, or pyelonephritis. Cholescintigraphy and cholesonography are frequently used for confirmation of suspected acute cholecystitis. Cholescintigraphy with ^{99m}Tc-iminodiacetic acid compounds has shown high accuracy in the diagnosis of acute cholecystitis (10). Unfortunately, in patients who have undergone prolonged fasting, received total parenteral nutrition, or who suffer from alcoholic liver disease, radionuclide biliary scans are often falsely positive for cystic duct obstruction (11).

The accuracy of ultrasound in the diagnosis of acute cholecystitis has been reported as quite low in hospitalized patients suffering from acute acalculous cholecystitis (12). Therefore, gallbladder aspiration with Gram stain and culture of the bile was proposed as an aid in diagnosing acute cholecystitis (13). It was postualated that in acute cholecystitis, bacteria and/or white blood cells could be found in the gallbladder aspirate, and the pathogens would be indentified in the bile culture. A positive Gram stain is defined as one in which 1 + bacteria or 1 + white cells are identified. A positive bile culture is defined as one demonstrating at least 1 + bacteriological growth. During a bile aspiration, a 20- to 22-gauge needle is passed transhepatically into the gallbladder under ultrasound control. Although the technique is simple, both the Gram stain of the bile and bile culture suffer from low sensitivity. While the specificities of Gram stains and culture are quite high (87%), the sensitivities of Gram stain and bile culture in predicting acute cholecystitis have been reported to be 48% and 38% respectively (8). Therefore, the shortcoming of this technique is that a negative diagnostic aspiration of the gallbladder bile does not exclude the diagnosis of acute cholecystitis.

In the largest series of ultrasound guided bile aspirations, most of the patients had received high-dose parenteral antibiotics before gallbladder aspiration and this may have rendered the bile cultures sterile (8). Additionally, surgical data suggest that the longer the duration of the acute cholecystitis, the higher the incidence of infected bile (14). It is postulated that the inflammatory response in acute cholecystitis will first occur in the gallbladder wall and only later within the bile itself. Therefore, if the gallbladder bile is aspirated early in the course of acute cholecystitis, the bile may be sterile. Alternatively, Gram stain has some advantages over bile culture in that the results are available immediately, while culture results are not available for 24 to 48 hours. In general, it is felt that bile aspiration from the gallbladder has a limited role in the diagnosis of acute cholecystitis, as a negative gallbladder bile aspirate does not exclude this condition (8).

However, there are certain circumstances in which gallbladder aspirate may be useful; for instance, in cases where purulent material is aspirated from the gallbladder. And in cases in which the gallbladder was surrounded by fluid, if bile is aspirated from the pericholecystic space, gallbladder perforation is indicated (Fig. 12.4). Postcholecystectomy aspiration and/or drainage of fluid from the gallbladder fossa may also be useful. Bile leakage may occur after a difficult cholecystectomy and ultrasound is an excellent method of guiding fluid aspiration and/or drainage (Fig. 12.5).

PERCUTANEOUS CHOLECYSTOSTOMY

Cholecystectomy is the accepted method of treatment of both chronic cholecystitis/cholelithiasis and acute cholecystitis. While elective cholecystectomy for chronic cholecystitis is associated with a low mortality rate (15), there are conflicting reports concerning the management of patients with acute cholecystitis, especially with reference to optimal time for intervention. Some surgeons prefer emergency cholecystectomy, while others advocate delaying cholecystectomy until the patient is less toxic. Emergency cholecystectomy has been shown to have a much higher mortality rate than elective cholecystectomy (16). While figures vary, the mortality rates for emergency cholecystectomy in the elderly are reported to be as high as 19% (17). The high mortality rate in the elderly patient undergoing cholecystectomy most certainly is a reflection of not only the cholecystitis, but the overall medical condition of these patients. Some patients with acute cholecystitis are ex-

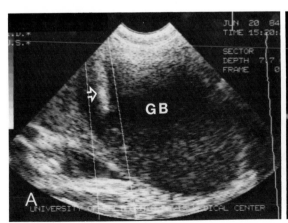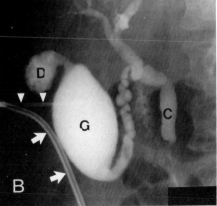

Figure 12.4. Diagnostic aspiration. **A,** A 22-gauge needle (*open arrow*) is inserted between the needle path guide into gallbladder (*GB*) for initial aspiration. Second aspiration demonstrated pericholecystic collection of bile and, therefore, catheters were placed. **B,** Fluoroscopic cholangiogram performed 48 hours later demonstrates one catheter inserted into the pericholecystic space (*arrows*). Cholecystostomy catheter (*arrowheads*) opacifies the gallbladder (*G*), a sealed perforation or diverticulum (*D*), and an otherwise normal biliary system (*C* = common bile duct). (Reproduced with permission from McGahan JP, Walter JP: Diagnostic percutaneous aspiration of the gallbladder. *Radiology* 155:619–622, 1985.)

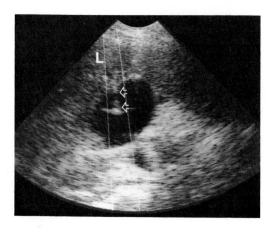

Figure 12.5. Post-cholecystectomy fluid aspiration. A needle (*open arrows*) is placed transhepatically into the gallbladder fossa for aspiration of a well-circumscribed fluid collection in this post cholecystectomy patient (*L* = liver).

tremely ill and, therefore, poor candidates for emergency cholecystectomy. These patients are very difficult to manage. Emergency cholecystostomy has been championed as a life-saving, although temporizing, procedure in the elderly, debilitated, or critically ill patient who presents too great a surgical or anesthesia risk for formal cholecystectomy. Surgical cholecystostomy is a simpler procedure than cholecystectomy and yet it too may be associated with high mortality because of the underlying medical problems in this group of patients (18, 19).

Surgical cholecystostomy may be associated with certain complications. In two separate series analyzing surgical cholecystostomy in high-risk patients, the reported surgical complication rate was 24% (18, 19). In Welch's series (18) of surgical cholecystostomies in an older patient population, 14 of the 59 patients (24%) had nonfatal complications. These included wound infections (six), subphrenic abscess (one) and one patient requiring cholecystectomy for bleeding from the gallbladder bed and one for bile peritonitis. In Jurkovich's review (19) published in 1988, the 24% complication rate included bile leakage after tube removal (one), inadvertent tube removal requiring replacement (four) and bile leakage into the subhepatic space (one). Therefore, some authors have proposed the use of percutaneous cholecystostomy as a safe alternative to

surgical cholecystostomy in the management of patients with acute cholecystitis (4, 20–26).

The literature regarding percutaneous cholecystostomy demonstrates that percutaneous catheter insertion is an effective and safe alternative to surgical cholecystostomy (7). A recent review of major published series of greater than 180 percutaneous cholecystostomies with 120 in patients suspected of having acute cholecystitis, indicates the complications are few. There was one reported death and not including pain as a complication, there were 14 other technical problems or complications (7%) in these 182 patients. Many of these technical problems were due to catheter dislodgment of early models designed without a securing device. There should be fewer problems in the future with the newer catheter designs. Certainly, the low morbidity rate of 7% compares well with the surgical complication rate for cholecystostomy of 24%.

A major advantage of ultrasound-guided cholecystostomy is that the procedure may be performed at the patient's bedside. Thus, critically ill patients need not be moved to surgery or to the radiology department. The catheter should include some type of securing device. One of a number of different catheters are currently in use, the Hawkins accordion catheter may be placed using a coaxial technique after initial puncture with a 22-gauge needle (21, 24–25). This catheter is self-retaining (Fig. 12.6, 21, 25).

The McGahan drainage catheter set has a distal Cope loop to prevent catheter dislodgment (Figs. 12.7 to 12.10, 24). The catheter is easily placed with ultrasound guidance using a transhepatic route. The catheter may be inserted by either the trocar method or guidewire exchange technique. Using the trocar method, the catheter may be placed by one individual. A fairly small-diameter catheter, adequate in size to decompress the inflamed gallbladder, may be easily placed via this method. The catheter fits over a stiffening cannula. A sharp inner stylet is placed within the cannula for insertion via the trocar method. The trocar catheter assembly is advanced transhepatically under ultrasound control into the gallbladder. The catheter is pushed from the cannula (Figs. 12.7 and 12.8). The Cope loop is reformed by tightening the attached string to secure the catheter within the gallbladder lumen.

In the guidewire exchange technique, the initial puncture needle is placed into the gallbladder. A guidewire is then advanced through the needle and coiled within the gallbladder. The needle is then removed and the guidewire is used as an anchor for passage of a dilator to widen the catheter tract. The catheter-cannula assembly is placed over the guidewire into the gallbladder. Once the catheter is within the gallbladder, the guidewire and the inner cannula are removed while the catheter is simultaneously advanced. The distal Cope loop of the catheter is re-formed to prevent catheter dislodgment (Figs. 12.9 and 12.10).

Using modern catheter systems, percutaneous cholecystostomy may be successfully performed with minimal complications. Bile leakage from the percutaneous cholecystostomy tract may be minimized by tamponade of the liver when the transhepatic route is used. Overmanipulation of the gallbladder when using the guidewire exchange technique should be avoided as this can cause life-threatening vagal reactions (27). Using the trocar method and a small-diameter catheter, we have encountered no patients with accompanying vagal reactions or cardiac collapse, even though these patients of-

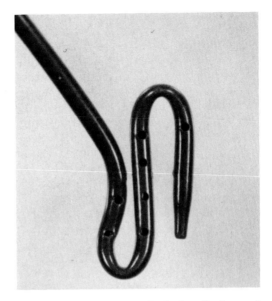

Figure 12.6. Drainage Catheter. Photograph of Hawkins accordion-type catheter that can be used for cholecystostomy. Once the catheter is within the gallbladder, the string is pulled to re-form the "accordion," thus preventing catheter dislodgment.

ten have major cardiac and respiratory problems (7, 24).

The major indication for percutaneous cholecystostomy at our institution is to decompress the acutely inflamed gallbladder prior to surgical cholecystectomy. To our surprise, we have found that percutaneous cholecystostomy is often a definitive treatment for patients with acute acalculous cholecystitis, avoiding the need for surgery. With the increased use of extracorporeal shockwave lithotripsy of the gallbladder, there may be increased need for ultrasound-guided percutaneous cholecystostomy to decompress the gallbladder in cases of mechanical obstruction of the cystic duct from gallstone fragments.

CHOLELITHIASIS: PERCUTANEOUS TREATMENT

A number of percutaneous techniques are currently being used or developed for treatment of cholelithiasis. These include contact stone dissolution, basket removal of cholelithiasis, and fragmentation of stones using percutaneously inserted lasers, ultrasound probes, and electrohydraulic or mechanical devices (28–31). A surgical cholecystostomy is required for mechanical extraction of gallstones. It is doubtful that the percutaneous transhepatic ultrasound-guided cholecystostomy will be used because of the large size of the sheath often needed for mechanical stone extraction. Calculi may then be aspirated, flushed, or removed with forceps or baskets through the sheath (28). Other methods of gallstone fragmentation include electrohydraulic lithotripsy, rotary mechanical devices, ultrasound probes, and laser (29–31). Percutaneous ultrasound-guided cholecystostomy may be utilized in these procedures, depending on the size of the instruments that will be used for access to the gallbladder.

At present, several agents, including methyltertiary-butyl ether (MTBE) have proven effective in contact dissolution of cholesterol gallstones. MTBE has been shown to be a more effective agent than other cholesterol agents such as mon-octanoin in contact dissolution of cholesterol gallstones (32–36). Usually, small catheters are placed into the gallbladder for stone dissolution. Stones may be dissolved with MTBE therapy within hours. Gentle agitation of MTBE causes more rapid stone dissolution, probably due to increased surface contact of the agent with the stone. The catheter may be placed using the combined sonographic-fluoroscopic method with the catheter in direct contact with the stones. MTBE is infused by hand or by a pump system for delivery of small aliquots of solvent, which are aspirated during each cycle. Balloons are placed in the cystic duct to block the flow of MTBE from the gallbladder and reduce parenteral absorption that may cause patient sedation. Other potential adverse effects of MTBE therapy include transient pain, hemolysis, and MTBE's propensity to dissolve certain catheter materials (36).

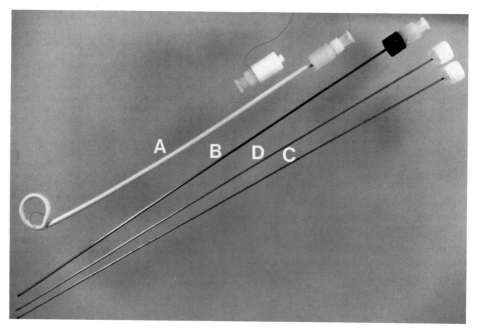

Figure 12.7. Drainage catheter. The McGahan drainage catheter is composed of four components, including a 25-cm long pigtail catheter with a Cope loop (**A**), a cannula (**B**), and an inner blunted obturator (**C**) used to straighten the catheter. Once the catheter and cannula are assembled together, the inner blunted obturator is removed and replaced with a sharp inner stylet (**D**) so that the catheter may be inserted via the trocar method. (Reproduced with permission from McGahan JP: A new catheter design for percutaneous cholecystostomy. *Radiology* 166:49–52, 1988.)

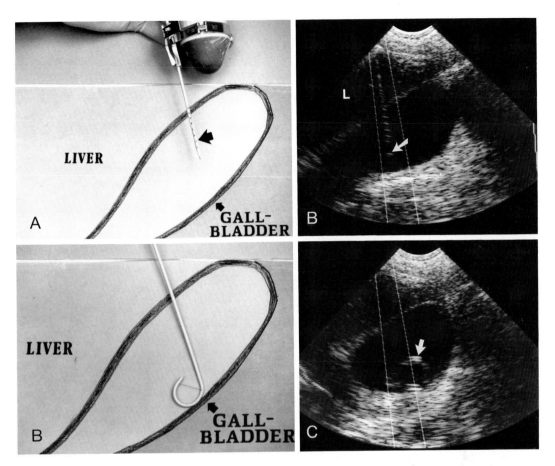

Figure 12.8. Cholecystostomy-trocar method. **A, B,** With sonographic guidance, a cholecystostomy catheter (*arrow*) is placed transhepatically via the trocar method into the gallbladder. *L* = liver. **C, D,** Once in the gallbladder, the stylet and the cannula are removed while the catheter is simultaneously advanced into the gallbaldder and the distal loop in the catheter (*arrow*) is reformed.

MTBE is not currently approved for marketing. Other solvents are being tested for dissolution of noncholesterol stones and combined therapy, such as contact stone dissolution and extracorporeal shockwave lithotripsy, is being used for treatment of gallstones.

Ultrasound-guided entry into the gallbladder may be useful for additional applications, such as percutaneous gallbladder ablation. Chemical cholecystectomy involves cystic duct occlusion (37), combined with transcatheter sclerosis of the gallbladder (38). This technique may be used in the future in patients too ill to undergo a surgical cholecystectomy.

In summary, ultrasound may be used to guide a number of percutaneous invasive gallbladder procedures including gallbladder biopsy, diagnostic cholecystography, and percutaneous cholecystostomy. Ultrasound may be used to guide catheter placement into the gallbladder for contact stone dissolution. Percutaneous ultrasound-guided techniques may be used to access the gallbladder for future applications including gallstone fragmentation and gallbladder ablation.

ACKNOWLEDGMENTS

Special thanks to Lou McHugh, Karen Anderson, and Edie Johnson for preparation of this chapter.

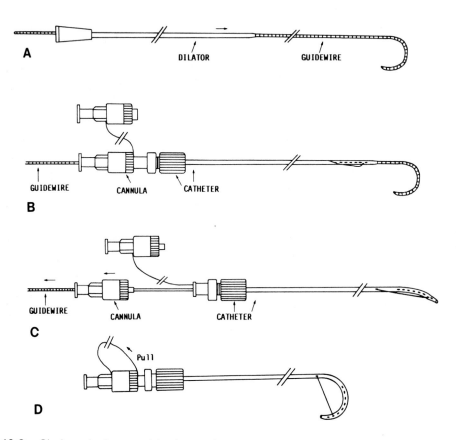

Figure 12.9. Cholecystostomy-guidewire exchange technique. **A,** After needle insertion and placement of a guidewire, a dilator is placed over the guidewire. **B,** The catheter/cannula assembly is then placed over the guidewire into the gallbladder. **C,** Once the catheter is in the gallbladder, the guidewire and inner cannula are removed while the catheter is simultaneously advanced. **D,** The Cope loop of the catheter is re-formed to prevent catheter dislodgment.

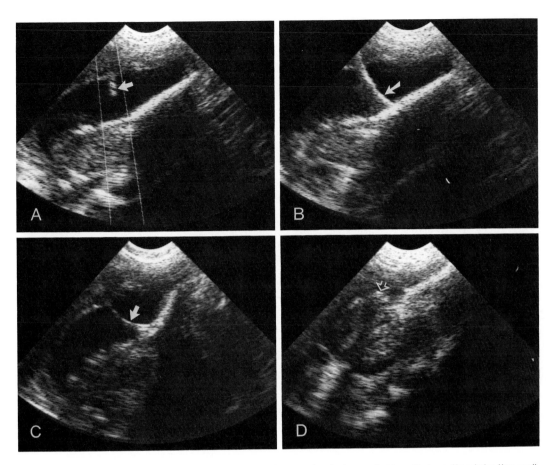

Figure 12.10. Cholecystostomy guidewire exchange technique. **A**, Needle insertion into the gallbladder (*arrow*). **B**, A guidewire is inserted and the dilator (*arrow*) is placed over the guidewire. **C**, Once the catheter/cannula is within the gallbladder, the guidewire and inner cannula are removed while the catheter is advanced (*arrow*). **D**, After complete aspiration of the gallbladder, only the echogenic catheter is visualized (*open arrow*).

REFERENCES

1. Schoenfield LJ, Lachin JM: Chenodiol (chenodeoxycholic acid) for dissolution of gallstones: the National Cooperative Gallstone Study. *Ann Intern Med* 95:257–282, 1981.
2. Glenn F, Dillon LD: Developing trends in acute cholecystitis and choledocholithiasis. *Surg Gynecol Obstet* 151:528–532, 1980.
3. Ranofsky AL: *Surgical Operations in Short-stay Hospitals: 1975.* Hyattsville, MD: National Center for Health Statistics, 1978 (Vital and Health Statistics, series 13, no. 34, DHEW; publication number PHS 78-1785).
4. VanSonnenberg E, Wittich GR, Casola G. Princenthal RA, Hofmann AF, Keightley A, Wing VW: Diagnostic and therapeutic percutaneous gallbladder procedures. *Radiology* 160:23–26, 1986.
5. Phillips G, Bank S, Kumari-Subaiya S, Kurtz LM: Percutaneous ultrasound-guided puncture of the gallbladder (PUPG). *Radiology* 145:769–772, 1982.
6. Warren LP, Kadir S, Dunnick NR: Percutaneous cholecystostomy: Anatomic considerations. *Radiology* 168:615–616, 1988.
7. McGahan JP, Lindfors KK: Percutaneous cholecystostomy: An alternative to surgical cholecystostomy for acute cholecystitis. *Radiology* 173:1989.
8. McGahan JP, Lindfors K: Acute cholecystitis: diagnostic accuracy of percutaneous aspiration of the gallbladder. *Radiology* 167:669–671, 1988.
9. McGahan JP, Gerscovich E, Lindfors KK: Gallbladder disease: Perspectives in diagnosis and treatment. *Radiology Report* 1:171–179, 1989.
10. Weissmann HS, Frank MS, Bernstein LH, Freeman LM: Rapid and accurate diagnosis of acute cholecystitis with 99mTc-HIDA cholescintigraphy. *AJR* 132:523–528, 1979.
11. Shuman WP, Gibbs P, Rudd TG, Mack LA: PIPIDA scintigraphy for cholecystitis: False positives in alcoholism and total parenteral nutrition. *AJR* 138:1–5, 1982.
12. Colletti PM, Ralls PW: Acute cholecystitis: An ultrasound diagnosis. In McGahan JP (ed): *Contro-*

versies in Ultrasound. New York, Churchill Livingstone, 1987, pp 77–97.

13. McGahan JP, Walter JP: Diagnostic percutaneous aspiration of the gallbladder. *Radiology* 155: 619–622, 1985.

14. Delikaris PG, Michail PO, Klonis GD, Haritopoulos NC, Golematis BC, Dreiling DA: Biliary bacteriology based on intraoperative bile cultures. *Am J Gastroenterol* 68:51–55, 1977.

15. Lewis RT, Allan CM, Goodall RG et al.: The conduct of cholecystectomy: incision, drainage, bacteriology and postoperative complications. *Can J Surg* 25:304–307, 1982.

16. Schwartz SI: Gallbladder and extrahepatic biliary system. In Schwartz SI, Shires GT, Spencer FC, Storer EH (eds): *Principles of Surgery*, ed. 4. New York, McGraw-Hill, pp 1307–1343, 1984.

17. Houghton PW, Jenkinson LR, Donaldson LA: Cholecystectomy in the elderly: A prospective study. *Br J Surg* 72:220–2, 1985.

18. Welch JP, Malt RA: Outcome of cholecystostomy. *Surg Gynecol Obstet* 135:717–720, 1972.

19. Jurkovich GJ, Dyess DL, Ferrara JJ: Cholecystostomy. Expected outcome in primary and secondary biliary disorders. *Am Surg* 54:40–44, 1988.

20. Eggermont AM, Lameris JS, Jeekel J: Ultrasound-guided percutaneous transhepatic cholecystostomy for acute acalculous cholecystitis. *Arch Surg* 120: 1354–1356, 1985.

21. Hawkins IF Jr: Percutaneous cholecystostomy. *Semin Intervent Radiol* 2:97–103, 1985.

22. Larssen TB, Gothlin JH, Jensen D, Arnesjo B, Soreide O: Ultrasonically and fluoroscopically guided therapeutic percutaneous catheter drainage of the gallbladder. *Gastrointest Radiol* 13:37–40, 1988.

23. Lohela P, Soiva M, Suramo I, Taavitsainen M, Holopainen O: Ultrasonic guidance for percutaneous puncture and drainage in acute cholecystitis. *Acta Radiol Diagn* 27:543–546, 1986.

24. McGahan JP: A new catheter design for percutaneous cholecystostomy. *Radiology* 166:49–52, 1988.

25. Pearse DM, Hawkins IF Jr, Shaver R, Vogel S: Percutaneous cholecystostomy in acute cholecystitis and common duct obstruction. *Radiology* 152: 365–367, 1984.

26. Vogelzang RL, Nemcek AA Jr.: Percutaneous cholecystostomy: Diagnostic and therapeutic efficacy. *Radiology* 168:29–34, 1988.

27. VanSonnenberg E, Wing VW, Pollard JW, Casola G: Life-threatening vagal reactions associated with percutaneous cholecystostomy. *Radiology* 151: 377–380, 1984.

28. Kerlan RK Jr, LaBerge JM, Ring EJ: Percutaneous cholecystolithotomy: Preliminary experience. *Radiology* 157:653–656, 1985.

29. Laffey KJ, Martin EC: Percutaneous removal of large gallstones. *Gastrointest Radiol* 11:165–168, 1986.

30. Lux G, Ell C, Hochberger J, Muller D, Demling L: The first successful endoscopic retrograde laser lithotripsy of common bile duct stones in man using a pulsed neodymium-Yag laser. *Endoscopy* 18: 144–145, 1986.

31. Martin EC, Wolff M, Neff RA: Casarella WJ. Use of the electrohydraulic lithotriptor in the biliary tree in dogs. *Radiology* 139:215–217, 1981.

32. Lee LL, McGahan JP: Dissolution of cholesterol gallstones: Comparison of solvents *Gastrointest Radiol* 11:169–171, 1986.

33. McGahan JP, Lee LL, Tesluk H, Nyland TG, Ruebner B, Schmidt B: Dissolution of gallstones using cholecystostomy tube in the pig. *Invest Radiol* 22:201–205, 1987.

34. McGahan JP, Tesluk H, Brock JM, Johnston R, Shaul DB: Dissolution of gallstones using methyl tertiary-butyl ether in an animal model. *Invest Radiol* 23:599–603, 1988.

35. May GR, Thistle JL: Percutaneous cholecystostomy for gallstone dissolution by methyl tert-butyl ether. *Radiology* 161 (P):90, 1986.

36. VanSonnenberg E, Hofmann AF: Horizons in gallstone therapy—1988. *AJR* 150:43–46, 1988.

37. Becker CD, Quenville NF, Burhenne HJ: Long-term occlusion of the porcine cystic duct by means of edoluminal radio-frequency electrocoagulation. *Radiology* 167:63–68, 1988.

38. Getrajdman GI, O'Toole K, LoGerfo P, Laffey KJ, Martin EC: Transcatheter sclerosis of the gallbladder in rabbits. A preliminary study. *Invest Radiol* 20:393–398, 1985.

13 Pancreas

PATRICE M. BRET

Percutaneous biopsy of focal lesions, drainage of pseudocysts, and percutaneous pancreatography are the main interventional procedures performed in the pancreas with ultrasound guidance. Accuracy of percutaneous biopsy in ductal adenocarcinoma varies from 65% to 100%. Thanks to the use of new needles, special cytological staining, and electron microscopy, pathologists can now routinely diagnose uncommon tumors such as variants of ductal adenocarcinomas, islet-cell, or cystic tumors. Although pancreatic biopsies are usually well-tolerated, severe complications, such as acute pancreatitis, can occasionally occur, especially after biopsy of "pseudo" tumors or small tumors. In the treatment of pancreatic pseudocysts, percutaneous aspiration alone has been abandoned because of the high recurrence rate. External drainage or transgastric drainage, with or without placement of a stent, are the current methods of percutaneous treatment of pancreatic pseudocysts and have demonstrated good results. Percutaneous pancreatography is an elegant technique of opacification of the pancreatic duct which can be used as a complement or an alternative to ERCP, when the latter is not technically possible or has only provided partial ductal opacification.

Percutaneous Biopsy of the Pancreas

Pancreatic carcinoma and pancreatitis are the most common diseases involving the pancreas. However, they have different prognosis and management. Pancreatic carcinoma is increasing in frequency and is now the fourth leading cause of death from cancer in men in the United States (1). Recent advances in cross-sectional imaging as well as in radioendoscopic techniques have made the detection of pancreatic cancer easier. However, no change has been made in the survival rate and, most of the time, only palliation can be offered to the patient. Distinction between pancreatitis and pancreatic carcinoma remains difficult as clinical, biochemical, and morphological criteria are not specific of one given disease. In addition, pancreatitis and pancreatic carcinoma are often associated, and pancreatitis may initially mask the malignant disease. Although pancreatic carcinoma is initially a focal process, diffuse involvement has been found in 27% of cases of pancreatic carcinoma, probably because of associated fibrosis and inflammation (2). Conversely, acute or chronic pancreatitis can present with a focal pancreatic abnormality (3). Until recently, the definitive diagnosis of a focal pancreatic lesion was made during laparotomy, and many patients were brought in the operating room for diagnostic purposes only. However, even during surgery distinction between pancreatitis and pancreatic carcinoma is difficult. The use of intraoperative biopsies of the pancreas is still controversial. Many surgeons avoid performing them whenever possible (4, 5). Their caution is based on the belief that direct pancreatic biopsy risks hemorrhage, fistulae, abscess formation, and pancreatitis. Other surgeons feel that a positive tissue diagnosis is essential before proceeding with a major surgical procedure such as pancreaticoduodenal resection. When treatment is based solely upon clinical criteria and palpation of the pancreas, the diagnostic error rate is 3% to 25% (1, 5). When an intraoperative biopsy is performed, a false negative result can be observed in as high as 30% of cases (5), especially with deep seated lesions. Complications for intraoperative pancreatic biopsies range from 5% to 10% (1, 4, 5). Nowadays, percutaneous biopsy of the pancreas can provide a tissue-proven diagnosis without surgery.

TECHNIQUE

Choice of a guidance modality

Pancreatic biopsies can be guided by ultrasound, computed tomography, or fluoroscopy. Fluoroscopy allows good visualization of the needle, but it requires either biplane imaging or rotating the patient on the side while the needle is in place in order to assess needle depth. Visualization of the lesion also requires contrast opacification of blood vessels or ducts by angiogram, transhepatic cholangiogram, percutaneous pancreatogram, or endoscopic retrograde cholangiopancreatogram. Also, an important drawback is the irradiation of both patient and operator. *Computed tomography* (CT) offers excellent image resolution of the lesion and of all other intraabdominal structures, including bowel, that are situated on the needle path. If contrast infusion is used, tumor vascularity can be assessed. However, CT-guided biopsy requires greater patient cooperation, and angulation of the needle is limited. Monitoring the progression of the needle is discontinued and the procedure involves a sizeable radiation dose to the patient. *Ultrasound* (US) is a simple, inexpensive guidance modality (Fig. 13.1). It images the tumor in three dimensions and most often the insertion of the needle can be followed throughout the procedure. Different patient positioning and needle angling are possible. Also, with ultrasound, the transducer compresses the abdominal wall and the abdominal cavity, thus reducing the distance between the skin and the lesion. This allows the use of shorter needles, which are easier to manipulate. However, structures along the path of the needle, such as bowel loops, are not as well seen as with CT. Biopsy of the pancreas with ultrasound guidance can be performed using special devices or biopsy transducers, but many radiologists use the freehand technique, which requires no special accessory (Figs. 13.2 and 13.3). The main limitation of ultrasound guidance is the presence of air in adjacent structures, which can obscure the pancreatic lesion. Factors such as patient morphotype, lesion size and location, equipment availability, and patient cooperation have to be considered in the choice of the method of guidance. In our experience, ultrasound is used in the majority of cases. CT guidance is mainly used when US has failed. In some rare cases, the lesion is not well shown either by US or CT. The biopsy can then be guided by fluoroscopy.

Access Route

Most pancreatic biopsies are performed with an anterior subxyphoid approach. Some lesions of the tail of the pancreas can be biopsied with a posterior approach. Transgression of the liver, stomach, small bowel, and some-

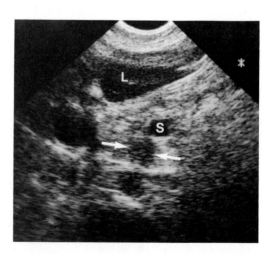

Figure 13.1. Tumor of the uncinate process. The lesion is visible on the ultrasound as a small hypoechoic mass (*arrows*) located posterior to the superior mesenteric vein (*s*). The best approach for biopsy is transhepatic (*L* = Liver).

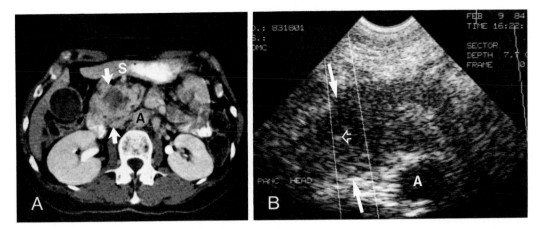

Figure 13.2. Pancreatic carcinoma. **A**, CT scan showing large inhomogeneous lesion in the head of the pancreas (*arrows*). The lumen of the stomach must be transgressed for this lesion to be biopsied through the anterior abdominal wall (*S* = stomach, *A* = aorta). **B**, Real-time ultrasonography with biopsy guide using a 22-gauge non-Teflon-coated needle showing just the tip of the needle (*open arrow*) in the enlarged pancreatic head (*between arrows*) corresponding to a pancreatic carcinoma (*A* = aorta). (Reproduced with permission from McGahan JP, Hanson F: Ultrasonographic aspiration and biopsy techniques. In Dublin AB (ed.): *Outpatient Invasive Radiologic Procedures.* Philadelphia, WB Saunders, 1989, pp 79–113.)

times colon commonly occurs during the placement of the needle. Celiac and mesenteric vessels, as well as the splenoportal confluence, are in the vicinity of most of the tumors of the head and the body and should be avoided during the placement of the needle whenever possible. If the patient presents with bile duct obstruction and significant dilatation of the intra- and extrahepatic bile ducts, the liver and the extrahepatic bile ducts should not be transgressed to decrease the risk of bile leakage.

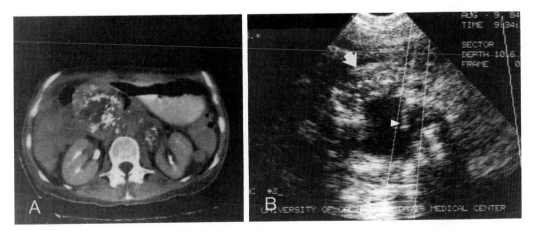

Figure 13.3. Pancreatic mass. **A**, CT scan showing calcified and enlarged head of the pancreas with central area of decreased density. **B**, A 22-gauge roughened needle being placed through the calcified head of the pancreas (*arrow*) with the tip of the needle (*arrowhead*) within the cystic portion of the mass. (Reproduced with permission from McGahan JP: Advantages of sonographic guidance. In McGahan JP (ed.): *Controversies in Ultrasound.* New York, Churchill Livingstone, 1987, pp. 249–267.)

Needles

The same needles that are used for any other biopsy in the abdomen are used for pancreatic biopsies. Most authors use 20- to 22-gauge needles in order to decrease the risk of complications. For several years, the most popular needles have been either the 15-cm Chiba needle or the 9-cm spinal needle, with both providing excellent cytological samples. More recently, a variety of needles (Wescott, SureCut, EZ, Rotex) has been introduced, all of which provide small cores of tissue suitable for conventional histology analysis. Finally, a preliminary use of the Biopty device has recently been reported in the pancreas (6). The Biopty needle is a modified Tru Cut needle with a distal hub of 2.5 cm that provides a long core biopsy. The needle is mounted on a gun that automatically advances the inner and outer parts of the needle at the time of the biopsy. The whole movement is performed almost instantaneously, and the sample quality is consistently better than that obtained with manual aspiration. Because of the speed of the movement, the biopsy itself is painless. At the moment, only 18-gauge needles are available with the Biopty devices. It is too early to know whether this system will prove to be safer than conventional aspiration biopsy techniques.

Aspiration

When an aspiration biopsy is performed, either of two methods of aspiration can be used. With the "dry" aspiration, a 20-ml plastic syringe is inserted into a "gun holder" that allows a strong and immediate suction. Back and forth movements of the needle are performed into the lesion during the aspiration. Usually, the suction is released during needle withdrawal. With the "wet technique," a 10-ml syringe containing 1 ml of normal saline is attached to the needle. During suction, the needle-syringe assembly is slowly advanced with a continuous rotary drilling motion. Aspirates can be smeared on slides without being crushed, thus preserving the cellular architecture. Some slides are air-dried to be stained with Giemsa, while others are fixed for Papanicolaou staining. Small fragments of tissue are fixed in formaline to be processed by the usual histologic techniques.

Another way of processing the specimens is to drop the contents of the needle and the syringe into a container of 50% alcohol solution that will be filtered or centrifuged before slides for cytology and cell block are obtained. Special stains can be used for the diagnosis of endocrine or other rare tumors. Stains can usually be performed on routine specimens as long as there is sufficient tissue. Electron microscopy can also be useful in some cases of rare pancreatic tumors. However, specimens have to be fixed in glutaraldehyde at the time of the aspiration. Some teams use the availability of a cytologist on site. In that case, slides are immediately stained with a commercial preparation (Diff-Quick Harleco, Gibbstown, New Jersey) or more recently, with toluedine blue, and a preliminary diagnosis can be obtained within 5 to 10 minutes. If the specimens are inadequate, more passes can be performed. When the diagnosis has been obtained, the procedure can be terminated. However, Miller and colleagues have found no improvement in results and complications from obtaining an immediate assessment of the specimens by a cytologist (7).

Cytology Results

In the field of percutaneous biopsies, the radiologist is the referring physician to the pathologist. He is the one who should provide the patient's clinical background, ask for special stainings, or decide to provide specimens for electron microscopy when necessary. For the best results, the radiologist should be aware of the various types of tumors which can be encountered in clinical practice, along with the pitfalls of the cytological diagnosis. The normal pancreatic aspirate consists of acinar cells and ductal structures. Ductal structures are seen as large sheets of a single layer of tightly bound cells with a scant cytoplasm and an oval nucleus with a dense chromatin. Acinar structures are well preserved even after passing through a 22-gauge needle. The nuclei of the acinar cells are round and eccentric with a pale birefringent and rich cytoplasma. Chromatin is regularly distributed. The wall of the nucleus is thin and the nucleolus is faint. The vast majority of pancreatic tumors arise from ductal cells: in *ductal adenocarcinomas*, the malignant cells have large, irregular, off-centered nuclei with little chromatin. Abnormal mitoses can often be seen. Cellular architecture is disorganized, with multiple layers of cells. A large number of variants of ductal adenocarcinoma can be identified on specimens. In *mucinous adenocarcinomas of the pancreas*, the carcinomatous cells float in a mucinous background. Mucin staining, such as periodic acid-Schiff and blue alcyan, are useful for the diagnosis. *Pleiomorphic giant cell carcinomas* (8) represent a highly malignant variant of ductal carcinoma of the pancreas with some similarity to sarcoma. The vascular spread is more common than the lymphatic spread. In histology and cytology, mononuclear and multinucleated pleomorphic malignant giant cells are present with an important mitotic activity. Electron microscopy has been found to be helpful in differentiating these tumors from other malignant or benign conditions in which giant cells can be found in aspirates from the pancreas. In a recent report, Silverman and colleagues (9) reported four cases of pleiomorphic giant cell carcinoma of the pancreas in which immunocytochemical studies were found to be instrumental in the diagnosis of the lesion. *Adenosquamous carcinomas of the pancreas* show an association of adenocarcinoma and lesions similar to an epidermoid tumor. The squamous element is thought to derive from metaplastic ductal epithelium. *Epidermoid carcinomas of the pancreas* are very rare and, in the presence of a squamous cell tumor of the pancreas, it is logical to consider the diagnosis of a pancreatic metastasis first rather than a primary epidermoid tumor (10). In a cadaver study, Kozuka and co-workers (11) have described *ductal hyperplasia of the pancreas* as a precancerous lesion or a lesion associated with in situ carcinoma. During percutaneous biopsies, these changes (atypical nuclei, secretory transformation of cells without definite signs of malignancy) can be seen either in association with typical changes of ductal adenocarcinoma or as isolated findings. When they are isolated, aspiration biopsy should be repeated.

Solid and papillary neoplasm of the pancreas (also called papillary cystic neoplasm, papillary epithelial neoplasm, low-grade papillary neoplasm, or papillary cystic carcinoma) represents a low-grade malignant tumor of the pancreas occurring in young women. Survival extending over 10 years has been reported after surgery. This justifies an aggressive treatment and, subsequently, an accurate preoperative diagnosis. These tumors are not specific in ultrasound or CT except for the frequency of hemorrhagic central zones (which can mislead toward the diagnosis of cystic pancreatic tumors) (Fig. 13.4). However, the cytologic findings are characteristic and a specific diagnosis can be established, especially when special stainings and electron microscopy are performed (12, 13); marked cellularity with monotonous cells is present with papillary arrangement and perivascular clustering of cells. Mucin and glycogen present in cystic tumors of the pancreas are absent, and Grimelius stain is negative for neuroendocrine granules, which helps in differentiating this entity from islet cell tumor. Electron microscopy shows an abundance of mitochondria and absence of neurosecretory or zymogen granules.

Islet cell tumors represent approximately 2% to 4% of all pancreatic tumors. However, their behavior is so different from that of exocrine malignant tumors that it is extremely important to make a specific diagnosis (Fig. 13.5, 14). Specimens are usually rich, with a monotonous population of cells that are either isolated or arranged in loose clusters and contain eccentric nuclei, and finely granular chromatin with small nucleoli. From a review of the literature in 1987, Bell (14) found 10 reported cases of percutaneous fine needle aspiration biopsy of endocrine tumors of the pancreas. Five aspirates were diagnostic of islet-cell tumors, two were suggestive of islet-cell tumors, one was suggestive of an epithelial neoplasm, and two were negative. However, it is probable that most of the cases stay unreported, and it is difficult to evaluate the actual accuracy of

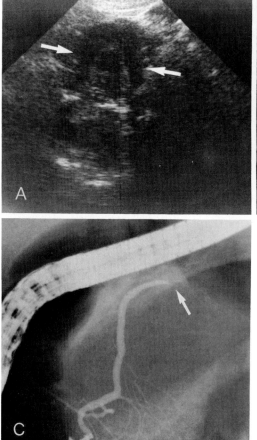

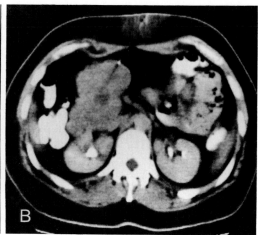

Figure 13.4. Solid and papillary neoplasm of the pancreas. **A,** Ultrasound shows a large solid mass (*arrows*) in the head of the pancreas with a cystic central area. **B,** CT demonstrates the same appearance. Biopsy was performed on the edge of the tumor to avoid central necrotic tissue. **C,** ERCP shows a complete block of the pancreatic duct (*arrow*). Biopsy allowed the specific diagnosis of solid and papillary tumor of the pancreas.

the technique. The differential diagnosis includes normal cellular constituents of the pancreas, well-differentiated adenocarcinoma of the pancreas, and lymphoma. In difficult cases, Grimelius staining, as well as immunohistochemical stains for neuron-specific enolases and polypeptide hormones can be helpful in establishing the diagnosis of islet-cell tumor and characterizing the type of secretion of the tumor.

Cystic tumors of the pancreas are now classified as microcystic adenomas, which are benign and usually made of multiple small cysts; and macrocystic mucinous adenomas and cystadenocarcinomas, which are malignant. It is felt that all cystadenocarcinomas derive from benign precursors (15). Several cases of mucinous cystadenocarcinomas of

the pancreas diagnosed by percutaneous aspiration biopsy have been reported (16–18). The diagnosis relies on the presence of intra- and extracellular mucin, which must be differentiated from necrotic debris sometimes seen in ductal adenocarcinomas. Special staining for mucin is of value in this regard. Differentiation between microcystic (serous) cystadenomas and mucinous cystadenomas is difficult on morphologic criteria only. However, special staining for glycogen (positive in microcystic adenoma) and mucin (positive in macrocystic adenoma) may be of help. Other authors have tried to correlate the values of the carcinoembryonic antigen, carbohydrate antigen, and elastase 1 with various types of cystic masses of the pancreas (19).

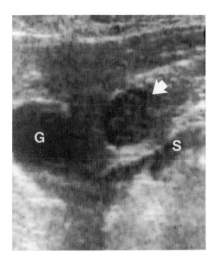

Figure 13.5. Islet cell tumor of the head of the pancreas. US shows a 2 cm well-limited round solid tumor in the head of the pancreas (*arrow*). Percutaneous biopsy allowed for the diagnosis of endocrine tumor of the pancreas. Patient was operated on and a tumor enucleation was performed instead of the initially planned Whipple's procedure (G = gallbladder, S = splenic vein).

RESULTS

Since 1975, multiple series of percutaneous biopsies of the pancreas have been reported (Table 13.1). The sensitivity in the diagnosis of pancreatic carcinoma varies from 64% to 100% according to the series, depending mainly on whether or not the authors have included nonconclusive results in their false-negative results (38). With such results, percutaneous fine-needle biopsy of the pancreas is an efficient alternative to diagnostic laparotomy if one takes in account the cost and morbidity of a surgical laparotomy. However, results of percutaneous pancreatic biopsies are consistently inferior to results obtained from biopsies taken elsewhere in the abdomen. The main reason for failed biopsies in pancreatic carcinomas is the common association between tumor and pancreatitis. Often, the inflammatory component of the tumor is sampled, leading to a false-negative result. Nonconclusive aspirations, which contain an inadequate amount of cells, are often the consequence of an aspiration in the squirrhous or necrotic components of the tumor. There has been no increase in accuracy of the biopsies in the latest reports when compared to initial series. The reason is that, as experience is gained, more small lesions, or lesions that are difficult to approach, are biopsied. The specificity of the percutaneous biopsies is 100% in most series, which indicates that no false-positive results are encountered. Although no definite difference in result has been shown with the use of different needles, the importance of obtaining tiny cores of tissue has been stressed by Wittenberg and co-workers (39). Indeed, histology and cytology are complementary, and the association of the two techniques increases the sensitivity (40). Until 1981, the main method of guidance used was fluoroscopic. From 1982 on, ultrasound and/or CT have been almost exclusively used. However, Hall and colleagues (36) have found that the combination of ultrasound and fluoroscopic guidance (during pancreatic duct opacification) increased their sensitivity in the diagnosis of pancreatic carcinoma from 67% to 75%.

In two series studying the clinical efficacy of pancreatic biopsies in clinical situations, results have shown a significant impact on patient management. Mitty and colleagues (28) found that among 43 patients with a pancreatic carcinoma who underwent a percutaneous biopsy of the pancreas, 30 were saved a laparotomy that would otherwise have been performed. In a prospective study on clinical efficacy of percutaneous fine-needle biopsies of abdominal lesions (including 27 pancreatic biopsies), we found that three laparotomies, one laparoscopy, four arteriograms, four endoscopic retrograde cholangiopancreatographies (ERCP) and four direct cholangiograms were cancelled because of the results of the biopsy (41). In terms of cost, the workup of a pancreatic mass was shown to be decreased by at least 35% when a percutaneous biopsy was undertaken, especially when it was performed early in the workup, as soon as a focal pancreatic lesion was detected. In terms of diagnostic value, the same study showed that in 75% of pancreatic lesions the correct diagnosis was strongly suggested by clinical

Table 13.1
Reported Results of Percutaneous pancreatic Biopsies

Year	Authors	Number of cases	Percent Success	Guidance
1975	Hancke et al. (20)	21	84	US
1975	Smith et al. (21)	6	83	US
1977	Haaga et al. (22)	10	70	CT
1978	Goldstein et al. (23)	21	73	US, Angiography
1978	Evander et al. (24)	52	64	Angiography
1978	McLoughlin et al. (25)	18	89	Angiography
1979	Yamanaka et al. (26)	22	86	US
1980	Ferrucci et al. (27)	21	86	US, CT, Fluoroscopy
1981	Mitty et al. (28)	43	86	US, Angiography
1982	Bret et al. (29)	90	77	US
1982	Hovdenak (30)	55	77	US
1982	Sundaram et al. (31)	16	68	CT
1983	Grant et al. (32)	15	100	US
1983	Schwerk et al. (33)	70	90	US
1983	Harter (34)	32	88	CT
1985	Hancke (35)	203	71	US
1986	Hall (36)	208	75	US & Fluoroscopy
1986	Hajdu (37)	126	97	US
1986	Fekete (38)	61	50	CT

and morphological studies prior to the biopsy. In these circumstances, the biopsy only provided a tissue-proven diagnosis. In the other 25% of cases, the exact diagnosis was not predicted before the biopsy. In those cases, the biopsy was instrumental in patient management.

Complications after percutaneous pancreatic biopsy are unusual. Traversing the gastrointestinal tract does not increase the risk of complications. Large vessels, such as the superior mesenteric artery, superior mesenteric vein, and inferior vena cava can easily be avoided since they are well visible in cross-sectional imaging. Also, dilated bile or pancreatic ducts should be avoided in order to decrease the risk of bile or pancreatic leakage. The major complication observed after percutaneous biopsy of the pancreas is acute pancreatitis. The risk seems to be related to the transgression of the normal pancreas since this complication mainly occurs after biopsy of small tumors or pseudo tumors in which the normal pancreatic tissue is traversed by the needle. In such cases, severe acute pancreatitis that can lead to patient's death has been reported (42). Mueller

and colleagues (43), reviewing 184 pancreatic biopsies, found five cases (3%) of severe pancreatitis. Four of the patients had to be operated on and one of them died. All five patients had lesions of less than 3 cm in diameter and three of them were finally shown to have normal pancreas. It is difficult to have an accurate estimate of the complication rate after percutaneous biopsy, since the incidence of complications is low and the largest published series does not exceed 200 to 300 patients. A large questionnaire survey presented in 1986 and 1988 (44, 45) on 60,000 abdominal biopsies showed 15 deaths, 5 of them occurring after pancreatic biopsies. However, the methodology used probably underestimated the rate of complications, because many of them occur in small series that are not reported. Also, data obtained through questionnaires are not as reliable as data collected in a regular series of patients. In another attempt to quantify the rate of complications, Livraghi and co-workers (46) compiled 11,700 cases of biopsy of abdominal lesions reported in the literature and found one case of fatal complication after biopsy of a normal pancreas. Seeding along the tract of the biopsy has also been reported in rare cases (47, 48) but is not frequent enough to be a significant problem in clinical practice.

Percutaneous Approach to Pancreatic Fluid Collections

The term of pancreatic pseudocyst has been initially applied to all pancreatic fluid collections. However, various types of pancreatic fluid collections should be considered: during an episode of acute pancreatitis, *intra- or extrapancreatic fluid collections* have no mature wall, and an internal surgical anastomosis at this time is hazardous. Also, a number of these collections disappear spontaneously. Fluid collections seen several weeks after an initial episode of acute pancreatitis have a mature fibrous wall—although it does not contain an epithelium—and deserve better the term of *pseudocyst*. Pancreatic *phlegmons* are characterized by enlargement of the pancreas due to edema and necrosis and inflammation of the peripancreatic tissues. Phlegmons are difficult to differentiate from pancreatic *abscesses*, especially at the initial phase. The optimal surgical treatment of an uncomplicated mature pseudocyst is internal drainage into the stomach, duodenum or small bowel (49). When surgery is done to treat acute fluid collections, most of the time an external drainage is performed. Differentiation of an acute fluid collection from a chronic pseudocyst can be achieved by several criteria, including delay between symptoms and patient's presentation, and morphological appearance of the pseudocyst with imaging techniques (50). Percutaneous treatment of pancreatic pseudocysts includes needle aspiration, external drainage, and transgastric drainage with possibility of inserting a stent between the pseudocyst and the stomach. Although percutaneous drainage is routinely used to drain almost any infected and noninfected fluid collection in the abdomen, percutaneous drainage of pancreatic fluid collections

is still controversial. In a recent surgical review of the treatment of pancreatic pseudocysts, percutaneous drainage is hardly mentioned and then only for the treatment of infected immature fluid collections (50).

However, recently vanSonnenberg and co-workers (50a) published his experience with percutaneous drainage of 101 pancreatic pseudocysts in 77 patients. These included 51 infected and 50 noninfected pseudocysts. Ninety-one of the 101 pseudocysts were cured by means of catheter drainage (90.1%) with slightly greater cures for the infected pseudocysts, 48 of 51 (94.1%), as compared to the noninfected pseudocysts, 43 of 50 patients (86%). Ultrasound was used for guidance of only seven of these patients, while CT was used in the remainder. In the majority of these patients, the transperitoneal or retroperitoneal route was utilized. It was their conclusion that percutaneous drainage is an effective front-line treatment for most pancreatic pseudocysts and that cure is likely if the fluid collections are drained adequately and a sufficient time is allowed for closure of the fistula from the pancreatic duct.

Why is there a difference between a fluid collection in the pancreas and an abdominal abscess? An abscess, in the absence of fistula, is an isolated pathologic process. When the fluid collection is drained and the cavity is sterilized, the patient is cured, while drainage of a pancreatic fluid collection does not treat the underlying pancreatitis. Before any treatment is attempted on a pseudocyst of the pancreas, and especially if a conservative treatment is planned, a complete workup should be obtained in order 1. To rule out other causes of fluid collections in the pancreas (cystic tumors, hematomas, necrotic tumors, abscesses of the pancreas) or around the pancreas (adrenal or renal cysts); 2. To evaluate the number, size, and locations of pseudocysts, as well as the status of the remaining pancreas and peripancreatic tissues; 3. To differentiate mature from immature pseudocysts; 4. To rule out infection [sterile, infected without systemic effects, infected with systemic effects, abscess (50)] hemorrhage, or other complications of the pseudocyst (bile duct or bowel obstruction).

The workup should include at least an ultrasound and a CT examination and, in some cases, an opacification of the pancreatic duct, in order to identify any ductal amputation or communication of the duct with the pseudocyst. When percutaneous drainage is contemplated, a diagnostic needle aspiration should always precede the drainage.

PERCUTANEOUS TREATMENT OF PSEUDOCYSTS

Methods of Guidance

Although ultrasound is extremely accurate in diagnosing pseudocysts of the pancreas, it does not provide as much information as CT about the access route of the catheter and the extension of pancreatitis at a distance from the pseudocyst. Therefore, although ultrasound combined with fluoroscopy is best suited to guide a drainage procedure, a CT examination should always be obtained prior to, or at the time of drainage. Other authors perform drainage with ultrasound guidance only or CT guidance only (51–53).

Needle Aspiration

A diagnostic needle aspiration is routinely performed prior to drainage to rule out a cystic tumor, or infection or an hemorrhage within the cyst. Ultrasound may be helpful to guide drainage (Fig. 13.6). Gram stain and culture, as well as fluid amylase level, are usually obtained. However, cytologic analysis of the fluid will not always allow differentiation between a pseudocyst and a cystic pancreatic tumor (54). When aspiration is used as a therapeutic procedure, at the end of the diagnostic aspiration, the needle is left in place and injection of contrast medium is performed to rule out a communication with the pancreatic duct. If the cyst communicates with the pancreatic duct, reaccumulation is likely to occur after needle withdrawal. If the cyst does not communicate with the pancreatic duct, aspiration alone has been advocated as a definitive treatment (55). However, the recurrence rate after aspiration is as high as 50 to 75%

(56–58). In Gandini's series (59) 15 out of 21 cases recurred shortly after aspiration. Repeated aspirations have been suggested to decrease the rate of failures, but repeated aspirations also increase the risk of infection of the cyst. Also the fistulous communication to the pancreatic duct may not be identified on initial injection of the pseudocyst, but may be seen 7–10 days following catheter drainage.

External Drainage.

Techniques used for external drainage of pancreatic pseudocysts are similar to those used for abscess drainage (Fig. 13.7). Either the trocar or the Seldinger method can be used. Catheter sizes range from 8 to 14 F, depending on the viscosity of the fluid. If necessary, sump catheters with a double lumen or 2 catheters can be inserted to improve drainage. Drainage is obtained by gravity. Irrigation is performed when fluid contents are of increased viscosity. Follow-up is obtained on the basis of the patient's clinical status, volume of catheter output,

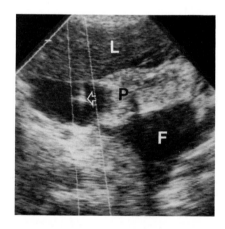

Figure 13.6. Pancreatic aspiration. Transverse scan demonstrating a 22-gauge needle (*arrow*) being passed transhepatically into a peripancreatic fluid collection. This and a second fluid collection (*F*) were aspirated with ultrasound (*L* = liver, *P* = pancreas). (Reproduced with permission from McGahan JP, Anderson MW, Walter JP: Portable real-time sonographic and needle guidance systems for aspiration and drainage. *AJR* 147: 1241–1246, 1986, © American Roentgen Ray Society.)

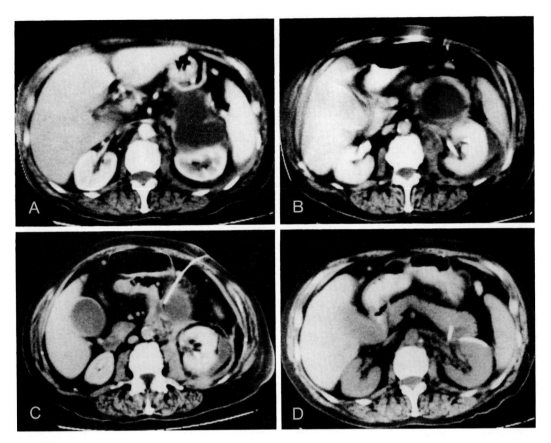

Figure 13.7. External drainage of an extra-pancreatic fluid collection. **A, B,** CT scan shows a large fluid collection in the region of the tail of the pancreas extending in the posterior pararenal and perirenal spaces. **C,** A 12 F catheter was placed under CT guidance with the trocar technique. Positioning of the tip of the catheter in the pararenal space was possible without transferring the patient to a fluoroscopy room. **D,** Control CT after a week of drainage: both the cyst in the tail and the posterior extension have disappeared.

and results of follow-up ultrasound, CT, and fistulograms. Ultrasound may be used for catheter drainage (Fig. 13.8). Dynamic CT or pulsed Doppler ultrasound may be used before drainage to exclude a potentially disastrous puncture of a pseudoaneurysm secondary to pancreatitis (Fig. 13.9). The average length of catheter stay is 3 weeks with extremes varying from 2 to 95 days (58, 59). However, in a recent series of 101 percutaneously drained pseudocysts, one patient required 102 days for drainage (50a). This patient had three pseudocysts that were completely cured. The authors cautioned against premature removal of catheters, which resulted in pseudocyst recurrence and drainage failure. Therefore, some authors (58) recommend to clamp the catheter for 48 hours and check for fluid reaccumulation before removing the catheter.

Transgastric Drainage

Initially, special care was taken to avoid transgressing the stomach when draining a pancreatic pseudocyst (Fig. 13.10). However, the close contact between the pseudocyst and the gastric cavity can preclude any extragastric approach to a pseudocyst. Also, experience with percutaneous gastrostomy has demonstrated the safety of catheter placement through the stomach (60). Finally, it was felt that interposition of the

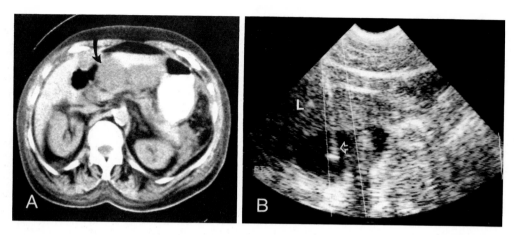

Figure 13.8. Pseudocyst drainage. **A,** CT scan demonstrating bilobed fluid collection (*curved arrow*) anterior to the pancreas and posterior to the fluid-filled stomach. **B,** Under sonographic control using the trocar technique and the transhepatic route, a catheter (*open arrow*) was placed into the pseudocyst, which was successfully percutaneously drained (*L* = liver). Courtesy of John P. McGahan M.D., Sacramento, California.

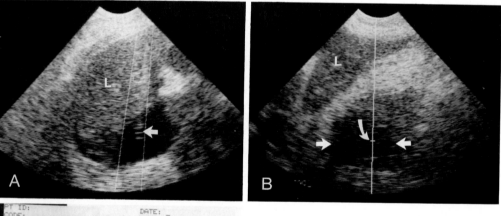

Figure 13.9. Pseudoaneurysm of the splenic artery. **A,** Longitudinal ultrasound showing an initial needle (*arrow*) placed transhepatically into a fluid collection (*L* = liver). **B,** Before aspiration of a second hypoechoic area (*arrows*) in the peripancreatic region, the Doppler cursor was placed centrally (*curved arrow*) **C,** Doppler tracing demonstrated a large amount of flow in this region and, therefore, no puncture was performed. This was surgically confirmed to represent a 4-cm pseudoaneurysm of the splenic artery with surrounding clot. (Reproduced with permission from McGahan JP, Anderson MW: Pulsed doppler sonography as an aid in ultrasound-guided aspiration biopsy. *Gastrointest Radiol* 12: 279–284; 1987, © Springer-Verlag.)

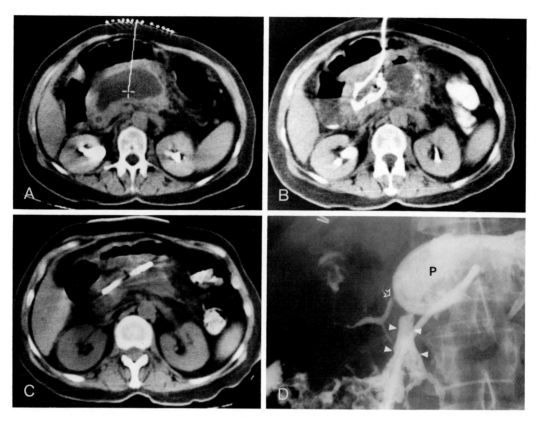

Figure 13.10. Transgastric drainage of a pseudocyst of the pancreas. **A,** CT of the pancreas demonstrates a large fluid collection in the body of the pancreas. **B,** With the trocar technique, a 12 F catheter is placed in the collection with a transgastric approach. **C,** Control CT after 1 week of drainage: the fluid collection has disappeared. **D,** Fistulogram in AP position done the same day as the control CT demonstrates opacification of the pseudocyst (*P*) with persistent communication with the pancreatic duct (*open arrow*) and a large posterior fistula between the cyst and the right colon (*arrowheads*) which was undiagnosed (or not present) on the initial examinations.

stomach between the pseudocyst and the entry site of the catheter on the skin could potentially decrease the risk of pancreaticocutaneous fistula. Prerequisite for transgastric drainage of a pseudocyst is a close contact between the stomach and the cyst. In cases of cysts arising from the body or tail of the pancreas, CT is useful for evaluating the distance between the posterior wall of the stomach and the pseudocyst (59). Distension of the stomach is achieved through a nasogastric tube or by effervescent granules. The entry site on the skin is chosen after ultrasound or CT localization of the left lobe of the liver and the transverse colon. Puncture is done either with a 5 F needle sheath or an 8 F trocar catheter (Meditech). Initially, the intragastric position of the needle or of the trocar is verified by injection of a small amount of contrast medium. Then the needle is further advanced in order to enter the pseudocyst. Some fluid is aspirated for amylase, cytology, Gram stain and culture. When initial aspiration has been made with a 18 G catheter needle, a guide wire is coiled in the cavity and dilatation of the tract performed up to 8 to 10 F before the final catheter is positioned.

Catheters are usually pigtail tubes with side holes within the pigtail. Drainage is obtained by gravity. Catheters are flushed daily with 5 to 10 ml of saline. Cystograms are obtained every 2 to 3 days. Ductal communication may not be demonstrated on initial opacification and may have to be searched for on several occasions. Catheters are maintained in place for 2 to 6 weeks. Patients can be discharged at the end of the acute episode. There are no large series available to assess the results of transgastric drainage versus external drainage or surgical internal anastomosis as a long term treatment modality. Table 13.2 summarizes the results reported in four recent series for a total of 30 cases (51, 52, 61, 62). Overall, four patients required surgery, three patients died, either from multiorgan failure or from causes unrelated to the drainage. One abscess developed after the drainage tube occluded in an outpatient. Also, a pseudoaneurysm of the splenic artery that developed and bled within a few days after transgastric drainage of a pseudocyst of the tail of the pancreas has been reported (63).

Cystogastrostomy

The principle of cystogastrostomy is that an internal stent can provide drainage as adequate as a transgastric drain. Hancke and Henriksen (64) advocate the use of combined ultrasound and endoscopic guidance while Bernardino and Amerson (65) have reported one case of successful placement of a stent with CT guidance. Whatever the method used, the technique is similar to that of a transgastric drainage. A transgastric puncture of the pseudocyst is performed either with the trocar technique or the Seldinger technique. With the trocar technique, a double pigtail stent is mounted on a needle. The needle is inserted in the pseudocyst, and a pusher allows the insertion of the stent into the pseudocyst. When the junction between the pusher and the stent is visible in the stomach, the stent is grasped with the endoscope while the needle and the pusher are removed. With the Seldinger technique, the tract is progressively dilated up to 8.3 F and the stent is positioned in a similar way to biliary stents. Twenty-two patients have been reported by Hancke with two technical failures. Four patients required surgery. There was no death. Stents were left in place an average of 3 months before being removed by gastroscopy. In all patients in whom the procedure was successful, the cyst collapsed within 24 hours. No complications were observed in this series, and no recurrence was observed during a 3- to 36-month period.

Endoscopy

When the pseudocyst bulges inside the gastric lumen, a cystogastrostomy can be performed endoscopically with a thermic probe (66, 67). Twenty cases of chronic pseudocysts treated with this method have been reported with a success rate of 90% and a complication rate of 20% (68). Initial results have also been reported in cases of infected and acute pancreatic fluid collections (69).

Infected Pancreatic Fluid Collections

In the category of infected pancreatic fluid collections, one must separate infected

Table 13.2
Transgastric Drainage of Pseudocysts of the Pancreas

Authors	Date	No. of	Results	Follow-up
Sacks et al. (52)	1988	8	1 pancreatic abscess requiring surgery. 1 unrelated death	5-25 months
Kuligowska et al. (61)	1985	3	1 death, 1 failure, 1 success	
Nunez et al. (51)	1985	7	no complication, no surgery	unknown
Matzinger (62)	1988	12	2 patients had surgery, 1 death, success in 8 cases	unknown

pseudocysts and simple pancreatic abscesses from complicated abscesses and phlegmons. Initial reports have shown comparable results of the external drainage in infected and noninfected pseudocysts (72, 73). In a more recent series of 38 infected fluid collections in 23 patients, Freeny and colleagues (70) reported a success rate of 65.2% (15 patients) without additional surgical treatment. In 10 patients, surgery was performed, although drainage had been successful in eight patients. Three complications occurred: one empyema of the chest and two hemorrhages. Average drainage duration was 29 days in the absence of pancreatic duct fistula and 96 to 104 days for patients with either a gastrointestinal or pancreatic duct fistula. VanSonnenberg and co-workers reported that the cure rate for the infected pseudocyst was 94% as compared to the noninfected pseudocyst cure rate of 86%. Additionally, the duration of drainage of the infected pseudocyst was 16.7 days as compared to the noninfected pseudocyst duration of drainage which was 21.2 days (50a). In complex abscesses and phlegmons, the major limiting factor to percutaneous drainage is pancreatic necrosis. Necrotic tissue requires surgical debridement. However, in these complex cases, combination of radiological and surgical procedures is often beneficial to the patient. Surgery is necessary to debride areas of necrosis and drain large areas of fluid collections, while residual or recurrent fluid collections can be managed more precisely by percutaneous drainage. Also, in emergency situations, an initial percutaneous drainage may have a temporizing positive effect on the patient's condition. Pancreatic abscesses can be drained either externally or via a transgastric approach. Frequently, multiple large-bore catheters up to 24 F in diameter are necessary. This type of aggressive combined approach requires a tremendous investment in time and procedures on the part of the surgeons and radiologists (close monitoring, multiple ultrasound and CT examinations, repeated catheter manipulations). In a group of 25 patients with complicated abscesses reported by Steiner

and colleagues (71), eight patients were successfully treated by catheter drainage only, 10 patients were improved by a catheter drainage followed by surgical debridement, and six had a percutaneous drainage procedure after initial surgery. One patient died early in the postprocedure period.

Percutaneous management of pseudocysts of the pancreas requires access to ultrasound, CT, and fluoroscopic facilities. Diagnostic aspiration should always precede therapeutic drainage. Whenever the clinical status of the patient allows it, a period of several weeks after initial symptoms should be given before any attempt at drainage is performed, since a significant number of acute pancreatic fluid collections disappear without treatment. Percutaneous drainage and surgical treatment of pancreatic pseudocysts are complementary techniques. Surgical cystogastrostomy or cystoenterostomy provides a more definitive treatment than percutaneous drainage. However, a percutaneous drainage does not carry the same rate of complications as surgery and can be offered if necessary at any stage of the inflammatory process. Percutaneous drainage can be reasonably proposed as an alternative to surgical external drainage, especially in acute fluid collections. Single-step drainage by aspiration should be abandoned because of the high rate of recurrence. Percutaneous drainage with a transgastric approach offers theoretical advantages whenever it is anatomically possible. Percutaneous cystogastrostomy is an elegant technique to drain pseudocysts into the gastric cavity, which provides an adequate temporary internal drainage. However, the communication between the cyst and the stomach is likely to close when the stent is removed, and long-term results have to be considered. Large or randomised series comparing short-term and long-term results of surgical external drainage versus percutaneous drainage, and percutaneous cystogastrostomy versus surgical anastomosis, still need to be obtained. In complicated pancreatic abscesses, a combined radiological and surgical approach provides the best patient care.

Pancreatic Duct Intervention

PERCUTANEOUS PANCREATOGRAPHY

Guidance

The initial step of a percutaneous pancreatogram is the placement of a needle in the pancreatic duct. Real-time ultrasound is the method of choice to guide needle placement since it demonstrates the pancreatic duct whether it is dilated or not (74, 75) and also allows continuous monitoring of the needle during its positioning. However, some authors have reported cases in which fluoroscopy has been used as a method of guidance, usually in patients presenting with calcified intraductal stones (76). CT can also demonstrate the normal and dilated pancreatic duct and be used as well as a method of guidance. The ideal setting is a real-time ultrasound unit in a fluoroscopy room: the puncture of the duct is performed under US guidance, and injection of contrast medium is done under fluoroscopic guidance.

Requirements for Percutaneous Pancreatography

Normal pancreatic ducts measure from 1 to 3 mm in diameter and are difficult to puncture. In most cases, percutaneous pancreatograms are attempted when the pancreatic duct measures over 5 mm in diameter. Patients are required to fast for 6 to 12 hours prior to the procedure since the needle may pass through the stomach. The procedure can be performed on an outpatient basis, but patients should fast for 6 hours after the procedure. Coagulation parameters are checked in the same way as for a pancreatic aspiration biopsy.

Technique

Twenty-two-gauge spinal needles or Chiba needles can be used for entering the duct. Since the pancreatic duct is relatively superficial, there is no need for a 15-cm Chiba needle, which is more difficult to ma-

nipulate than spinal needles. The entry site on the skin is usually the midline in the subxyphoid region. The duct is entered in the body of the pancreas where it is more anterior. After local anesthesia, the needle is introduced with the freehand technique or using a biopsy transducer. No special attempt is made to avoid traversing the stomach or the bowel during the procedure. However, in case of bile duct obstruction, the needle tract should avoid going through the liver parenchyma because of the risk of bile leakage. When the tip of the needle is visible in the pancreatic duct, the needle is carefully connected to a flexible tube to avoid needle dislodgement and a light aspiration is performed until reflux of pure pancreatic juice is obtained. Depending on the degree of duct dilatation, 1 to 10 ml of pancreatic juice are aspirated and sent to the laboratory for amylase and lactoferrine assays. The opacification is performed by injecting 10 to 20 ml of water-soluble hexaiodinated contrast medium. No injection should be performed unless a free reflux of pancreatic juice is present. Injection is continued until the entire pancreatic duct and the papilla are opacified. However, when the duct is severely dilated, more pancreatic juice is aspirated before injecting large amounts of contrast medium to avoid hyperpressure in the ductal system. Multiple spot films are performed during the course of contrast medium injection. When a stenosis of the pancreatic duct is demonstrated, a percutaneous fine-needle biopsy can be performed under fluoroscopic control in the area of stenosis to obtain a tissue diagnosis (Fig. 13.11). At the end of the procedure, the contrast medium is aspirated before removing the needle in order to decrease the risk of extravasation. In cases of pseudocysts, injection is made first in the cystic lesion. In a number of cases, this results in opacification of both the pseudocyst and the pancreatic duct (Fig. 13.12). A complete pancreatogram can be obtained if the communication is wide open. If no communication is demonstrated, the pancreatic duct is punctured as described above. At the time of injection, an attempt is again made to opacify the cyst, but the injection is

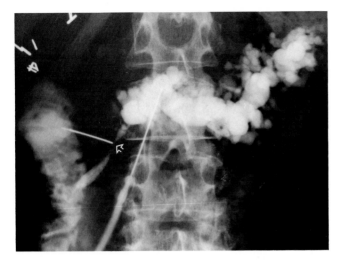

Figure 13.11. Pancreatic carcinoma. Percutaneous pancreatography was obtained with combined US and fluoroscopic guidance. During the procedure, a percutaneous biopsy was performed at the level of the stenosis. (*open arrow*).

stopped if the patient experiences pain. In cases of pseudocysts, particular attention should be given to the appearance of the fluid aspirated from the cyst or from the pancreatic duct. Indeed, on two occasions, we encountered what were thought to be communicating pseudocysts of the pancreas that turned out to be mucinous cystic tumors of the pancreas widely communicating with a severely dilated pancreatic duct mimicking chronic pancreatitis with pseudocysts. Only the macroscopic appearance of the pancreatic fluid suggested the diagnosis of cystic tumors of the pancreas.

Results

Since 1979, several cases or short series of percutaneous pancreatograms have been reported (76–81). Recently, two series of respectively 28 (82) and 75 (83) cases have been reported with a rate of success of 89% in each series. The diameter of the duct varied from 3 to 15 mm in one series (82) and averaged 12 mm in the other series (83). The

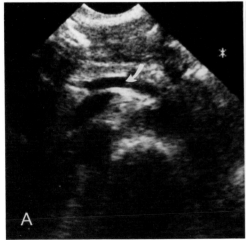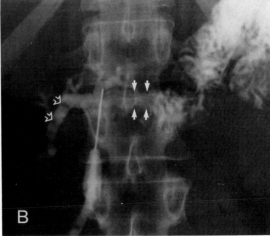

Figure 13.12. Percutaneous opacification of a pancreaticojejunostomy. **A,** US shows persistent pancreatic duct dilatation (*curved arrow*) after surgery for pancreatitis. **B,** Percutaneous pancreatogram shows recurrent pancreaticolithiasis (*open arrows*) with widely patent anastomosis (*arrows*).

main cause of failure was the small size of the duct: in Lees's series (83), out of eight failed attempts, the duct measured less than 3 mm in four cases and less than 6 mm in the other four. In our series of 28 cases (82), causes for failure included two cases of lack of cooperation due to dyspnea and agitation, and one case of chronic pancreatitis in which the pancreatic parenchyma was so hard that it could not be punctured. Complications included one case of septicemia caused by *Escherichia Coli* that resolved with antibiotics (83), and one case of bile leakage secondary to the transgression of a dilated left intrahepatic bile duct in a patient with a tumor of the head of the pancreas (82). No leakage of pancreatic juice along the needle tract was reported, probably because of the small size of the needle used. The same criteria as in endoscopic retrograde cholangiopancreatographies (ERCP) are used to differentiate chronic pancreatitis from pancreatic carcinomas. In Lees's series (83), a complete obstruction of ducts was highly suggestive of pancreatic carcinoma, although it was present in as many as 8% of patients with chronic pancreatitis. Atrophy of side branches at less than 1 cm in length was visible in 89% of patients with pancre-

atic carcinomas versus 8% of patients with chronic pancreatitis. Ectasia of collateral branches was more often seen in patients with chronic pancreatitis than in patients with carcinoma of the pancreas.

Indications for Pancreatic Duct Opacification

In most instances, a complete pancreatic workup can be obtained with US, CT, and percutaneous fine-needle biopsy only. Opacification of the pancreatic duct is justified only when results of US and CT are doubtful, or nondiagnostic, or when a provisional diagnosis of cancer has been made but the lesion is difficult to localize for biopsy, or when surgery is contemplated, especially in case of chronic pancreatitis (84).

Endoscopic Cannulation versus Percutaneous Puncture

ERCP is currently the method of choice for pancreatic duct opacification (see Table 13.3). However, the percutaneous approach is simpler and cheaper since it requires neither extensive training of the operator nor endoscopic equipment. Pure pancreatic juice is almost invariably obtained with the percuta-

Table 13.3.
Comparison of ERCP and Percutaneous Pancreatograms To Opacify the Pancreatic Duct

ERCP	Percutaneous Pancreatogram
Advantages	
Success rate independent of duct size	Provides pure pancreatic juice
Allows bile duct as well as pancreatic duct opacification	No extensive training required
Allows direct visualization and biopsies of the ampulla	Gives information proximal to a stenosis
Carries less risk of hemorrhage or perforation	Usually provides more complete opacification
	No ductal hyperpressure
	Possible after a Whipple's procedure
Drawbacks	
Provokes hyperpressure in the duct	Possible only if duct is dilated
Risk of pancreatitis if cannulation is difficult	Only pancreatic duct is opacified
Requires more training for the operator	Risk of hemorrhage and perforation
Biopsy of stenoses more difficult	
Aspiration of pure pancreatic juice more difficult	
When complete stop no information proximal to stop	
Not possible after gastrojejunostomy procedure	

neous approach. Also, aspiration of pancreatic fluid decreases the pancreatic duct pressure and the risk of parenchymal extravasation. The injection is done directly into the duct, which gives more flexibility to obtain adequate filling of the ductal system: pancreatic side branches can fill better, and the distal segment of a stenosis is often opacified. The endoscopic approach is not possible after a Whipple's procedure and may be difficult after a gastrojejunostomy, in case of ectopic or endodiverticular papilla, or of pancreas divisum; this does not affect the rate of success of the percutaneous approach (Fig. 13.12; 85). On the other hand, ERCP provides a direct visual examination of the papilla with the possibility of taking biopsies. Both bile ducts and the pancreatic duct can be opacified in the same session and the rate of success of the examination is not related to the size of the pancreatic duct. In fact, ERCP and percutaneous pancreatograms can supplement each other: in case of a complete stop, especially in the head of the pancreas, the information provided by ERCP may be incomplete or equivocal. In that situation, percutaneous opacification of the duct proximal to the stenosis can be helpful for diagnosis and preoperative workup. For Lees and colleagues (83), the sensitivity of a fine-needle biopsy of the pancreas is increased if a combination of methods of guidance (ultrasound and percutaneous pancreatograms) is used. Although a percutaneous biopsy can be performed immediately after ERCP, the rapid clearing of the contrast medium from the duct often makes ERCP difficult to use for biopsy guidance. During percutaneous pancreatography, one can always inject more contrast medium into the pancreatic duct should it be necessary. ERCP is the method of choice of opacification of the pancreatic duct whenever the duct is not dilated, or when opacification of the bile ducts is also necessary. The percutaneous approach should be used when ERCP is not possible, has failed, or is nondiagnostic. When the pancreatic duct is dilated and a focal lesion is suspected, the percutaneous approach should also be preferred for biopsy localization. In chronic pancreatitis, opacification of the pancreatic duct is usually obtained prior to surgery, and the percutaneous approach should be chosen if the pancreatic duct is dilated.

PANCREATIC DUCT DRAINAGE

Only one case of pancreatic duct drainage through a percutaneous approach has been reported so far (86). In the case published, good clinical results were obtained by placing an 8 F external drainage in an obstructed pancreatic duct. In most cases, pancreatic duct drainage is obtained endoscopically by sphincterotomy of the ampullary part of the pancreatic duct with or without endoscopic placement of pancreatic stents (87, 88).

In conclusion, the combined development of cross-sectional imaging and interventional techniques has dramatically modified the approach to pancreatic diseases. The diagnosis of a pancreatic disease is no longer obtained through a surgical procedure but by a combination of imaging tests and biopsy. Because rare but severe complications of biopsy can occur in patients with small lesions or benign conditions, biopsies of these lesions must be performed cautiously. In the treatment of pancreatic fluid collections, especially in cases of infection, percutaneous and surgical procedures are complementary.

REFERENCES

1. Gudjonsson B, Livstone EM, Spiro HM: Cancer of the pancreas. Diagnostic accuracy and survival statistics. *Cancer* 42: 2494–506, 1978.
2. Wittenberg J, Simeone JF, Ferruci JT, Muller PR, vanSonnenberg E, Neff CC: Non-focal enlargement in pancreatic carcinoma. *Radiology* 144: 131–135, 1982.
3. Silverstein W, Isikoff MB, Hill MC, Barkin J: Diagnostic imaging of acute pancreatitis: Prospective study using CT and sonography. *AJR* 137: 497–502, 1981.
4. Beazley RM: Needle biopsy diagnosis of pancreatic cancer. *Cancer* 47: 1685–1687, 1981.
5. Lee, Y-TN: Tissue diagnosis for carcinoma of the pancreas and periampullary structures. *Cancer* 49: 1035–1039, 1982.
6. Lees WR, Rode J: 18 SWg cutting biopsy of the pancreas in RSNA 1986 abstract book.
7. Miller DA, Carrasco CH, Katz RL, Cramer FM, Wallace S, Charnsangavej C: Fine needle aspiration biopsy: The role of immediate cytologic assessment. *AJR* 147: 155–158, 1986.
8. Pinto MM, Monteiro NL, Tizol DM: Fine needle aspiration of pleiomorphic giant-cell carcinoma of the pancreas. *Acta Cytol* 30: 430–434, 1986.
9. Silverman JF, Dabbs DJ, Finley JL, Geisinger KR:

Fine needle aspiration biopsy of pleomorphic (giant-cell) carcinoma of the pancreas. Cytologic, immunocytochemical and ultrastructural findings. *Am J Clin Pathol* 89: 714–720, 1988.

10. Kolbusz R, Reyes CV, Hakky M, Gradini R: Asymptomatic esophageal squamous cell carcinoma masquerading as a rare primary pancreatic carcinoma. Diagnosis by percutaneous fine needle aspiration. *Acta Cytol* 32: 399–402, 1988.

11. Kozuka S, Sassa R, Taki T, et al.: Relation of pancreatic duct hyperplasia to carcinoma. *Cancer* 43: 1418–1428, 1979.

12. Foote A, Simpson JS, Stewart RJ, Wakefield JSJ, Buchanan A, Gupta RK: Diagnosis of the rare solid and papillary epithelial neoplasm of the pancreas by fine needle aspiration cytology; Light and electron microscopy of a case. *Acta Cytol* 30: 519–522, 1986.

13. Chen KTK, Workman RD, Efird TA, Cheng AC: Fine needle aspiration cytology diagnosis of papillary tumor of the pancreas. *Acta Cytol* 30: 523–527, 1986.

14. Bell DA: Cytologic features of islet-cell tumors. *Acta Cytol* 31: 485–492, 1987.

15. Compagno J, Oertel JE: Microcystic neoplasms of the pancreas with overt and latent malignancy (cystadenocarcinoma and cystadenoma): A clinicopathologic study of 41 cases. *Am J Clin Pathol* 69: 573–580, 1978.

16. Vellet D, Leiman G, Mair S, Bilchik A: Fine needle aspiration cytology of mucinous cystadenocarcinoma of the pancreas. Further observations. *Acta Cytol* 32: 43–48, 1988.

17. Emmert GM, Bewtra C: Fine needle aspiration biopsy of mucinous cystic neoplasm of the pancreas: A case study. *Diagn Cytopathol* 2: 69–71, 1986.

18. Fond A, Bret PM, Bretagnolle M, Thiesse F, Marion D, Dubreuil A: Apport de l'èchographie et de la ponction guidèe percutanèe au diagnostic des tumeurs kystiques du pancrèas. A propos de 14 observations. *J Belge Radiol* 67; 277–284, 1984.

19. Tatsuta M, Iishi H, Ichii M, Noguchi S, Yamamoto R, Yamamura H, Okuda S: Values of carcinoembryonic antigen, elastase 1, and carbohydrate antigen determinant in aspirated pancreatic cystic fluid in the diagnosis of cysts of the pancreas. *Cancer* 57: 1836–1839, 1986.

20. Hancke S, Holm HH, Koch F: Ultrasonically guided percutaneous fine needle biopsy of the pancreas. *Surg Gynecol Obstet* 140: 361–364, 1975.

21. Smith EH, Bartrum RJ, Chang YC, et al.: Percutaneous aspiration biopsy of the pancreas under ultrasonic guidance. *N Engl J Med* 292: 825–828, 1975.

22. Haaga JR, Reich NE, Havrille TR, Alfide RJ: Interventional CT scanning. *Radiol Clin N Am* 15: 449–456, 1977.

23. Goldstein H, Zornoza J: Percutaneous transperitoneal aspiration biopsy of pancreatic masses. *Dig Dis* 23: 840–843, 1978.

24. Evander A, Ihse I, Lunderquist A, Tylen U, Akerman M: Percutaneous cytodiagnosis of carcinoma of the pancreas and bile duct. *Ann Surg* 188: 90–92, 1978.

25. McLoughlin MJ, Ho CS, Langer B, McHattie J, Tao LC: Fine needle aspiration biopsy of malignant le-

sions in and around the pancreas. *Cancer* 41: 2413–2419, 1978.

26. Yamanaka T, Kimura K: Differential diagnosis of pancreatic mass lesion with percutaneous fine needle aspiration biopsy under ultrasonic guidance. *Dig Dis* 24: 694–699, 1979.

27. Ferrucci JT, Wittenberg J, Muller PR, Simeone JF, Harbin WP, Kirkpatrick RH, Taft PD: Diagnosis of abdominal malignancy by radiologic fine needle aspiration biopsy. *AJR* 134: 323–330, 1980.

28. Mitty HA, Efremidis SC, Yeh HC: Impact of fineneedle biopsy on management of patients with carcinoma of the pancreas. *AJR* 137: 1119–1121, 1981.

29. Bret PM, Fond A, Bretagnolle M, Barral F, Labadie M: Percutaneous fine needle biopsy (PFNB) of intra-abdominal lesions. *Eur J Radiol* 2: 322–328, 1982.

30. Hovdenak N, Lees WR, Pereira J, Beilby JOW, Cotton PB: Ultrasound guided percutaneous fine-needle aspiration cytology in pancreatic cancer. *Br Med J* 285: 1183–1184, 1982.

31. Sundaram M, Wolverson MK, Heiberg E, Pilla T, Vas WG, Shields JB: Utility of CT guided abdominal aspiration procedures. *AJR* 139: 1111–1115, 1982.

32. Grant EG, Richardson JD, Smirniotopoulos JG, Jacobs NM: Fine-needle biopsy directed by real-time sonography: Technique and accuracy. *AJR* 141: 29–32, 1983.

33. Schwerk WB, Durr HK, Schmitz-Moormann P: Ultrasound guided fine needle biopsies in pancreatic and hepatic neoplasms. *Gastrointest Radiol* 8: 219–225, 1983.

34. Harter LP, Moss AA, Goldberg HI, Gross BH: CT guided fine needle aspirations for diagnosis of benign and malignant disease. *AJR* 140: 363–367, 1983.

35. Hancke S, Holm HH, Koch F: Ultrasonically guided punture of solid pancreatic masses lesions. In Holm HH, Kvist Kristensen J et al.: *Interventional Ultrasound.* Copenhagen, Munksgaard, pp 100–105, 1985.

36. Hall-Craggs MA, Lees WR: Fine-needle aspiration biopsy: Pancreatic and biliary tumors. *AJR* 147: 399–403, 1986.

37. Hajdu EO, Kumari-Sabaiya S, Philips G: Ultrasonically guided percutaneous aspiration biopsy of the pancreas. *Sem Diag Path* 3: 166–175, 1986.

38. Fekete PS, Nunez C, Pitlik DA: Fine needle aspiration biopsy of the pancreas. A study of 61 cases. *Diagn Cytopathol* 2: 301–306, 1986.

39. Wittenberg J, Mueller PR, Ferrucci JT, et al.: Percutaneous core biopsy of abdominal tumors using 22 gauge needles: Further observations. *AJR* 139: 75–80, 1982.

40. Chagnon S, Cochan D, Priollet B, Jacquenod P, Vilgrain V, Blery M: Intèrêt de la cytoponction associèe á la microbiopsie dans les masses solides du pancrèas. *J Radiol* 68: 733–736, 1987.

41. Bret PM, Fond A, Casola G, Bretagnolle M, Bret P, Germain-Lacour MJ, Labadie M, Buffard P: Abdominal lesions: A prospective study of clinical efficacy of percutaneous fine needle biopsy. *Radiology* 159: 345–346, 1986.

42. Evans WK, Ho CS, McLoughlin MJ, Tao LC: Fatal necrotizing pancreatitis following fine needle aspi-

ration biopsy of the pancreas. *Radiology* 141: 61–62, 1981.

43. Mueller PR, Miketic LM, Simeone JF, Silverman SG, Saini S, Wittenberg J, Hahn PF, Steiner E, Forman BH: Severe acute pancreatitis after percutaneous biopsy of the pancreas. *AJR* 151: 493–494, 1988.

44. Smith EH: Hazard of fine needle aspiration biopsy. *Ultrasound Med Biol* 10(5): 629–634, 1984.

45. Smith EH: Is percutaneous biopsy a hazard? An update (abstr.). Presented at the annual meeting of the Radiologic Society of North America, Chicago, December 1987.

46. Livraghi T, Damascelli B, Lombardi C, Spagnoli I: Risk in fine needle abdominal biopsy. *JCU* 11: 77–81, 1983.

47. Bergenfeldt M, Genell S, Lindholm K, Ekberg O, Aspelin P: Needle tract seeding after percutaneous fine needle biopsy of pancreatic carcinoma. *Acta Chir Scand* 154: 77–79, 1988.

48. Rasleigh HJC, Russell RCG, Lees WR: Cutaneous seeding of pancreatic carcinoma by fine needle aspiration biopsy, *Br J Radiol* 59: 182–183, 1986.

49. Bradley EL, Clements JL, Gonzalez AC: The natural history of pancreatic pseudocysts: A unified concept of management. *Am J Surg* 137: 135–141, 1979.

50. Mullins RJ, Malangoni MA, Bergamini TM, Casey JM, Richardson JD: Controversies in the management of pancreatic pseudocysts. *Am J Surg* 155: 165–172, 1988.

50a.VanSonnenberg E, Wittich GR, Casola G, et al.: Percutaneous drainage of infected and noninfected pancreatic pseudocysts: Experience in 101 cases. *Radiology* 170: 757–761, 1989.

51. Nunez D Jr., Yrizarry JM, Russel E, Sadighi A, Casillas J, Guerra JJ Jr., Hutson DG: Transgastric drainage of pancreatic fluid collections. *AJR* 145: 815–818, 1985.

52. Sacks D, Robinson ML: Transgastric percutaneous drainage of pancreatic pseudocysts. *AJR* 151: 303–306, 1988.

53. Ho CS, Taylor B: Percutaneous transgastric drainage for pancreatic pseudocyst. *AJR* 143: 623–625, 1984.

54. Isaacs P, Pinder C, Jourdan M, Filipe I, Sladen G: Therapeutic aspiration of pseudocysts: A cautionary tale of the pancreas. *Am J Gastroenterol* 81: 1087–1090, 1986.

55. VanSonnenberg E, Wittich GR, Casola G et al.: Complicated pancreatic inflammatory disease: Diagnostic and therapeutic role of interventional radiology. *Radiology* 155: 335–340, 1985.

56. Barkin JS, Smith FR, Pereiras R Jr, Isikoff M, Levi J, Livingstone A, Hill M, Roger AI: Therapeutic percutaneous aspiration of pancreatic pseudocysts. *Dig Dis Sci* 26: 585–586, 1981.

57. Hancke S, Pedersen JF: Percutaneous puncture of pancreatic cysts guided by ultrasound. *Surg Gynecol Obstet* 142: 551–552, 1976.

58. Torres WE, Evert MB, Baumgartner BR, Bernardino ME: Percutaneous aspiration and drainage of pancreatic pseudocysts. *AJR* 147: 1007–1009, 1986.

59. Gandini G, Grosso M, Bonardi L, Cassinis MC, Regge D, Righi D: Results of percutaneous treatment of sixty-three pancreatic pseudocysts. *Ann Radiol* 31: 117–122, 1988.

60. Ho C-S: Percutaneous gastrostomy for jejunal feeding. *Radiology* 149: 595–596, 1983.

61. Kuligogowska E, Olson WL: Pancreatic pseudocysts drained through a percutaneous transgastric approach. *Radiology* 154: 79–82, 1985.

62. Matzinger FRK, Ho C-S, Yee AC, Gray RR: Pancreatic pseudocysts drained through a percutaneous transgastric approach: Further experience. *Radiology* 167: 431–434, 1988.

63. Quinn SF, Finnery R, Rosemurgy A, Pieck CG: Splenic artery pseudoaneurysm after placement of percutaneous transgastric catheter for a pancreatic pseudocyst. *AJR* 151: 495–496, 1988.

64. Hancke S, Henriksen FW: Percutaneous pancreatic cystogastrostomy guided by ultrasound scanning and gastroscopy. *Br J Surg* 72: 916–917, 1985.

65. Bernardino ME, Amerson JR: Percutaneous gastrocystostomy: A new approach to pancreatic pseudocyst drainage. *AJR* 143: 1096–1097, 1984.

66. Kozarek RA, Brayko CM, Harlan J, Sanowski RA, Cintora I, Kovac A: Endoscopic drainage of pancreatic pseudocysts. *Gastrointest Endosc* 31: 322–327, 1985.

67. Bucchi KN, Bowers JH, Dixon JA: Endoscopic pancreatic cystogastrostomy using the ND:YAG laser. *Gastrointest Endosc*32: 112–114, 1986.

68. Sahel J, Bastid C, Pellat B, Schurgers P, Sarles H: Endoscopic cystoduodenostomy of cysts of chronic calcifying pancreastitis: A report of 20 cases. *Pancreas* 2: 37–44, 1987.

69. Sahel J, Bastid C, Sarles H: Dèrivation endoscopique des pseudokystes et abcés au cours des pancrèatites aigues. *Gastroenterol Clin Biol* 431–435, 1988.

70. Freeny PC, Louis JP, Traverso LW, Ryan JA: Infected pancreatic fluid collection: Percutaneous catheter drainage. *Radiology* 167: 435–441, 1988.

71. Steiner E, Mueller PR, Hahn PF, Saini S, Simeone JF, Wittenberg J, Warshaw AL, Ferrucci JT Jr: Complicated pancreatic abscesses: Problems in interventional management. *Radiology* 167: 443–446, 1988.

72. Gerzof SG, Johnson WC, Robbins AH, Spechler SJ, Nabseth DC: Percutaneous drainage of infected pseudocysts. *Arch Surg* 119: 888–893, 1984.

73. Karlson KB, Martin EC, Fankuchen EI, Mattern RF, Schultz RW, Casarella WJ: Percutaneous drainage of pancreatic pseudocysts and abscesses. *Radiology* 142: 619–624, 1982.

74. Parulekar SG: Ultrasonic evaluation of the pancreatic duct. *J. Clin. Ultrasound* 8: 457–463, 1980.

75. Weinstein DP, Weinstein BJ: Ultrasonic demonstration of the pancreatic duct: An analysis of 41 cases. *Radiology* 130: 729–734, 1979.

76. Zimmon DS: Percutaneous pancreatography: Case report and presentation of technique. *Gastroenterology* 77: 1101–1104, 1979.

77. Makuuchi M, Bandai Y, Ito T, Wada T: Ultrasonographically guided percutaneous transhepatic cholangiography and percutaneous pancreatography. *Radiology* 134: 767–770, 1980.

78. Bret PM, Fond A, Bretagnolle M, Labadie M, Descos L, Lambert R, Brette R, Bret P, Buffard P: La wirsungographie transcutanèe sous repèrage

èchographique en temps rèel. *JEMU* 2: 133–136, 1981.

79. Ohto M, Karasawa E, Tsuchiya Y, Kimura K, Saisho H, Ono T, Okuda F: Ultrasonographically guided percutaneous contrast medium injection and aspiration biopsy using a real-time puncture transducer. *Radiology* 136: 171–176, 1980.

80. Matter D, Spinelli G, Warter P: Ultrasonically guided percutaneous pancreatography. *J Clin Ultrasound* 11: 401–404, 1983.

81. Cooperberg PL, Cohen MM, Graham M: Ultrasonographically guided percutaneous pancreatography: Report of two cases. *Am J Roentgenol* 132: 662–663, 1979.

82. Matter D, Bret PM, Valette PJ, Fond A: Pancreatic duct: US-guided percutaneous opacification. *Radiology* 163: 635–636, 1987.

83. Lees WR, Heron CW: US-guided percutaneous pancreatography: Experience in 75 patients. *Radiology* 165: 809–813, 1987.

84. Wong DC, Schuman BM, Grodsinsky C: The value of endoscopic retrograde cholangiopancreatography in the surgical management of chronic pancreatitis. *Am J Gastroenterol* 73: 353–356, 1980.

85. Matter D, Adloff M, Warter P: Ultrasonographically guided percutaneous opacification of a pancreaticojejunostomy. *Radiology* 148: 218, 1983.

86. Gobien RP, Stanley JH, Anderson MC, Vujic I: Percutaneous drainage of pancreatic duct for treating acute pancreatitis. *AM J Gastroenterol* 141: 795–796, 1983.

87. Huibregts K, Schneider B, Vrij AA, Tytgat GNJ: Endoscopic pancreatic drainage in chronic pancreatitis. *Gastrointest Endosc* 36: 9–15, 1988.

88. McCarthy J, Geenen JE, Hogan WJ: Preliminary experience with endoscopic stent placement in benign pancreatic diseases. *Gastrointest Endosc* 34: 16–18, 1988.

14 Percutaneous Gastrostomy

Gerhard Wittich
Eric vanSonnenberg
Hans Jantsch

Surgical gastrostomy was described by Egeberg in 1841 (1). Early experience demonstrated a fairly significant mortality rate. With refinement in surgical techniques, complications have become less frequent, but they are still appreciable; possible complications include pneumonia, peritonitis, shock, pulmonary aspiration, catheter dislodgement, and hemmorhage. These problems are attributable in part to the poor condition of the patients in whom the procedure is performed. Frequently they are debilitated, undernourished, and poor operative risks. Surgical gastrostomy performed under general anesthesia thus is a high risk in some patients, and the alternative—surgical gastrostomy under local anesthesia—is associated with poor surgical exposure and lack of patient cooperation. Surgical gastrostomy requires general anesthesia in 23% to 66% of patients, has a morbidity of 7% to 15.7% and an operative mortality of 2% to 6% (2–4).

Percutaneous gastrostomy is routinely performed under local anesthesia with mild intravenous sedation, has a morbidity of less than 8%, and no procedure-related fatal complication has been reported (5–13). The main indication is enteric feeding in patients with malignant tumors obstructing the upper alimentary tract or with uncorrectable dysphagia secondary to neurological disorders such as stroke. Another common indication is gastric or intestinal decompression in patients with partial small bowel obstruction (9–11). Percutaneous gastrostomy can be performed by a radiologist or an endoscopist. The endoscopic technique implies percutaneous puncture of the stomach after insertion of a gastroscope. A guidewire is then advanced through the needle, grasped under endoscopic control, and pulled back through the esophagus and mouth. A tube is fed over the guidewire through the esophagus into the stomach and is pushed and pulled through the anterior gastric and abdominal wall. This is a simple, safe, and fast procedure which does not require radiologic imaging. It has two disadvantages. First, it is often not feasible in patients with high-grade malignant obstruction of the hypopharynx or the esophagus. Second, jejunal placement of catheters, which is desirable in patients with gastroesophageal reflux and a tendency for aspiration, may be difficult without fluoroscopic and radiological support.

Radiological gastrostomy can be performed both in patients with and without significant obstruction of the esophagus. In addition, it is usually easy to advance a catheter through the pylorus into the jejunum for enteric feeding or the decompression of the small bowel.

Technique

Radiological gastrostomy is essentially a fluoroscopic technique. Fluoroscopic guidance is important in localizing the transverse colon, which should not be trangressed. The

193

transverse colon is identified radiographically by gas or by water-soluble contrast medium. Distension of the stomach greatly facilitates percutaneous placement of a catheter. We have used several techniques; the most common and efficient is distension of the stomach by air after advancing the nasogastric tube into the stomach. In cases of high-grade obstruction of the esophagus, the use of a curved-tip catheter and a floppy-tip or J-shaped guidewire may be required to cross the stricture and to advance the catheter into the stomach. Optimal distension can be achieved by using an intragastric balloon attached to the tip of a nasogastric tube. A balloon distended by dilute contrast material provides an excellent target for puncture of the stomach, and is very helpful if single-stick trocar technique for placement of a gastrostomy tube is intended (Fig. 14.1). Thus, percutaneous gastrostomy can be performed under sonographic guidance alone (Fig. 14.2) and it can be performed at the bedside. Balloon disten-

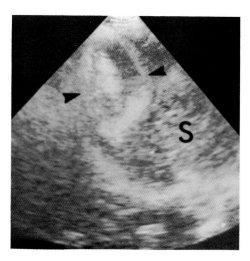

Figure 14.2. Intragastric balloon—sonographic guidance. Parasagittal sonogram in left upper quadrant of a dog demonstrates an intragastic balloon (*arrowheads*) that has been partially distended with 50 cc of water. The stomach (S) contains additional water for optimal distension. This method is partially helpful for trocar puncture under sonographic guidance (Reproduced with permission from Van-Sonnenberg E et al.: Percutaneous gastrostomy and gastroenterostomy: 2. Clinical experience. *AJR* 146:581–586, 1986, © American Roentgen Ray Society.)

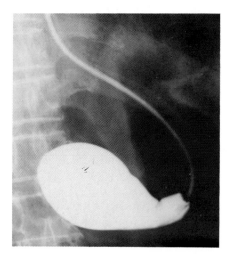

Figure 14.1. Intragastric balloon support—fluoroscopic guidance. A balloon has been attached to the tip of a nasogastric tube. The balloon distended by contrast material represents an easy target for percutaneous puncture under fluoroscopic guidance. (Reproduced with permission from VanSonnenberg E et al.: Percutaneous gastrostomy and gastroenterostomy: 2. Clinical experience. *AJR* 146: 581–586, 1986, © American Roentgen Ray Society.)

sion however, has a few disadvantages. In patients with obstructing head and neck tumors, attempts to pass a nasogastric tube with a large deflated balloon at its tip may compromise the upper airways and may be technically impossible. In these situations, partial distension of the stomach can be achieved by encouraging the patient to swallow water-soluble contrast material and carbon dioxide-releasing granules. If this is contraindicated because of potential aspiration in the airways, fine-needle puncture of the stomach and injection of contrast material may be necessary.

Glucagon (0.5 to 1 mg intravenously) is routinely used to augment gastric distension, unless this is achieved by a balloon. Glucagon reduces gastric peristalsis and thereby reduces the escape of air through the pylorus into the duodenum.

The site of skin puncture is determined by

the anatomic position of the distended stomach, the transverse colon, and the inferior margin of the liver as outlined by ultrasonography. The inferior epigastric artery—which is of concern for percutaneous punctures in the lower abdomen—is divided into multiple small branches above the umbilicus. These vessels have a diameter of 1 mm or less, and are therefore insignificant for percutaneous intervention in the upper abdomen, unless they serve as major collateral pathways in patients with aortic occlusion.

Xylocaine is used for local anesthesia, a skin nick is made with a No. 11 scalpel blade, and the soft tissues are dissected bluntly and deeply. We have used the trocar technique in conjunction with intragastric balloon support for single-stick insertion of a gastrostomy tube. However, our standard procedure now is the Seldinger technique starting with puncture of the stomach distended by air, using an 18-guage needle. We now routinely use three or four T-fasteners for fixation of the stomach to the anterior abdominal wall. This technique has several advantages: coaxial dilatation and insertion of 16 F feeding tubes (Fig. 14.3) can easily be achieved, whereas larger dilators and catheters have a tendency to push away the gastric wall, rather than entering the stomach, if the stomach is freely mobile within the peritoneal cavity. Second, the puncture needle can easily be directed into the gastric antrum and guidewires and catheters can be suc-

cessfully manipulated through the pylorus into the duodenum and jejunum. Without gastric fixation this is possible, although guidewires have a tendency to recoil in the gastric fundus (Fig. 14.4). Thirdly, gastric fixation reduces the likelihood of leakage of gastric contents into the peritoneal cavity.

After catheter insertion, we use the nasogastric tube for gastric decompression and remove it within 24 hours.

Role of Ultrasonography

Ultrasonography has two potential functions in assisting percutaneous gastrostomy: preprocedure localization for parenchymal organs in the upper abdomen and direct sonographic guidance for needle puncture of the stomach.

Preprocedure Localization of Parenchymal Organs

The inferior margin of the left lobe of the liver is typically located between the anterior abdominal wall and a variable portion of the gastric antrum and corpus (Fig. 14.5 A). It is important to realize that the position of the lesser curvature of the stomach as outlined by a plain radiograph of the abdomen or by fluoroscopy usually is not identical with the inferior margin of the left lobe of the liver. The latter can readily be localized by ultrasonography. Thus, we routinely ap-

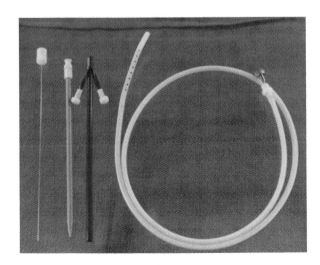

Figure 14.3. Instruments used for percutaneous gastrostomy. This set consists of an 18-gauge needle, a 16 F dilator with peel-away sheath and a soft 16 F feeding tube with sufficient length for transgastric intubation of the jejunum. (Reproduced with permission from VanSonnenberg E et al.: Percutaneous gastrostomy and gastroenterostomy: 2. Clinical experience. *AJR* 146:581–586, 1986, © American Roentgen Ray Society.)

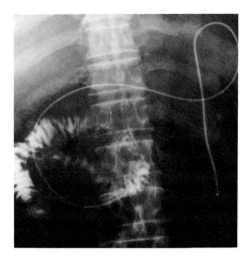

Figure 14.4. Percutaneous gastrojejunostomy. After successful puncture of the stomach, a guidewire and catheter have been advanced through the pylorus into the duodenum and the first jejunal loop. Note coiling of the catheter in the gastric fundus. This does not preclude successful canalization of the pylorus but makes this more difficult. (Reproduced with permission from VanSonnenberg E et al.: Percutaneous gastrostomy and gastroenterostomy: 2. Clinical experience. *AJR* 146:581–586, 1986, © American Roentgen Ray Society.)

ply sonographic localization of the liver and mark the caudal edge of the left lobe on the patient's skin prior to selecting the puncture site for gastrostomy (Fig. 14.5 B) Other abnormalities that might influence the selection of the optimal puncture site, such as the presence of splenomegaly or an abdominal aortic aneurysm, are readily detectable by ultrasonography. Although it is not reported in the literature, we consider inadvertent puncture of the left lobe of the liver a potential complication of radiological percutaneous gastrostomy. This can easily be avoided by sonographic localization prior to needle puncture.

Direct Sonographic Guidance for Needle Puncture of the Stomach

We have performed laboratory studies on cadavers demonstrating the feasibility of sonographic puncture of the stomach (8). This was done after inserting a balloon attached

to the tip of a nasogastric tube through the esophagus into the stomach and then distending the balloon with fluid. The purpose of this procedure was to evaluate the feasibility of sonographic guidance for bedside percutaneous gastrostomy. We prefer fluoroscopic guidance for the reasons outlined above. And we have not yet performed percutaneous gastrostomy exclusively under sonographic guidance in patients.

In one patient, we attempted direct percutaneous jejunostomy using sonographic guidance. While fluid-filled bowel loops could be outlined sonographically, we were unable to insert a guidewire and a catheter into the lumen of these nondilated, freely mobile bowel loops. We have performed several successful direct jejunostomies under fluoroscopic guidance using intraluminal balloon support. We have also been successful in gaining direct access to the retroperitoneal portion of the duodenum and to jejunal loops that were fixed by adhesions.

Through gastrostomy access, feeding may be accomplished in the stomach, the duodenum, or the jejunum. We prefer small bowel position of the catheters for three reasons. 1. Alimentation can be initiated immediately after placement of the tube—particularly if the chance of gastric leakage is eliminated by fixation of the stomach with T-fasteners. 2. The possibility of gastroesophogeal reflux is minimized, which is of particular importance in patients with swallowing disorders. 3. There is an extra measure of anchoring and safety with the more distally seated catheter. Gastroenterostomy tubes also may be used for enteric decompression in patients with chronic partial small bowel obstruction, as with advanced ovarian carcinoma.

Complications

Percutaneous gastrostomy has few complications. We have observed dislodgment of the catheter into the peritoneal cavity in 4% of patients. This caused local peritonitis in one patient who was treated surgically. In the remaining patients, this was detected

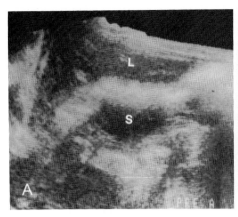 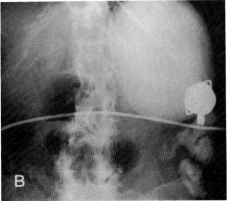

Figure 14.5. Preprocedure localization of the optimal skin entrance site for percutaneous gastrostomy. **A**, Left parasaggital sonogram outlines the fluid-filled stomach (*S*) posterior to the left lobe of the liver (*L*). The inferior margin of the liver was marked on the patient's skin. **B**, Radiograph demonstrates the inferior margin of the liver (curved metal rod) as determined by ultrasonography. It also indicates the position of the transverse colon and of an intragastric balloon distended by dilute contrast material. This patient had received intraperitoneal chemotherapy for advanced ovarian carcinoma. (Reproduced with permission from VanSonnenberg E et al.: Percutaneous gastrostomy and gastroenterostomy: 2. Clinical experience. *AJR* 146:581–586, 1986, © American Roentgen Ray Society.)

before feeding was initiated and was corrected by reinsertion of a catheter into the stomach and jejunum. The problem of tube dislocation has been eliminated since the routine use of T-fasteners for fixation of the stomach to the anterior abdominal wall. A small amount of hemorrhage into the stomach has been observed in a few patients who did not require further treatment. We have observed major respiratory distress in one patient due to sedation and attempts at passing a nasogastric tube and balloon past a high-grade obstruction of the hypopharynx. No fatal complications have occurred.

Summary

Percutaneous gastrostomy and gastroenterostomy for feeding or enteric decompression is a safe and effective radiological method. The routine use of T-fasteners has eliminated the risk of tube dislodgment in our experience. Ultrasonography plays a limited—but not unimportant—role in assisting percutaneous gastrostomy. We recommend preprocedure localization of the inferior edge of the liver prior to fluoroscopic puncture of the stomach. Potentially, sonographic guidance might be useful for bedside gastrostomy by trocar puncture of a distended intragastric balloon.

ACKNOWLEDGEMENT

Our appreciation to Alice Mullins and Deborah Suslovic for preparation of the manuscript.

REFERENCES

1. Egeberg CA: Om behandlingen af impenetrable stricturer i madroret (oesophagus). *Norsk Mag Laegevidensk* 2:97–107, 1841.
2. Wasiljew BK et al.: Feeding gastrostomy: Complications and mortality. *Am J Surg* 143:194–195, 1982.
3. Miller RE et al.: Percutaneous endoscopic gastrostomy—procedure of choice. *Ann Surg* 204: 543–546, 1986.
4. Ruge J, Vasquez RM: An analysis of the advantages of STAMM and percutaneous endoscopic gastrostomy. *Surg Gynecol Obstet* 162:13–16, 1986.
5. Gauderer MWL et al.: Gastrostomy without laparotomy: A percutaneous endoscopic technique. *J Pediatr Surg* 15:872–875, 1980.
6. Ponsky JL et al.: Percutaneous endoscopic gastrostomy: Review of 150 cases. *Arch Sur* 118:913–914, 1983.
7. Ho C et al.: Percutaneous gastrostomy for enteral feeding. *Radiology* 156:349–351, 1985.
8. VanSonnenberg E et al.: Percutaneous gastrostomy and gastroenterostomy: 1. Techniques derived from laboratory evaluation. *AJR* 146:577–580, 1986.

9. VanSonnenberg E et al.: Percutaneous gastrostomy and gastroenterostomy: 2. Clinical experience. *AJR*146:581–586, 1986.
10. Malone JM et al.: Palliation of small bowel obstruction by percutaneous gastrostomy in patients with progressive ovarian carcinoma. *Obstet Gynecol* 68: 431–433, 1986.
11. Wittich GR, et al.: Percutaneous gastroenterostomy. *Radiologe* 5:221–224, 1987.
12. Wills JS, Oglesby JT: Percutaneous gastrostomy. *Radiology* 167:41–43, 1988.
13. Brown AS et al.: Controlled percutaneous gastrostomy: Nylon T-fastener for fixation of the anterior gastric wall. *Radiology* 158:543–545, 1986.

15 Urinary Tract

DANIEL J. LINDSAY
EDWARD A. LYONS
CLIFFORD S. LEVI

Introduction

With the advances recently made in all of the imaging modalities of the genitourinary system, many disease entities and their extent can be diagnosed sooner and more accurately. In particular, current imaging modalities can be used to direct the acquisition of material for biochemical, bacteriologic, cytologic, or histologic analysis. Ultrasound alone or in combination with other imaging modalities has a role in the diagnosis and treatment of genitourinary infections, neoplasms, and both traumatic and surgical complications. Although dependent upon local expertise, ultrasound is often uniquely suited to interventional procedures because of its biologic safety, low cost, portability, and capacity to display both the instrumenting device and the pathologic process.

Renal Cystic Masses:

Suspected space-occupying renal masses are a common problem. Eighty to eighty-five per cent of asymptomatic space occupying lesions represent simple renal cysts (1). Ultrasound has a 90% to 98% confidence level in detecting renal cysts (2–4).

The sonographic criteria for a simple cyst are:

1. No internal echoes;
2. Smooth well defined walls;
3. Good posterior acoustic enhancement;
4. No solid component;
5. No thick septa.

If a renal cyst meets the criteria for a simple renal cyst and the patient is asymptomatic, no further investigation need be performed.

If the patient is symptomatic or the criteria for a simple cyst cannot be met, ultrasound can be used to easily guide the percutaneous placement of a small (20- to 22-gauge) needle for diagnostic aspiration of cyst fluid. Cystic masses that should be avoided because the diagnosis can be made without resorting to aspiration biopsies include calyceal diverticula, arteriovenous malformations, and vascular aneurysms (Fig. 15.1; 2) Calyceal diverticular often have a characteristic appearance on ultrasound, computed tomography (CT), or plain film radiology. Conventional pulsed or color Doppler analysis, contrast-enhanced CT or nuclear medicine renal scans may be helpful in diagnosing arteriovenous malformations and vascular aneurysms. Indications for percutaneous aspiration of a simple cyst include a cyst with:

1. Thick or irregular wall;
2. Wall calcification;
3. Internal echoes or septations;
4. Conflicting imaging results;
5. Solid mass arising from the wall.

The purpose of the aspiration is to differentiate a simple cyst of atypical appearance from an infected or malignant cystic lesion.

199

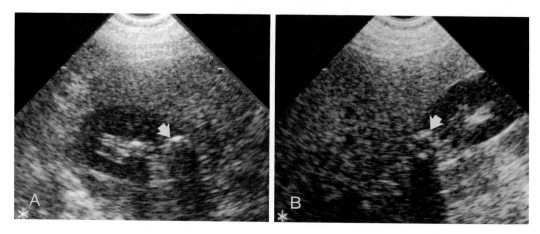

Figure 15.1. Transverse **A**, and oblique **B**, images of the kidney demonstrating a renal artery aneurysm (*arrows*) simulating a peripherally calcified renal cyst.

TECHNIQUE

Ultrasound-guided percutaneous fine-needle aspiration is a relatively simple procedure. The patient is positioned in a supine, prone, or oblique position to facilitate the most direct access to the renal cyst. If possible, a subcostal location for needle entry is marked on the skin. A subcostal posterolateral approach is preferred because the needle tract remains retroperitoneal in location, avoiding the peritoneal cavity or pleural space. It is important to avoid breaching the pleural space or peritoneal cavity at all times but especially if there is suspicion of an infected renal cyst. The needle entry point is marked and the skin is cleansed with an antiseptic solution. A local anesthetic is instilled into the subcutaneous and intradermal tissues. If the lesion is superficial and easily accessible, local anesthetic may not be necessary. The patient is then requested to suspend respiration and, with aseptic technique, a 22-gauge thin-walled needle is directed into the cyst under ultrasonic guidance. If the cyst is large and superficial, the needle can be positioned into the cyst utilizing the skin mark and the predetermined depth. If the cyst is less accessible, direct needle visualization is preferred during cyst puncture.

Two variations of real-time needle guidance are used. The first is a commercially available biopsy guide on the transducer. A disadvantage of this technique is that a 20- or 22-gauge needle can deflect outside the imaging plane of the transducer (Fig. 15.2). In addition, the needle is relatively fixed, not allowing for needle movement with patient respiration. An alternative approach as explained in prior chapters, is the freehand method of needle guidance. This allows for continued visualization with needle deflection and respiratory movement. Very few

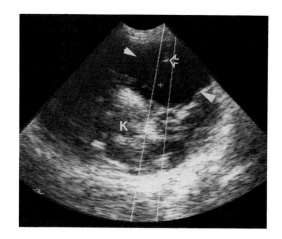

Figure 15.2. Renal cyst aspiration. Renal cyst puncture was performed in this symptomatic patient using a biopsy guidance attachment. The echogenic needle (*open arrow*) is noted between the biopsy guidance attachment passing into the renal cyst (*arrowheads*) (K = kidney). Courtesy of John P. McGahan, M.D., Sacramento, California.

complications occur as a result of a percutaneous aspiration with a 20- or 22-gauge needle. Potential complications include infection, pneumothorax, and bleeding, which is usually manifested as mild transient hematuria. The fluid from a simple cyst is usually clear or, if bloody, clears rapidly with aspiration.

Investigation of aspirated cyst fluid includes culture and sensitivity, lipids (Sudan stain), LDH, protein, and glucose. A small amount of protein ($<2.5g/dl$) and LDH (<25.5 mU/liter) may be obtained from simple cysts (5, 6). LDH is known to be associated with renal neoplasms and may be a specific tumor marker (7). However, the single most valuable test performed on the aspirated fluid is cytology (8). In a hemorrhagic cyst, the confidence level of cytology predicting a benign lesion is 80% to 85% (1). If there is only a limited amount of fluid aspirated, cytology is the investigation of choice because it is also helpful in identifying cellular material characteristic of an infected cyst. It is important to remember that although the occurrence is uncommon, cytologic analysis can occasionally be falsely positive for malignancy (8). There is a very high retrieval rate of malignancy in all types of abnormal renal cysts, with the exception of multiloculated cysts, hematomas, and cystic nephromas (1). Although common in the past, installation of contrast material into the cyst postaspiration to define the architecture of the wall is now seldom performed.

In specific clinical settings, some patients can benefit from drainage of simple renal cysts. Simple cysts can cause pain (9) and have been associated in the pathogenesis of hypertension (9, 10). Percutaneous aspiration in a patient who is experiencing pain will help to determine if there is a causal relationship between the two. In patients with increasing hypertension and large renal cysts or documented elevated serum renin levels, percutaneous cyst drainage may have long-term therapeutic benefits (10–12). Renal cysts often recur after aspiration, but there has been recent reported success in the ablation of renal cysts with the instillation of sclerosing agents (13–15). In the future,

ablation of renal cysts may become an accepted part of the management of symptomatic renal cysts. In the situation of an infected cyst or carbuncle, percutaneous aspiration and drainage is part of currently accepted management when combined with appropriate antibiotics (Fig. 15.3; 16).

Solid Renal Masses

Angiography, ultrasound, computed tomography, nuclear medicine, magnetic resonance imaging, and percutaneous aspiration biopsy all have a role in the investigation of solid parenchymal renal masses. These modalities should be used in combination so that pseudotumors, such as an hypertrophied column of Bertin or lobar nephronia are not biopsied or surgically removed. The vast majority of neoplastic renal masses can be accurately diagnosed with current imaging modalities without resorting to percutaneous aspiration or core biopsy (1). The conventional management of a solid renal mass is nephrectomy with preservation of an intact Gerota's fascia. Appropriate surgical and clinical management, however, may require the additional information provided by percutaneous aspiration biopsy (Figs. 15.4 and 15.5). These situations include differentiation of primary renal neoplasms from metastases or the diagnosis of an extensive tumor prior to administration of chemotherapy or vascular embolization (17). Percutaneous aspiration biopsy is also helpful in the diagnosis of lymphoma, chloroma, fibroma and lipoma (1). For instance obtaining a diagnosis of lymphoma of the kidney may change therapy from surgery to systemic treatment with chemotherapy.

TECHNIQUE

The technique of percutaneous aspiration of a solid renal mass is similar to that described for renal cyst aspiration, on page 200. Unlike renal cyst aspiration however, a wide variety of needles are used in different centers to obtain aspirated material for cytology or core specimens. Needle selection

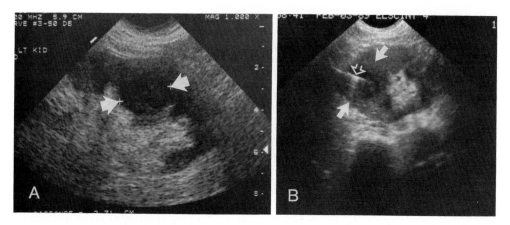

Figure 15.3. Renal carbuncle in a febrile patient. **A,** Hypoechoic mass (*arrows*) demonstrates internal echoes that are secondary to purulent material. **B,** Using the freehand method, a needle is inserted (*open arrows*) percutaneously into this renal carbuncle (*arrows*). A drainage catheter was left in place.

depends upon patient age, nature of suspected lesion, biopsy site, and radiologist's preference. Material aspirated with a 20- or 22-gauge needle is usually sufficient to characterize the nature of a solid renal mass (1). Air-dried slide specimens fixed at the time of the biopsy can help the cytopathologist in establishing the diagnosis of renal lymphoma. Although tumor seeding along the needle tract is exceedingly rare, some techniques still further decrease the risk of seeding in suspected neoplastic cystic or

solid masses. Erick K. Lang has described a modification of conventional cyst puncture technique in which an 18-gauge Seldinger needle is introduced into the perirenal space. Aspiration of the lesion is then performed with a 22-gauge needle introduced through the sheath. After removal of the 22-gauge needle, distilled water can then be injected through the 18-gauge sheath to lyse potentially implantable tumor cells (1). Core specimens can also be obtained with cutting 20-gauge needles provided the radiologist is

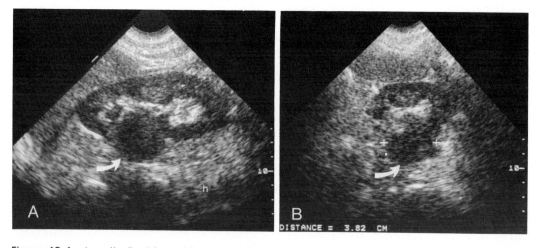

Figure 15.4. Longitudinal **A,** and transverse **B,** scans demonstrating a solid renal mass (*curved arrow*) in a patient with a known gastrointestinal primary neoplasm. Biopsy was performed to differentiate primary renal malignancy from metastases.

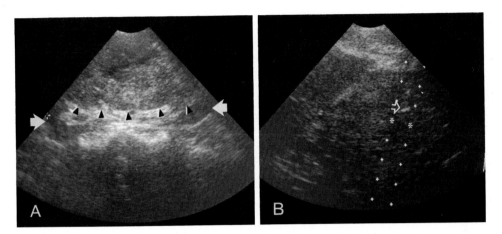

Figure 15.5. Renal cell carcinoma. **A,** Longitudinal ultrasound demonstrating large mass (*arrowheads*) that compresses the remaining normal kidney (*between arrows*). **B,** Using a needle guide attachment a small-bore needle (*open arrow*) is placed into this renal mass, which revealed renal cell carcinoma. Courtesy of John P. McGahan, M.D., Sacramento, California.

experienced. Although the risks of hemorrhage are higher with larger cutting needles, large cores of tissue are sometimes needed for histologic characterization. This is especially true in suspected lymphoma where a large amount of tissue is often needed to diagnose and subtype the tumor. The bowel can be punctured with a 22-gauge needle with relative impunity, but it must be avoided when a larger cutting needle is used. The pleura should always be avoided although the potential for pneumothorax is much greater with larger-bore needles. Platelet count, prothrombin time, and partial thromboplastin time should be measured before a large-core biopsy is performed. Anticoagulants should not be started for at least 12 hours after a biopsy (18). After a large-core needle biopsy, a limited ultrasound examination can be performed to assess for renal, subcapsular, perirenal, or collecting system hematomas (Fig. 15.6). Vital signs should be monitored for approximately 6 hours after the procedure.

Occasionally, it is difficult to determine if a mass in the upper pole of the kidney is renal or adrenal in origin (Fig. 15.7). As only 50% of patients with pheochromocytomas have the classic vascular episodes (18), 24-hour urinary vanillylmandelic acids or cat-

echolamines can help in detecting pheochromocytomas. Despite all precautions, however, an adrenal pheochromocytoma may be inadvertently biopsied. Although inadvertent percutaneous biopsy of a pheochromocytoma may be uneventful, manipulation of pheochromocytomas can result in both hypertensive and paradoxical hypotensive reactions (19–21). Should an acute hypertensive crisis occur, 5 mg of phentolamine administered intravenously can rapidly normalize the blood pressure. Intravenous titration of a solution contain-

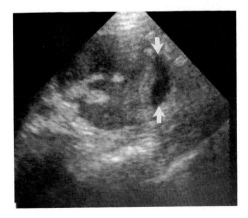

Figure 15.6. Transverse image of the kidney demonstrating a subcapsular hematoma (*arrows*) that occurred after a renal biopsy.

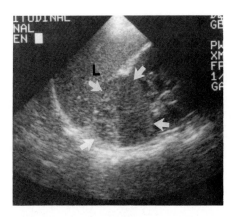

Figure 15.7. Longitudinal scan of the right upper quadrant of the abdomen demonstrating an apparent upper pole renal mass (*arrows*) that was in fact adrenal in origin (*L*=liver).

ing 20 mg of phentolamine in 500 cc of 5% dextrose in water is used to maintain a stable blood pressure. Aliquots of 1 mg of intravenous propranolol is used to control adrenaline-induced cardiac arrhythmias or paradoxical hypotensive episodes. Propranolol should not be used in isolation, however, because of the risk of paradoxical hypertension. Physicians performing aspiration biopsies must be familiar with the management of hypertensive crises.

Parenchymal Abnormalities

Conventional renal imaging modalities, when combined with renal function studies and biochemistry, can be very accurate in diagnosing renal parenchymal abnormalities. Histologic examination of the renal parenchyma may be necessary, however, to determine the exact cause and extent of diminished renal function and thus to facilitate management.

Complications of renal core biopsy include renal, subcapsular, perirenal and collecting system hematomas, urinary leaks and fistulas, AVMs, and arteriocalyceal fistulas (22–26). Ultrasound can be used to direct the core-biopsy needle to avoid the renal pedicle and collecting system. When a

biopsy of the native kidney is performed, a posterior approach is used to biopsy the lateral aspect of the lower pole of the kidney (Fig. 15.8). The technique of renal core biopsy is similar to that described for the biopsy of a solid renal mass, above.

Percutaneous Nephrostomy

Percutaneous nephrostomy is a simple, effective method of creating temporary supravesicular urinary diversion. The procedure is effective in the management of patients with urinary tract obstruction, leaks, or fistulas (Figs. 15.9 and 15.10). Percutaneous nephrostomy also provides access to the urinary system for endourologic procedures. Goodwin and colleagues originally described a technique for percutaneous nephrostomy in 1959 (27). More recently, ultrasound has gained wide acceptance as either the initial or the primary imaging modality of choice for the placement of a percutaneous nephrostomy drainage tube (28–30; Fig. 15.10).

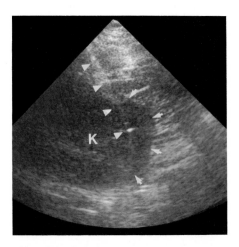

Figure 15.8. Renal core biopsy. 16-gauge needle (*arrowheads*) was placed percutaneously under freehand ultrasound guidance with the tip of the needle noted within the lower pole of the kidney (*arrows*), (*K* = kidney). Courtesy of John P. McGahan, M.D., Sacramento, California.

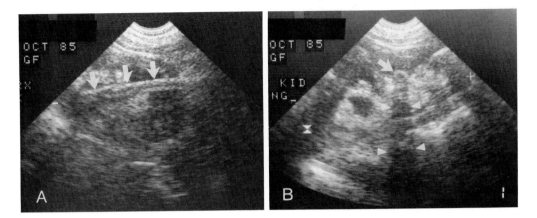

Figure 15.9. Transverse **A**, and longitudinal **B**, scans demonstrating a percutaneous nephrostomy tube (*arrows*) positioned in the renal collecting system. There is no evidence of hydronephrosis or perirenal fluid collections. Note distal acoustic shadowing (*arrowheads*) helping to identify the tube on the longitudinal scan.

TECHNIQUE

As in any interventional procedure, normal clotting parameters should be confirmed and the patient should be on appropriate antibiotic coverage. Many techniques are commonly employed in the placement of percutaneous nephrostomy tubes. Ultrasound is proposed by some authors as being the imaging modality of choice for identification of the dilated renal collecting system and placement of the nephrostomy tube (28). Depending upon local expertise, ultrasound is used in isolation or in conjunction with fluoroscopy for percutaneous nephrostomy tube placement. If the procedure is performed with the assistance of fluoroscopy, the patient is placed in a prone position and ultrasound is used to locate the renal pelvis. Calculation of the depth and direction of the nephrostomy approach is made and, utilizing a modified Seldinger technique, a 22-gauge needle is inserted through a posterior calyx into the renal pelvis (Fig. 15.10). Although ultrasound can usually identify bowel adjacent to the kidney, a posterolateral approach is used to avoid puncture of the colon. An opening

pressure can be measured at this time to help confirm if obstruction is the cause of the hydronephrosis. This may be of particular value in a dilated collecting system in a

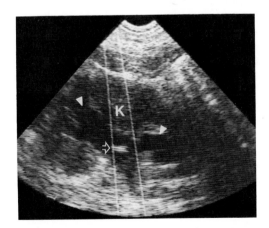

Figure 15.10. Nephrostomy. Using the biopsy guidance attachment, a needle is passed into the hydronephrotic kidney (*K*) with the needle tip (*open arrow*) visualized within the renal collecting structures (*arrowheads*). Nephrostomy tube was then placed under fluoroscopic control using the guidewire exchange technique. Courtesy of John P. McGahan, M.D., Sacramento, California.

transplanted kidney (31). A guidewire with a flexible tip is then inserted into the renal pelvis and the needle is removed.

There are several modifications used for the guidewire exchange technique. These would include initial puncture with a thin-wall 18-gauge needle. The advantage of this approach is that the needle accepts a 0.038-inch guidewire. However, the 18-gauge needle or an 18-gauge long dwell is more traumatic as an initial needle puncture than a 22-gauge needle. Therefore, some advocate use of a coaxial system with initial needle puncture within a 22-gauge needle and an 18-gauge needle placed coaxially over the 22-gauge needle. The theoretical advantage of use of a small-bore needle for initial puncture is to minimize renal trauma. Finally, there are several commercially available systems that will allow initial puncture with a 22-gauge needle through which a small guidewire is placed. A dilator system that will allow passage of a larger guidewire (0.038) may be used for the guidewire exchange technique.

The percutaneous nephrostomy tract is then successively dilated to accommodate a nephrostomy drainage catheter. It is important that the guidewire selected have a flexible tip and a nonflexible shaft. The nonflexible portion of the guidewire should be positioned so that it is in the renal parenchyma. This facilitates dilation of the nephrostomy tract and tube placement. Nephrostomy tract dilation and nephrostomy tube insertion can be monitored either sonographically or fluoroscopically.

After decompression of the collecting system, contrast material is instilled through the nephrostomy tube to ensure adequate communication with the renal pelvis and to document any contrast extravasation. Many institutions use ultrasound alone in placing nephrostomy tubes, but it is recommended that a nephrostogram always be performed after the procedure. The nephrostomy tube is then either sutured to the skin surface or fixed with some other retention device (for example, Mylar disc). If it is anticipated that the nephrostomy tube may be in place for a long time, then a silicone nephrostomy tube should be considered because of its flexibility and greater patient tolerance (28).

An alternative and less common percutaneous nephrostomy technique is the use of one of the commercially available trocar nephrostomy sets. With this technique, under aseptic conditions, a trocar is inserted directly into the renal pelvis and an overlying sheath is advanced into the collecting system. This technique is generally faster than the modified Seldinger technique, although it is also more traumatic. Both the modified Seldinger technique and the trocar technique can be safe with experienced practitioners, but the modified Seldinger technique is more commonly practiced.

FETAL HYDRONEPHROSIS

With the advent of high-resolution real-time ultrasound, the identification of oligohydramnios and fetal hydronephrosis can be made. Oligohydramnios can result in fetal pulmonary dysmaturity that has a very high perinatal mortality. Prenatal urinary diversion techniques have been performed in utero in an attempt to decompress the fetal urinary system into the amniotic cavity. Ultrasound has been used to direct the placement of the diversion tubes into the dilated fetal bladder, ureter, or renal pelvis. Although there are many reports in literature of prenatal fetal urinary diversions, the complications are high and the management of these fetuses remains controversial. Before a urinary diversion procedure is performed, an accurate prenatal diagnosis of the site and cause of the fetal hydronephrosis is necessary. Recent articles, however, have demonstrated the difficulty of accurately diagnosing the correct cause of fetal hydronephrosis (32). In addition, complication rates are high with those procedures and only a limited number of fetuses have received documented improvement (33). Although ultrasound-guided placement of urinary diversion tubes may prove useful, a prospective study is needed to document what benefit can be anticipated before these procedures will be widely accepted.

Perinephric Fluid Collections

The location of perinephric and retroperitoneal fluid localization has been well described in the literature. The anatomic location of these fluid collections makes them most amenable to a retroperitoneal route of percutaneous drainage (34, 35; Fig.15.11) Computed tomography provides the most precise information with regard to the anatomic location of perinephric fluid collections because of its better resolution of fat and ability to differentiate bowel from gas containing abscesses. It may be difficult for ultrasound to define the extent of perinephric and retroperitoneal fluid collections and occasionally locate adjacent bowel. Despite these limitations, however, in experienced hands, ultrasound can provide rapid anatomic delineation of the fluid collection and guide catheter insertion. Fluid collections that occur in the perirenal and retroperitoneal space include abscesses, urinomas, lymphoceles, and hematomas. It may be difficult to differentiate between these collections without percutaneous aspiration. Perirenal urinomas can be readily treated with percutaneous drainage provided that no urinary obstruction is present.

Lymphoceles can also occur in the perinephric space, and are particularly prone to develop in post-renal-transplant patients. It has been estimated that up to 50% of renal transplant patients develop perirenal fluid collections; a large percentage of which are lymphoceles (36). Small asymptomatic perirenal fluid collections in the post transplant patient should be followed sonographically and not aspirated, because many of these collections will resolve spontaneously (37). If the fluid collection is complex or symptomatic, a percutaneous aspiration can be performed to determine its nature. As a general rule, lymphoceles should not be repeatedly drained percutaneously because of the risk of infection or the rare complication of fluid and electrolyte depletion (38). Although there are reports of successful use of sclerotherapy in the management of lymphoceles (39, 40), its use in perinephric locations has not been well established. Conventional management of lymphoceles is surgical intraperitoneal marsupialization. The only well-established indication for external drainage of a lymphocele is infection (40).

TECHNIQUE

For simple aspiration of perinephric fluid collections, the procedure follows the same principles as renal cyst aspiration. If place-

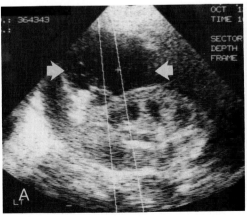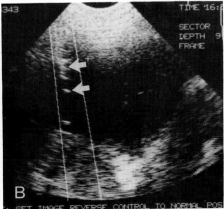

Figure 15.11. **A**, Ultrasonographic demonstration of a large perinephric abscess (*arrows*). **B**, Needle is placed (*arrows*) into the perinephric abscess using ultrasound biopsy guidance attachment. The needle was exchanged for a drainage catheter. Courtesy of John P. McGahan, M.D., Sacramento, California.

ment of an external drainage catheter is indicated, the size of the drainage catheter should be 8 F or larger depending upon the viscosity of the fluid to be drained. Establishment of an intravenous line and the administration of intravenous analgesics or sedatives prior to the procedure is often helpful in reducing patient pain and anxiety. The location of bowel, vascular structures, and pleural and peritoneal spaces must be noted prior to needle insertion. The subcutaneous, intradermal, and intervening tissues are infiltrated with xylocaine to provide local anaesthesia. A small incision is made and a needle is inserted into the fluid collection under ultrasonic guidance. A small amount of fluid is aspirated and sent for appropriate biochemical, cytologic, and bacteriologic investigations.

One of several different needle systems may be used for initial needle puncture, that is, 22- to 18-gauge coaxial system. After placement of the needle, a flexible tip 0.038-inch J wire is inserted through the needle into the cavity. The needle is then removed leaving the guidewire in place. Successfully larger dilators and eventually a drainage catheter are inserted over the guidewire. There are many available drainage catheters but those selected should be pliable and radiopaque. Many of these are outlined in the initial chapter and elsewhere throughout the text. There are a number of commercially available systems. These should have a catheter and cannula that can pass over a 0.038-inch guidewire. The cannula maintains the rigidity of the drainage tube to facilitate passage of the tube over the guidewire. The sideholes of the catheter should be confirmed to lie inside the cavity after insertion. The catheter is then sutured or fixed to the skin with a surface adhesive device. Saline irrigation of the catheter is performed on a routine basis to assist in drainage and maintain patency of the catheter. Although acetyl cystine is not commonly used, some authors have advocated its use to reduce the viscosity of high-viscosity fluid collections thereby improving drainage (35). If the fluid collection is large, multiseptated, or contains very viscous fluid, insertion of multiple catheters is advocated to ensure adequate drainage. An attempt should be made to completely drain the fluid collection (especially if it is an abscess) at the time of drainage tube insertion (18). The cavity size should be monitored on a biweekly basis with ultrasound, CT or fluoroscopy to ensure improvement.

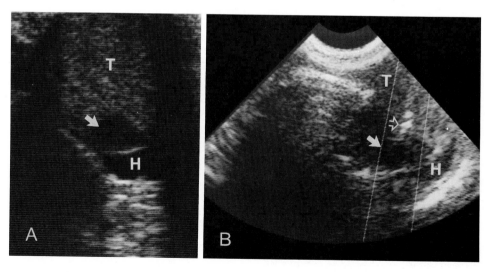

Figure 15.12. Testicular lymphoma. **A,** Ultrasound of the testes (*T*) demonstrating small hydrocele (*H*) and hypoechoic nodule noted within the testes (*arrow*). **B,** After a cutaneous nerve block using an ultrasound needle biopsy guide, the needle was placed (*open arrow*) into this hypoechoic testicular lymphoma (*arrow*). Courtesy of John P. McGahan, M.D., Sacramento, California.

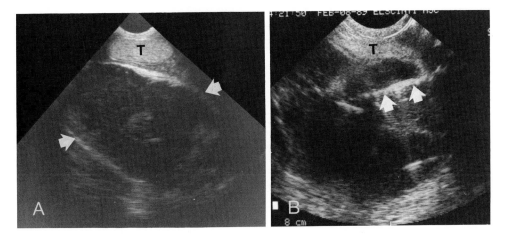

Figure 15.13. Testicular abscess. **A,** Longitudinal scan demonstrating testicle (*T*) and a large abscess posterior to the testicle (*arrows*). **B,** Using the freehand method, a trocar percutaneous drainage catheter (*arrows*) was placed into the abscess cavity.

Scrotal Masses

Scrotal and testicular abnormalities can be divided according to infectious, vascular (testicular torsion), traumatic, or neoplastic origin. Management of testicular and scrotal masses often depends upon the ability to differentiate the anatomic location of the mass. Ultrasound is readily suited to the visualization of small parts, such as the testicle and scrotal contents. the conventional management of primary testicular masses is usually surgical excision. In the past, characterization of a scrotal mass was often made at the time of surgery or upon histiopathologic examination of an excised scrotal mass or testicle. When combined with the clinical assessment, however, ultrasound can usually differentiate a testicular from a scrotal abnormality, often obviating the need for surgical exploration. Ultrasound can, as in other areas of the body, direct the percutaneous aspiration biopsy of both cystic and solid masses. This is useful when it is clinically necessary to differentiate primary from metastatic testicular tumors or when there is confusion between a neoplastic or inflammatory process (Figs. 15.12 and 15.13). Ultrasound can also be used in the placement of percutaneous drainage catheters in scrotal abscesses. The principles of diagnosis and abscess management are as previously described. Figure 15.13 demonstrates a large, complex, predominantly cystic scrotal abscess that was successfully managed with percutaneous catheter drainage. Ultrasound provides excellent visualization of testicular and scrotal masses and will undoubtedly provide an increasing role in the percutaneous diagnosis and management of infectious and neoplastic scrotal masses.

REFERENCES

1. Lang EK: Rental cyst puncture studies. *Urol Clin N Am* 14:91–102, 1987.
2. Morteza KE, Orlando FG, Morgantown WV: Comparison of various methods of diagnosis of renal cystic masses. *South Med J* 76:341–348, 1983.
3. Lingard DA, Lawson TL: Accuracy of ultrasound in predicting the nature of renal masses. *J Urol* 122:724, 1979.
4. Pollack HM, Banner MP, Arger PH, et al.: The accuracy of grey-scale renal ultrasonography in differentiating cystic neoplasms from benign cysts. *Radiology* 143:741, 1982.
5. Clayman RV, Williams RD, Fraley EE: Medical intelligence. *N Engl J Med* 300:72–74, 1979.
6. Lang EK, Johnson B, Chance HL, et al.: Assessment of avascular renal mass lesions. *South Med J* 65:1–10, 1972.
7. Phillips GN, Kumari-Subaiya S: Rental Cyst Puncture: LDH as a tumor marker. Presented at annual meeting of The Radiological Society of North America, Chicago, 1986.
8. Amis ES, Cronan JJ, Pfister RC: Needle puncture of cystic renal masses: A survey of the society of uroradiology. *AJR.* 1148:297–299, 1987.
9. Bennett WM, Elzinga L, Golper TA, et al.: Reduction of cyst volume for symptomatic management

of autosomal dominant polycystic kidney disease. *J Urol* 17:620–622, 1987.

10. Luscher TF, Wanner C, Siegenthaler W, et al.: Simple renal cyst and hypertension: cause or coincidence. *Clin Nephrol* 26:91–95, 1986.

11. Babka JC, Cohen MS, Sode J: Solitary renal cyst causing hypertension. *N Engl J Med* 291:343, 1974.

12. Churchill D, Kimoff R, Pinski M, et al.: Solitary intrarenal cyst: Correctable cause of hypertension. *Urology* 6:485, 1975.

13. Okaso A, Yamamoto H, Asari T, et al.: A new treatment of simple renal cyst: Percutaneous instillation of minocycline hydrochloride into simple renal cyst. *Hinyokika Kiyo* 33:1162–1166, 1987.

14. Wernecke K, Heckemann R, Rehwald U: Therapeutic results of ultrasonically guided kidney cyst punctures. *ROFO* 143:553–556, 1985.

15. Higashi Y, Kawamura J, Yoshida O, et al.: Percutaneous cyst puncture. *Hinyokika Kiyo* 31:1275–1279, 1985.

16. Kaver I, Merimsky E, Shilo R, et al.: Conservative approach in treating renal carbuncle. *Israel J Med Sci* 21:157–162, 1985.

17. Hattery RR, Williamson B, Stephens DH, et al.: Computed tomography of renal abnormalities. *Radiol Clin N Am* 15:401–418, 1977.

18. Murphy FB, Bernardino ME: Interventional computed tomography. *Cur Prob Diagn Radio* 17:125–154, 1988.

19. Cassola G, Nicolet V, vanSonnenberg, et al.: Unsuspected pheochromocytomwa: Risk of blood-pressure alterations during percutaneous adrenal biopsy. *Radiology* 159:733–735, 1986.

20. Hessel SJ, Adams DF, Abrams HL: Complications of angiography. *Radiology* 138:273–281, 1981.

21. Lembke T, Greenberg H: Cystic pheochromocytoma with inadvertent biopsy and glucagon administration. *Can Assoc Radiol J* 38:232–233, 1987.

22. Roa KV: Urologic complications associated with a kidney transplant biopsy: Report of 3 cases and review of the literature. *J Urol* 135:768–770, 1985.

23. Leonard JC, Nanney SM, Tytle T: Arteriovenous fistula secondary to renal biopsy. *Clin Nuc Med* 11:284, 1986.

24. Benoit G, Bellamy J, Charpentier B, et al.: Arteriocalyceal fistula after grated kidney biopsy. *Urology* 24:487–490, 1984.

25. Sulahudeen AK, Sellars L, Srinivasa LN, et al.: Extrarenal arteriovenous fistula. *Nephron* 37:64–65, 1984.

26. Cooper PH, Maisey MN, Shaw P: Arteriovenous fistula following renal transplant biopsy. *Br J Radio* 57:181–183, 1984.

27. Man DW, Hendry GM, Hamdy MH: Percutaneous nephrostomy in pelviureteric junction obstruction in children. *Br J Uro* 55:356–360, 1983.

28. Juul N, Nielson V, Torp-Pedersen S: Percutaneous balloon catheter nephrostomy guided by ultrasound: Results of a new technique. *Scand J Urol Nephrol* 19:291–294, 1985.

29. Pedersen H, Juul N: Ultrasound-guided percutaneous nephrostomy in the treatment of advanced gynecologic malignancy. *Acta Obstet Gynecol Scand* 67:199–201, 1988.

30. Stanley P, Bear JW, Reid BS: Percutaneous nephrostomy in infants and children. *AJR* 141:473–477, 1983.

31. Bennett LN, Voegeli D, Crummy A, et al.: Urologic complications following renal transplantation: Role of interventional radiologic procedures. *Radiology* 160:531–536, 1986.

32. Sholder AJ, Maizels M, Depp R, et al.: Caution in antenatal intervention. *J Urol* 139:1026–1029, 1988.

33. Elder JS, Duckett JW, Snyder HM: Intervention for fetal obstructive uropathy: Has it been effective? *Lancet* 2(8566):107–10, 1987 Oct. 31.

34. Gerzof SG, Gale ME: Computed tomography and ultrasonography for diagnosis and treatment of renal and retroperitoneal abscesses. *Urol Clin N Am* 9:185, 1982.

35. Rosen RJ, Roven SJ: Percutaneous drainage of abscesses and fluid collections. *Urology* 23:54–58, 1984.

36. Silver TM, Campbell D, Wicks, JD, et. al.: Peritransplant fluid collections. *Radiology* 138:145–151, 1981.

37. Letourneau JG, Day DL, Fienberg SB: Ultrasound and computed tomographic evaluation of renal transplantation. *Radio Clin N Am* 25:267–279, 1987.

38. Roney PD, Wellington JL: Traumatic lymphocoele following renal transplantation. *J Urol* 134:322–323, 1985.

39. Pope AJ, Ormiston MC, Bogod DG: Sclerotherapy in the treatment of a recurrent lymphocoele. *Postgrad Med J* 58:573–574, 1982.

40. Ridge JA, Manco-Johnson M, Weil R: Ultrasonic diagnosis of infected lymphocele after kidney transplantation. *Eur Urol* 3:31–34, 1987.

16 Guided Aspiration Biopsy with Transvaginal Sonography

ARTHUR C. FLEISCHER
CARL M. HERBERT
ROBERT L. BREE

Introduction

Sonography, due to its capability to delineate the location of needles placed within the body in real time, has multiple applications that involve precise guidance for interventional procedures. This application is particularly useful in the pelvis where pelvic structures can be sonographically accessed either across the vagina, through a distended urinary bladder, or through the rectum. For each of these approaches, sonography can provide a means for real-time delineation of the location of a biopsy or aspiration needle.

This chapter will describe the techniques and advantages of sonographically guided interventional procedures in the pelvis as well as discuss some of the potential complications. The use of transvaginal probes that have attachable needle guides will be emphasized.

Instrumentation and Technique

There are currently various transvaginal probes that can be used for aspiration biopsy guidance. The three major types of transvaginal transducer probes include mul-

tielement curved linear array, single-element mechanically sectored, and multielement phased array. The field of view of these probes typically covers an 80° to 100° sector and depth of up to 10 cm. Of these, the multielement large-aperture arrays that afford the greatest line density and field of view are preferred (Fig. 16.1).

Each of these transducer probes has its own set of advantages and limitations. First, a relatively small probe is desirable for transvaginal guidance and aspiration so that there is ample maneuverability. For deeper structures, probes that offer deeper penetration, which may necessitate a relatively lower frequency transducer and an adjustable focus or magnified view in order to achieve the greatest line density, are preferred.

Probably the most important aspect of the instrumentation used for transvaginal aspiration guidance is the attachable needle guide. On most probes, the needle guide is flush to the end of the probe shaft. The needle guide insures a needle path that is within the incidental beam. The projected needle path is displayed on the video output monitor of the ultrasound unit (Fig. 16.2). The scanner should have a display that shows the needle path clearly and should be equipped with a video cassette recorder. In

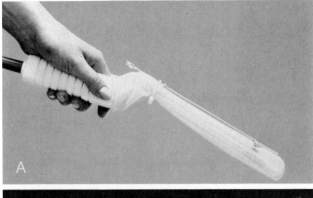

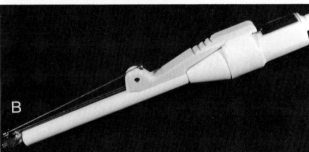

Figure 16.1. Transvaginal probes and needle guides. A, Multielement curved linear-array transvaginal probe with needle guide attached over a condom. The needle guide is flush with the shaft of the probe. B, Single-element mechanical-sector transvaginal probe with an attached needle guide.

mechanically sectored transducers, the needle guide must be angled relative to the shaft of the probe. This creates some inconvenience in that the needle guide may touch the urethral area causing some discomfort to the patient. This occurs when the probe and its needle guide are placed in an anterior position for posteriorly directed aspiration. This situation is relatively rare since in most aspirations, the probe/needle guide is directed laterally within the vagina.

As with other biopsy needles, it is helpful to have a needle with a scored tip for transvaginal aspiration. This afford greater echogenicity and therefore enhances the ability to locate the tip of the needle (Fig. 16.3). The needle should fit snugly into the biopsy needle guide; the significant space within the needle hole may contribute to inaccurate needle placement.

For transvaginal aspirations, the probe should be covered by a condom and local

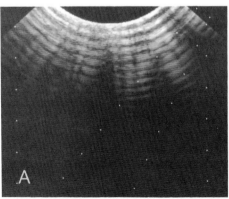

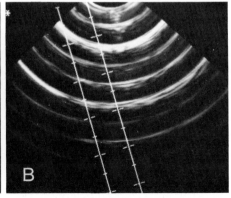

Figure 16.2. Needle path display. A, the two lines of cm dots show projected needle path. B, Projected needle path is between the two slanted, graduated lines.

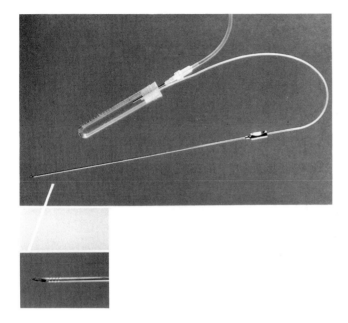

Figure 16.3. Needle used for follicular aspiration. The magnified image shows the scored tip that facilitates sonographic delineation.

anesthesia should be administered. The probe itself can be used to manipulate the structure being scanned so that it is in the closest proximity to the transducer. This is particularly helpful in follicular aspiration where the ovary can be trapped in the ovarian fossa by manipulating the probe (Fig. 16.4).

FOLLICULAR ASPIRATION

There are several methods of sonographic guidance for follicular aspirations (Fig. 16.5). They vary according to the approach used for aspiration and the type of scanning used for guidance. The most common include:

1. Transvaginal aspiration and guidance;
2. Transurethral-transvesical aspiration with transabdominal guidance;
3. Percutaneous transvesical aspiration with transabdominal guidance.

There have been only a few randomized studies to determine which approach results in the highest pregnancy rate (1). Although there is controversy as to whether or not the pregnancy rate is affected by the approach used, it is clear that the approach should be tailored to each patient's anatomy. For example, a transvesicular approach may be needed for patients with ovaries that are anteriorly located whereas transvaginal approaches are preferred in women whose ovaries are located in the cul-de-sac. In general, if the ovary is greater than 3 cm from the transvaginal probe, it may be better accessed by an alternative approach.

The difficulty in controling the several variables that determine successful pregnancy should not be underestimated. These include the etiology of infertility, the type of medications used for ovulation induction, the number and quality of the retrieved oocytes, the fertilization and cleavage rate, and the state of endometrial development at implantation.

Most in vitro fertilization (IVF) centers use the transvaginal approach, although some use the periurethral-transvesical approach. The advantages of the transvaginal approach include the need for only mild sedation and local anesthesia, high patient acceptance, and low complication rate. Some studies have reported high fertilization and pregnancy rates for the periurethral-transvesical approach and except for transient hematuria, no significant complications are reported (2, 3).

For transvaginal follicular aspiration there are some data that suggest that preoperative

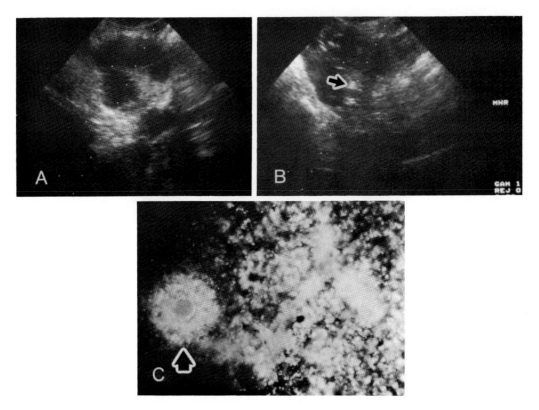

Figure 16.4. Follicular aspiration. **A**, preaspiration, a mature follicle is lined up in the beam path as depicted by the cm dots. **B**, During aspiration, the multiple interfaces arising from the scored needle tip (*arrow*) are seen within the follicle. **C**, Picture of a retrieved ovum with surrounding cluster of granulosa cells (*arrow*).

antibiotic coverage decreases the possibility of infection from the procedure (4). Since the vagina contains various bacterial flora, one theoretic concern is the possibility of contamination. However, the actual incidence of this seems to be very low.

Transvaginal Approach

Immediately prior to transvaginal aspiration, the vagina should be cleansed with a sterile saline solution. Once the desired area is lined up with the beam path, the needle can be passed through the vagina under constant sonographic visualization. Passing through areas where the larger uterine vessels lie to either side of the cervix and laterally towards the pelvis sidewalls where the iliac vessels course should be avoided (Fig. 16.6). If multiple follicles are present, the needle does not have to be withdrawn to-

tally from the vagina between advances. It is best placed in the proximal portion of the ovary where the follicle is first aspirated.

Once the proper advancement of the needle is achieved, mild negative pressure (100 mm Hg) is applied for aspiration; the follicular fluid is then transferred into a test tube (Fig. 16.3). Although most practitioners use a manual technique for achieving the proper amount of needle advancement, some authors advocate the use of a spring-loaded device (5). The contents of the test tube are then examined under a microscope for the presence of an ovum (Fig. 16.4). Most follicular aspirations involve flushing the follicle with a buffered solution several times in order to obtain any ovum that may be floating within the follicle.

One should be careful not to confuse the short-axis view of a pelvic vessel for a ma-

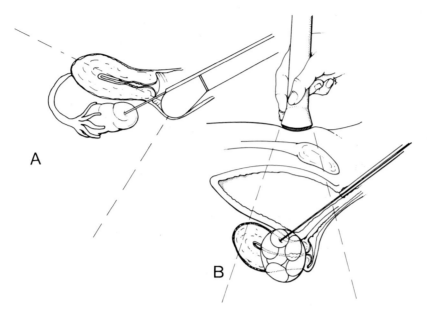

Figure 16.5. Types of ultrasound guidance for follicular aspiration. **A,** Ovarian follicular aspiration and guidance utilizing the transvaginal approach. **B,** Transurethral and transvesical approach using the needle guidance system shown in Figure 16.1A.

ture follicle (Fig. 16.6). If a vessel is entered, the needle should be withdrawn as soon as possible. External pressure on the area can be applied by using the probe as a form of ballotment. Similarly, some hydrosalpinges may mimic the sonographic appearance of a mature follicle (Fig. 16.6**B**; 5).

Transabdominal sonography can be used to guide follicular aspiration using the transurethral approach. For this procedure, the needle is placed within the tip of a Foley catheter that is passed through the urethra. Once the Foley and needle are within the urinary bladder, the needle is popped out from the end of the catheter and directed through the posterior bladder wall and into the follicle. While follicles can be aspirated successfully, this procedure causes more patients discomfort than the transvaginal route when the needle passes through the innervated bladder wall.

The success rate for transvaginal, transvesicular, and laparoscopic ovum retrieval seem to be comparable (1; Table 16.1). However, major advantages of the transvaginal route include lack for the need of general anesthesia and high patient acceptance.

These factors substantiate this as the method of choice for follicular aspiration.

In a recently reported large series of patients undergoing transvaginal ultrasound-directed oocyte collection for IVF, a 98.7% rate of success was documented. In addition, the high (80%) fertilization rate associated with this technique was greater than those resulting from laparoscopic ovum retrieval reported in a previous series. This study also described the incidence of complications that could be attributed to transvaginal aspiration (6).

The complications that were reported included three pelvic abscesses and three pelvic hematomas. The abscesses were successfully treated by aspiration of their contents followed by instillation of antibiotics combined with a course of intravenous antibiotics. The authors advocate the use of intraoperative antibiotics particularly in patients with known endometriosis (6). The three patients with pelvic hematomas were managed conservatively and there was no significant fall in the hemaglobin level in any case. Five patients experienced vaginal bleeding immediately postprocedure that

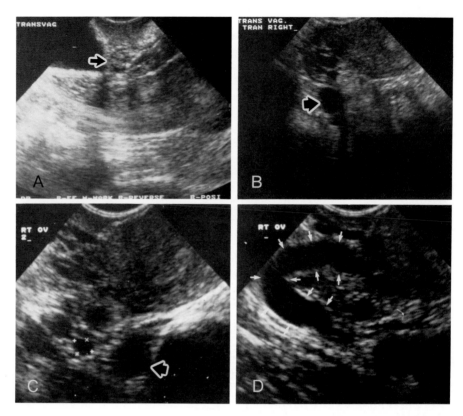

Figure 16.6. Ultrasound mimics. **A**, Uterine vessels (*arrow*) adjacent to the cervix. These vessels should be avoided during aspiration. **B**, Iliac vein (*arrow*) immediately posterior to the right ovary. **C**, A hydrosalpinx appearing initially as a rounded structure mimicking a mature follicle (*arrow*). **D**, Same patient showing the fusiform configuration of a typical simple hydrosalpinx (*arrows*).

required insertion of a vaginal pack. One patient suffered a 200 ml blood loss immediately after withdrawal of the aspirating needle and required suturing.

Table 16.1
Results of Ovum Pickup by Three Methods[a]

	Laparoscopic	Transvesical	Transvaginal
Oocytes Recovered/Patient	6.4 +/− 0.9	6.2 +/− 0.3	5.7 +/− 0.6
Oocytes Recovered/Follicle (%)	93.0	86.0	82.0
Fertilization Rate (%)	73.6	72.3	70.9
Cleavage Rate (%)	82.6	79.4	81.6
No. Embryos Transferred	3.9 +/− 0.6	3.2 +/− 6.4	3.6 +/− 0.3
Pregnancy Rate/Pickup (%)	23.7	22.3	21.6
Pregnancy Rate/Transfer (%)	26.6	26.7	25.9
Pregnancy rate/Cycle (%)	20.2	22.6	21.1

[a]From Feldberg D, Goldman JA, Ashkenazi J, Shelef M, Dicker D, Samuel N: Transvaginal oocyte retrieval controlled by vaginal probe for in vitro fertilization: A comparative study. J Ultrasound Med 7:339–343, 1988.

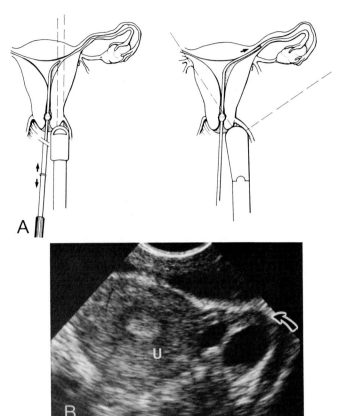

Figure 16.7. Other applications of transvaginal/sonographic (*TVS*) guidance. **A,** Diagram of TVS guidance of transcervical catheterization of the left tube for Gamete Intrafallopian Tube Transfer procedure. **B,** Normal proximal left tube (*arrow*) on TVS (U=Uterus).

OTHER APPLICATIONS

In the patient undergoing embryo transfer a cystic mass such as a follicular cyst may be present in the follicular phase of the cycle and may interfere with eventual oocyte retrieval, particularly if a transvaginal route is used. These masses can be aspirated transvaginally in the early part of the cycle so that follicle stimulation and subsequent follicular aspiration can be optimized (Fig. 16.8).

Transvaginally guided aspiration can also be utilized for completely cystic adnexal masses and for biopsy of some selected pelvic masses that are thought to be benign. In elderly patients, or those at high risk for surgery because of pelvic adhesions, a transvaginal approach for aspiration of cystic pelvic masses is preferable. The sonographic findings that favor benignancy are a smooth wall, lack of internal echoes, and lack of papillary excrescences or tumor nodules. Most, if not all, completely cystic masses can be aspirated through the transvaginal route (Fig. 16.9). Some cystic masses, particularly in younger women, will reoccur following aspiration if there is inflammatory or hormonal stimulation (Fig. 16.10). Other masses with higher risks of malignancy should only be aspirated if no surgical approach is possible (7). We have performed diagnostic procedures on ovarian masses in high-risk patients; all the masses had benign characteristics with ultrasound and benign cytologic features. Patients with a prior history of gynecologic neoplasms and suspected recurrence can be biopsied with a transvaginal approach with ease and safety (8, 9). The cystic contents of the uterus in a patient with a recurrent endometrial carcinoma with cervical stenosis may also be aspirated using the transvaginal approach.

Theoretic complications of transvaginal aspiration include inadvertent aspiration of an ovarian tumor with subsequent perito-

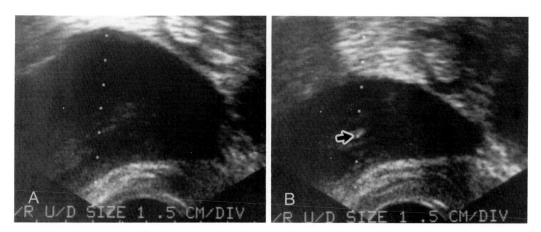

Figure 16.8. **A,** Transvaginal scan (image oriented with vagina at bottom) on an IVF patient early in the cycle demonstrates a large cystic mass in the pelvis. The patient had a history of endometriosis and an endometrioma is suspected. Since it was felt that this mass would interfere with the aspiration procedure, it was elected to aspirate the mass prior to beginning the next menstrual cycle. **B,** Scan performed during aspiration demonstrates needle within the partially collapsed mass (*arrow*). The row of dots indicates the position of the needle guide. The mass was completely aspirated during that cycle.

neal spread, aspiration of an abscess with spread of septic fluid intraperitoneally, and aspiration of dermoid cysts or endometriomas with intraperitoneal spread of their contents, which may cause peritonitis. The actual incidence of these complications has not been documented and awaits further experience with a large series of patients.

Availability of an operating room suite for surgical management for these complications must be maintained.

Patients with suspected pelvic abscesses are also good candidates for transvaginal aspiration either for diagnosis or definitive treatment (10; Fig. 16.11). Transvaginal sonography can also be used for guided aspi-

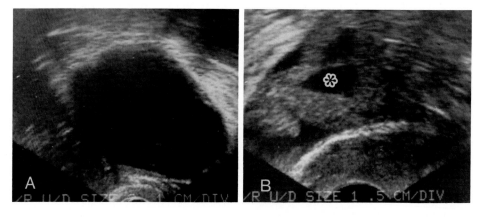

Figure 16.9. An elderly woman was found to have a cystic pelvic mass on routine transabdominal ultrasound. Her surgical risk factors were high and transvaginal aspiration was suggested. **A,** Transvaginal scan shows larges cystic pelvic mass which contains no internal echoes. The chance of this being a benign cyst is very high. **B,** Scan obtained following aspiration demonstrates a small amount of residual fluid within the cyst (*). The surrounding echogenic tissue indicates that the mass is ovarian in origin. Cytologic evaluation of the fluid yielded benign cells.

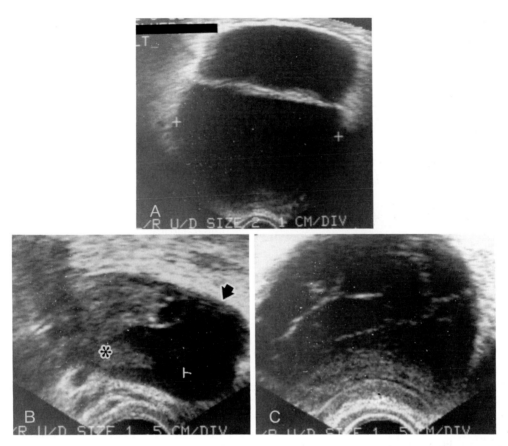

Figure 16.10. A young woman with recurrent ovarian cysts was scanned during an episode of acute pelvic pain. **A,** Transvaginal scan demonstrates a large cystic pelvic mass with a septation within it. **B,** Transvaginal aspiration was performed and the scan following the aspiration shows a small amount of residual fluid within the mass (*arrow*). When collapsed the mass appears to emanate from the ovary (*). **C,** Scan obtained 5 days later demonstrates recurrence of the mass, which is now multiloculated. The pain recurred and the mass required surgical removal.

ration of cul-de-sac fluid in patients with suspected ruptured ectopic pregnancies. For this indication, an appropriate pocket of fluid is identified and entered under real-time sonography. Culdocentesis is indicated in patients with emergent clinical findings and suspicion of ectopic pregnancy. The aspiration of free nonclotted blood indicates a high probability of ruptured ectopic pregnancy and can actually decrease the time between patient presentation and surgery.

Transvaginal sonography may be employed for the transvaginal placement of drainage catheters for nonsurgical treatment of tubo-ovarian abscesses (TOA). Most importantly, a TOA must be clearly distin-

guished from a simple hydrosalpinx by demonstration of the abscess cavity located within the ovary.

Transvaginal sonography can also be used for guidance of catheters into the area of the proximal tubal ostia for Gamete Intrafallopian Tube Transfer (GIFT) techniques (11). Prior to this procedure, one should evaluate carefully where the endometrium invaginates into the area of the proximal tubal ostia. The catheter is then manipulated to allow passage out into the tubal isthmus. The proximal portion of the uterine tube can be delineated in some patients, particularly if it is surrounded by intraperitoneal fluid (Fig. 16.7).

REFERENCES

1. Feldberg D, Goldman JA, Ashkenazi J, Shelef M, Dicker D, Samuel N: Transvaginal oocyte retrieval controlled by vaginal probe for in vitro fertilization: A comparative study. *J Ultrasound Med* 7:339–343, 1988.
2. Parsons J, Booker M, Goswamy R, et al.: Oocyte retrieval for in vitro fertilization by ultrasonically guided needle aspiration via the urethra. *Lancet* 1 (May 11, 1985):1076, 1985.
3. Wisanto A, Braeckmans P, Camus M, Devroey P, Khan I, Staessen C, Smitz J, Van Wasberghe L, Van Steirteghem AC: Perurethral ultrasound-guided ovum pickup. *J In Vitro Fertilization Embryo Transfer* 5(2):107–111, 1988.
4. Dellenbach P, Nisand I, Moreau L, Feger B, Plumere C, Gerlinger P: Transvaginal sonographically controlled follicle puncture for oocyte retrieval. *Fertil Steril* 44(5):656–662, 1985.
5. Kemeter P, Feichtinger W: Transvaginal oocyte retrieval using a transvaginal sector scan probe combined with an automated puncture device. *Hum Reproduction* 1(1):21–24, 1986.
6. Baber R, Porter R, Picker R, Robertson R, Dawson E, Saunders D: Transvaginal ultrasound directed oocyte collection for in vitro fertilization: Successes and complications. *J Ultrasound Med* 7:377–379, 1988.
7. deCrespigny LCH, Robinson HP, Davaren RAM, Fortune DW: Ultrasound guided puncture for gynecologic and pelvic lesions. *Aust and NZ J Obstet Gynecol* 25:227–229, 1985.
8. Nash JD, Burke TW, Woodward JE, et al.: Diagnosis of recurrent gynecologic malignancy with fine needle aspiration cytology. *Obstet Gynecol* 71:333–337, 1988.
9. Ganjej P, Nadji M: Aspiration cytology of ovarian neoplasms. *Acta Cytol* 28:329–332, 1984.
10. Nosher JL, Winchman HK, Needell GS: Transvaginal pelvic abscess drainage with US guidance. *Radiology* 165:872–873, 1987.
11. Jansen RPS, Andersen JC: Catheterization of the fallopian tubes from the vagina. *Lancet* 2:309–310, 1987.
12. Strickler RC, Christianson C, Crane JP, Curato A, Knight AB, Yang V: Ultrasound guidance for human embryo transfer. *Fertil Steril* 43(1):54–61, 1985.

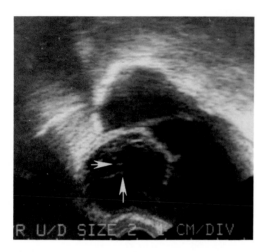

Figure 16.11. Pelvic abscess. A multiloculated cystic mass was found in a patient with fever and pelvic pain. A pelvic abscess was suspected and a transvaginal scan demonstrates a multiloculated cystic mass with a portion of the mass containing internal echoes and septations (*arrows*). This mass was aspirated and thin purulent material was removed. The abscess completely collapsed following aspiration, without immediate recurrence.

Sonography has been used for catheter placement in embryo transfer (12) to monitor the location of the embryo-loaded catheter relative to the fundal portion of the uterine lumen as it is placed transvaginally. Theoretically, this ensures transfer of the embryo to the proper intrauterine location.

In conclusion, sonography, particularly with transvaginal scanning, is a useful means of guiding and/or biopsy of pelvic structures. It is extensively used for follicular aspiration, but is also useful for aspiration/biopsy of selected pelvic masses.

17 Prostate and Other Transrectally Guided Biopsies

ROBERT L. BREE

The use of ultrasound to detect prostatic carcinoma and guide biopsies has received much attention in the radiologic and urologic literature in recent years. There has also been attention in the lay press because of ultrasound's potential as a screening examination similar to mammography for breast cancer. To date, however, data have not supported widespread use of ultrasound in screening for prostatic carcinoma, although some studies have shown improvement in lesion detection over digital rectal examination (1–4). This chapter will briefly review the role of transrectal prostate sonography with the focus on prostate biopsy. This will include a description of various techniques and equipment available for prostate biopsy. Review of the results and complications and a description of other pelvic biopsy procedures will also be presented.

Prostate Imaging

The transrectal approach to prostate sonography has emerged as the preferred route over transabdominal techniques primarily because of significant improvements in equipment design and development of high-frequency (> 5 MHz) near-field focused transducers. As the probe is placed in close contact with the prostate, it allows increased resolution as compared to the transabdominal technique. Scanning is typically performed in a recumbent lateral decubitus position following careful cleaning of the probe (as described in prior chapters) and covering it with a condom. Single-plane, biplane, and multiplane probes are commercially available (Fig. 17.1).

NORMAL ANATOMY

There is currently no standardized orientation for sonographic imaging of the prostate. In this chapter, even though some equipment will not allow reverse orientation at real-time, most images will be shown as in Figure 17.2. The prostate is divided into three major glandular zones—transition, central, and peripheral. There is also one nonglandular region, the anterior fibromuscular stroma. The urethra and the ejaculatory ducts pass through these zones. The urethra is divided into a proximal portion that extends from the bladder neck to the verumontanum, and a distal portion that extends from the verumontanum to the external sphincter.

The transition zone is located in a periurethral position superior to the verumontanum. Prior to the development of benign prostatic hyperplasia (BPH), it constitutes approximately 5% of the prostatic glandular tissue. The transition zone is the main site of origin of benign prostatic hyperplasia, while 10% to 20% of prostate carcinomas originate from this region.

A histologically silent area, the central zone, constitutes approximately 25% of the prostatic glandular tissue. The central zone narrows to an apex in the region of the veru-

221

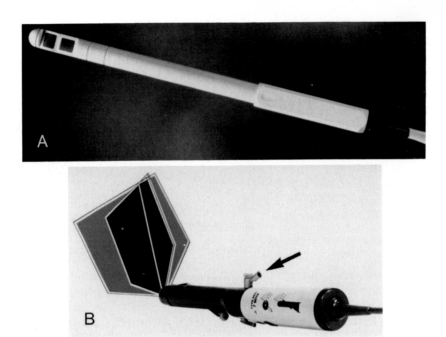

Figure 17.1. Transrectal probes. **A,** A biplane probe is illustrated. Sagittal and axial planes can be alternated easily with a switch on the console. **B,** Multiplane transrectal probe that allows imaging in longitudinal, transverse, and any oblique plane. A needle guide (*arrow*) runs through the transducer shaft allowing the water path to remain inflated during biopsy procedures. (**A,** courtesy of General Electric, Milwaukee, Wisconsin; **B,** courtesy Bruel and Kjaer, Marlborough, Massachusetts)

montanum. The echogenicity of the central zone is normally greater than that of the peripheral zone. While the central zone occupies 25% of the glandular tissue, it is the site of origin of only 5% to 10% of prostate carcinomas.

The peripheral zone constitutes 70% of the prostatic glandular tissue. The peripheral zone comprises the posterior, lateral, and apical aspects of the prostate and is the origin of 70% of prostate carcinoma (5–7). Superior and posterior to the prostate gland are the seminal vesicles (Fig. 17.2).

SONOGRAPHIC APPEARANCE OF PROSTATE CANCER

Small prostate carcinomas detected in the peripheral zone are almost uniformly anechoic or hypoechoic relative to the surrounding peripheral zone (Fig. 17.3). As carcinomas enlarge in the peripheral zone, they tend to grow longitudinally along the peripheral zone and are protected from entering the transition zone by the surgical

capsule bordering the peripheral zone anteriorly and medially. However, the interface separating the peripheral from the central zone is easily traversed by cancers. Therefore, peripheral zone cancers can directly extend into the central zone. Most tumors in the peripheral zone tend to become hypoechoic. Yet not all hypoechoic nodules are carcinomas and some small cancers may be isoechoic with the rest of the prostate and, therefore, not detectable. As tumors become more extensive, usually larger than 1.5 cm, the echogenicity often changes, becoming isoechoic, mixed,, or even hyperechoic. These large cancers may create diagnostic problems because of the difficulty in differentiating cancer from benign process and because of tumor infiltration into areas of BPH (8–10; Fig. 17.4).

Particular diagnostic difficulty can be expected when large diffuse cancers infiltrate into the entire peripheral zone, creating a uniformly hypoechoic appearance (Fig. 17.5). Frequently, prostate carcinoma is

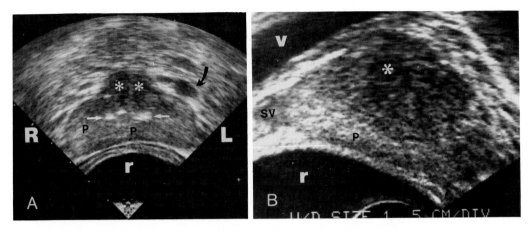

Figure 17.2. Normal prostate sonogram. **A.** Axial examination of the prostate. The prostate gland is normal in size and has a uniform echodensity aside from a few bright areas (*arrows*) representing corpora amylacea near the junction of the peripheral zone (*P*) and transition zone (*asterisks*). The curved arrow points to a periprostatic vein. **B,** Sagittal sonogram through the right lobe of the prostate demonstrating peripheral zone (*P*) encompassing most of the image. A small portion of the transition zone and anterior fibromuscular stroma is denoted by the *asterisk*. At the cephalic end of the gland is the seminal vesicle (*SV*). A large vein (*V*) coarses anterior. *r* = water-filled balloon in rectum.

multifocal, creating lesions in separate areas, some of which may be isoechoic and not perceptible sonographically. Asymmetry and capsular bulge may be the only clues to the presence of cancer (5).

LESION DETECTION PREDICTIVE VALUES AND SCREENING

Ultrasound has a definite place in the detection of prostate cancer as evidenced by a significant number of papers devoted to lesion detection and the appearances of prostate cancer. The role of ultrasound in relation to digital rectal examinations has been studied. There is some indication that ultrasound is superior to digital rectal examination in screening for prostate cancer, but the yield is low and the cost savings with ultrasound moderate (2–4). Because of the impossibility of proving the validity of a negative ultrasound examination, the specificity and negative predictive values of prostate ultrasound cannot be evaluated (3). Newer data suggest that a positive predictive value for combined ultrasound and prostate specific antigen (PSA) of about 80%. PSA acts in concert with ultrasound in

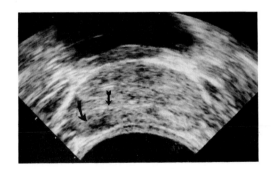

Figure 17.3. Small prostate carcinoma. Transverse sonogram through the prostate demonstrates a small hypoechoic mass (*curved arrow*), which is nonpalpable. Biopsy revealed adenocarcinoma. Mass is contained within the peripheral zone, which is separated from the transition zone by a well-defined surgical capsule (*arrow*).

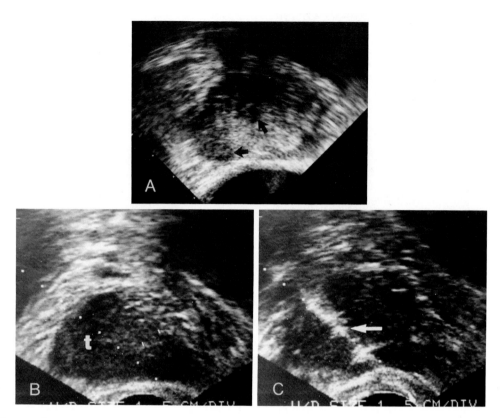

Figure 17.4. Large prostate carcinoma with biopsy. **A,** Transverse sonogram demonstrating extensive tumor (*arrows*) represented as hypoechoic areas in the peripheral zone extending into the transition zone. **B,** Sagittal examination prior to biopsy. The area of tumor (*t*) is extensive. The small white dots represent the direction of the biopsy needle using a biopsy guide. The distance between each dot is 5 mm. **C,** Frozen image during the biopsy shows the needle (*arrow*) having traversed the tumor along the path of the guidelines.

predicting which patients could most benefit from biopsy (11–13).

Prostate Biopsy

While controversy still surrounds the exact role of prostate ultrasound, one of the most significant contributions of transrectal prostate imaging in the diagnosis and management of prostate cancer is the use of ultrasound-guided biopsy techniques. In this section, the results of nonguided techniques will be reviewed; transrectal and transperineal techniques compared; cytologic and histologic methods analyzed; and ultrasound guided techniques and complications discussed.

CONVENTIONAL BIOPSY TECHNIQUES

Transperineal and transrectal blind biopsy techniques have been performed by urologists for many years. A palpable nodule or indurated gland is the primary diagnostic indication for the biopsy. With the transperineal approach, a finger is placed in the rectum and the needle is guided into the nodule by palpating its path through the perineal tissues.

Using the transrectal approach, the needle is passed into the nodule adjacent to the palpating finger, sometimes with a finger-tip guide. With larger needles, such as a 14-gauge core-needle, the advantage of transperineal biopsy is fewer septic complica-

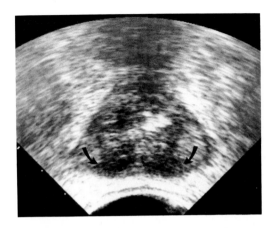

Figure 17.5. Diffuse carcinoma of the prostate. The peripheral zone is diffusely infiltrated with hypoechoic neoplasm (*arrows*). In such cases, where the peripheral zone is uniformly hypoechoic, its abnormality may only be appreciated by comparison with the transition zone that should normally be less echogenic.

tions, but its disadvantages are decreased accuracy and the need for extensive local or general anesthesia. With transrectal biopsy, anesthesia problems are fewer, accuracy is greater, but prophylactic antibiotic coverage and rectal preparation are required (14).

Fine-needle techniques with a transrectal approach using cytologic evaluation have been proposed as safer and more comfortable outpatient procedures for biopsy of the prostate (15–16). The accuracy of these techniques versus large-needle procedures varies, with false-negative or false-positive rates from 0% to 30% (14–16). A disadvantage of cytologic techniques is the problem with designating a Gleason grade (degree of dedifferentiation) to the specimen, an important prognostic feature only available histologically. Recent work has shown an approximately 80% correlation between cytological grading of prostate carcinoma with Gleason grading (17). Gleason grading is subjective and can vary from one pathologist to another. A combination of cytology and histology has been described using a modified Menghini needle (21 gauge) with histologic yields above 80% and sensitivity of over 70% for adequate tissue cores (18). The advent of the automatic Tru-cut needle has now obvi-

ated the need for other needle techniques, although these needles are more applicable to ultrasound-guided biopsy below.

Irrespective of the approach or needle used, conventional techniques have a yield of carcinoma ranging from 25% to 50% with most series well below 50%. These are patients with palpable nodules, a condition naturally yielding higher positive results than pure screening procedures. A small number of false-negative biopsies have occurred (14) in patient populations who have repeat biopsies performed.

ULTRASOUND-GUIDED BIOPSY

The use of transrectal ultrasound for biopsy guidance has received attention in the literature since 1978, when Holm and Gammelgaard (19) described their experience with a transperineal approach utilizing an axial rotating scanner. Other authors have advocated the use of a linear-array probe with a transperineal approach (20–24). Recently, transrectal needle techniques have been described, utilizing sector probes and a needle approach running parallel to the probe or through a tunnel in the probe (25–28). In addition to biopsy, these probes can be used for drainage procedures, cryosurgery, or insertion of radioactive seeds. The transrectal or transperineal approach can also be used to perform other biopsies in the perineal area.

Equipment

Almost every ultrasound manufacturer producing transrectal probes for the prostate has adapted the equipment to perform biopsy procedures. Originally, the stress was on the transperineal approach and, in that instance, a guide is placed near the base of the probe, allowing for needle placement parallel to the probe through the perineum when the probe is in the rectum (Fig. 17.6). This approach has its advocates because of its inherent safety, but it has more recently been overshadowed by the transrectal technique.

Many manufacturers have introduced guidance systems for transrectal biopsy that allows the needle to enter the prostate paral-

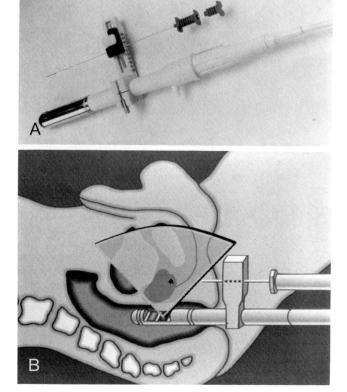

Figure 17.6. Guidance system for transperineal biopsy. A biplane probe is fitted with a guidance system allowing placement of the needle at an appropriate level anterior to the rectum following medial-lateral localization of the lesion. **A** demonstrates a needle traversing the guidance system. The technique is illustrated in **B**, with the needle entering the perineum. In the sagittal plane, the needle can be followed into the prostate. (**A**, courtesy Diasonics, Milpitas, California; **B**, courtesy General Electric, Milwaukee, Wisconsin).

lel to the probe or through the probe, and enter the lesion with direct sonographic guidance, penetrating the rectal mucosa (Figs. 17.1**B** and 17.7).

Needle selection for biopsies will often depend upon the approach chosen and the guidance system used. As with unguided biopsies, the use of core needles versus fine needles for aspiration of cells depends on the needs of the surgeon and/or therapist for grading and staging.

The needle now considered superior for core biopsy because of its relatively small diameter and ease of use is an automatic Tru-cut needle available in an 18-gauge diameter (29). This needle, and others like it, is triggered by a mechanical firing device or gun, which is constructed with strong springs and performs the biopsy automatically. The inner needle advances 23 mm producing a 17-mm tissue core. The outer needle then cuts the tissue core and fixes it into the beveled chamber of the inner needle. The entire process occurs in a fraction of

a second and is perceived as a single motion by both patient and physician (Fig. 17.8; 25, 27–29).

We have used the following aspiration-cytology technique to assess the ability of cytology to diagnose and grade prostate cancer. A syringe holder allows suction to be placed on an aspiration needle, preferably with a roughened tip, with one hand while the transducer to be held with the other hand facilitating performance by a single operator. The histologic and cytologic biopsies can be performed through the biopsy guide at the same sitting.

Patient Preparation

With the increasing availability of diagnostic scanning of the prostate in an ambulatory setting, many patients will have a biopsy performed with little or no prior warning in an outpatient setting. Patients receiving therapeutic doses of anticoagulants, aspirin, or other platelet adhesion in-

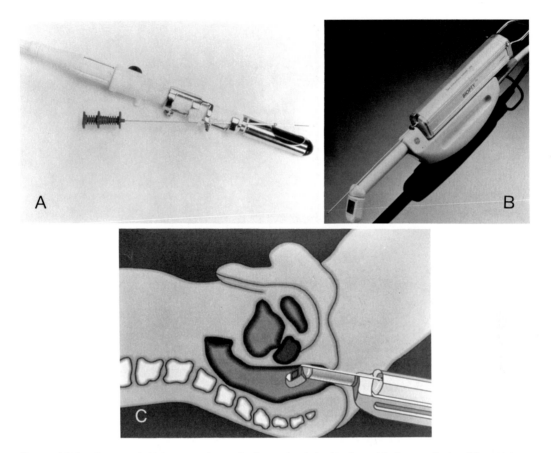

Figure 17.7. Transrectal biopsy systems. Systems depicted in **A** and **B** demonstrate different transrectal biopsy systems that can visualize the needle running parallel to the shaft of the probe. The biplane system (**A**) allows the angle to be changed according to the position of the lesion relative to the probe. The system in **B** utilizes an angled crystal scanning in the sagittal plane. **C**, The position of the probe and the needle relative to one another in the rectum. Electronic guidelines are placed on the monitor based on the position of the needle guide relative to the probe. (**A**, courtesy Diasonics, Milpitas, California; **B** and **C**, courtesy General Electric, Milwaukee, Wisconsin).

hibitors should be told to discontinue use for at least 1 week. Any evidence of active infection in the lower urinary tract is a contraindication for biopsy. The incidence of infection with transperineal biopsy is extremely low and antibiotic coverage usually is not considered essential with that approach (26, 17). It is now considered appropriate to administer antibiotics before and after a transrectal biopsy. A useful compound for this procedure is noroxin, (Norfloxacin, Merck, Sharp & Dohme, West Point, PA.), because of its rapid absorption and high blood level. When given 1 hour before and the evening after a transrectal biopsy, it provides adequate antibiotic coverage (28). It has been our practice to administer a neomycin enema prior to a transrectal biopsy in order to further minimize septic complications. As with any biopsy technique, informed consent should be obtained, keeping in mind that bleeding is a common complication and that serious complications are extremely rare (30). Because many of the patients will be elderly, it is important to ask that a companion be available to accompany the patient from the hospital or office.

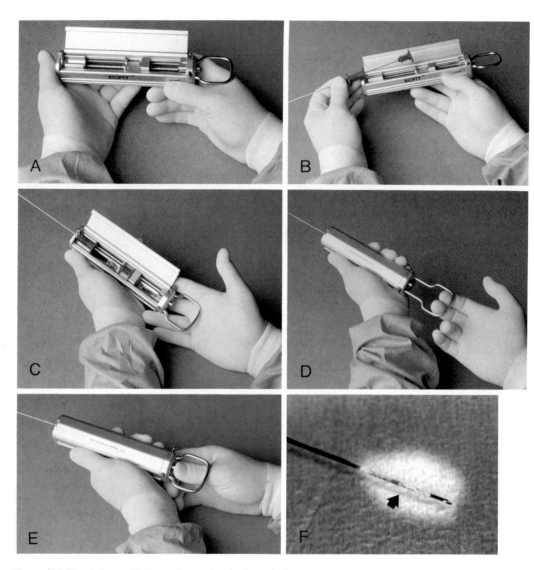

Figure 17.8. Automatic Tru-cut needle device. **A**, Two-stage spring biopsy gun that greatly facilitates the performance of prostate biopsies. It has also been utilized for kidney and other soft tissue biopsies. The specially devised needle fits into two grooves in the handle (**B**) and the cover is ready to be closed (**C**). The device is cocked (**D**) and the biopsy performed by pressing a button at the tip of the gun (**E**). **F**, A typical specimen (*arrow*). Note the distal 5 mm of the needle does not contain the specimen. The specimen is contained between 5 and 23 mm from the needle tip. (Courtesy Bard Urological, Covington, GA).

Transperineal Technique

Following initial localization of a lesion with the standard decubitus scanning position, the patient is placed in a lithotomy position, or the decubitus position can be maintained. It is possible to perform the biopsy with a longitudinal probe alone, an axial probe alone, or with the use of a biplane probe. Switching between axial and sagittal probes during the biopsy is very cumbersome in our experience.

Utilizing the axial probe alone is the most difficult approach because the needle is not visualized until it reaches the plane of the lesion. If the needle does not follow a true path, it may have to be completely reinserted. This technique is not recommended.

The sagittal or biplane approach is considered the optimum for a transperineal biopsy. After the probe has been inserted, a sagittal image is obtained and the lesion located. Using either a guide attachment or a freehand approach, a position in the perineum relative to the midline and parallel to the probe is selected. The anteroposterior distance from the rectum can be measured or selected from the guidelines on the video monitor of the ultrasound unit when a biopsy guide is used. Local anesthetic is placed in the skin and, utilizing a 22-gauge needle, the perineum is infiltrated rather generously including the prostatic capsule. Proper local anesthesia will greatly reduce patient discomfort. The biopsy needle is then inserted and, with the longitudinal orientation, the shaft of the needle can be seen to enter the prostate and approach the lesion. If a Tru-cut needle is used, either manual or automatic, the needle tip should be at least 5 mm proximal to the lesion. When biplane equipment is used, the axial orientation can now be chosen to see if the needle tip is oriented in the lesion in a medial-lateral plane, a more difficult orientation to ascertain on the longitudinal image. The Tru-cut biopsy can then be performed (Fig. 17.9; 19-21, 23, 24, 27). Cytological biopsy may be performed with standard techniques as described in preceding chapters.

Transrectal Technique

The transrectal technique for biopsy has recently become popular because of its relative ease and the development of transrectal guidance systems compatible with the automatic Tru-cut needle device. This approach is less cumbersome, is easier to perfect, and produces less patient discomfort. It does have a minimally higher septic complication rate, but this is offset by its improved accuracy in placing the needle in the lesion (25–28). The physician beginning to perform these procedures will probably choose the transrectal approach, but should also be familiar with the transperineal technique for special situations.

The biopsy is performed in the decubitus position without anesthesia. Premedication is optional. It may be appropriate to swab the anal and perineal area with iodine solu-

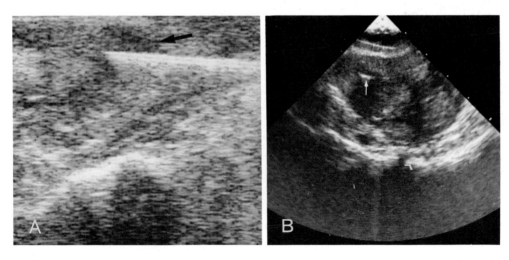

Figure 17.9. Transperineal biopsy. **A**, The sagittal sonogram demonstrates the needle having extended through the hypoechoic lesion (*arrow*) following the biopsy procedure. In the sagittal plane it is sometimes difficult to identify the exact point of the needle tip in a medial-lateral direction. **B**, When available, a biplane probe is useful to determine the exact position of the needle (*arrow*). The images are rectal side up, as was seen at the time of biopsy showing the inability of some instruments to invert the realtime image.

tion. The probe is cleaned and covered with a sterile sheath. A sterile guide is then placed over the probe. The lesion is localized and the guidelines for the needle are lined up with the lesion. The needle is advanced to the appropriate position proximal to the lesion. In the case of the Biopty gun (Bard Urological, Covington, GA.), the needle tip should be 5 mm proximal to the edge of the lesion such that after the 25-mm firing distance, the lesion is between 5 mm and 20 mm from the starting point. It is also important to position the needle so it does not reach beyond the confines of the prostate anteriorly into the periprostatic venous plexus. In most instances, the lesions are lo-cated in the peripheral zone near the rec-tum. It is important to allow the needle to penetrate the rectal wall before performing the biopsy, avoiding rectal wall damage (Figs. 17.4 and 17.10).

The vast majority of patients have a pres-sure sensation on performance of the bi-opsy, without overt pain. The automatic Tru-cut needles are particularly pain-free bi-opsy devices.

When cytologic biopsy is performed, the standard suction technique should be uti-lized with a rapid back and forth motion of the needle through the lesion. The suction should be released before the needle is re-moved from the prostate.

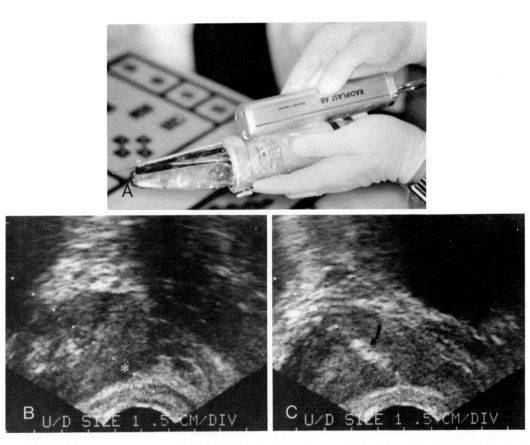

Figure 17.10. **A,** The sagittal transrectal biopsy probe has been covered with a sterile drape and the guide mechanism has been attached. The biopsy device is loaded and the needle inserted through the guide showing its relative position to the probe. **B,** Sagittal image of the prostate dem-onstrating a lesion (*asterisk*) at the apex of the gland. The guidelines show the path of the needle. The needle is placed approximately 5 to 7 mm proximal to the lesion usually just penetrating the rectal wall. **C,** Image obtained following insertion of the needle shows the needle tip having trav-ersed the lesion (*arrow*).

End-firing probes may have a slight advantage over side-viewing probes, allowing biplane imaging and guidance in either coronal oblique or longitudinal oblique planes (28). We have found these end-firing probes useful in obtaining specimens from the apex of the gland because the needle can be placed parallel to the direction of the probe, and does not have to enter from below the prostate (Fig. 17.11). In all other areas of the prostate, the side-viewing probes are preferred because of the true longitudinal image and the improved visualization of the needle in the lesion. The necessity for angling the probe anteriorly with the end-firing design increases patient discomfort, however (25, 28).

The Biopsy Specimen

Generally, with either the transperineal or transrectal technique, two to three core biopsies are obtained from the lesion. It has become our practice to perform a single biopsy with the core needle through a normal area in the contralateral lobe of the prostate. In our series of transrectal and transperineal biopsies, a single cytological specimen was obtained from the lesion. When cytology alone is being utilized, at least three aspirations should be obtained from the lesion.

The discovery of neoplasm in both lobes of the prostate has been reported, adding to the accuracy of staging and help in deciding on appropriate therapy (25).

The tissue cores from the prostate are placed in formalin, separating the biopsy sites. The core often has a sticky consistency and may be difficult to transfer to a jar. We have found a plastic needle cover to be useful in performing this maneuver (Fig. 17.12).

Cytologic specimens are processed by the usual slide smear technique. When aspirations are performed in a hospital, it is very helpful to have a cytology technologist handle the specimen. In an office setting, an appropriate cytology smear technique can be developed in concert with the laboratory that will interpret the results (16).

The histologic specimens from the automatic Tru-cut needles, even though these are 18-gauge needles, have provided uniformly excellent diagnostic information. Gleason grading is almost always possible and benign diagnoses can be made with confidence. Cytology results have usually centered on the presence or absence of cancer. Some cell grading can be done. Other authors have reported success in correlating cytologic grade to Gleason grade (16–18, Fig. 17.13).

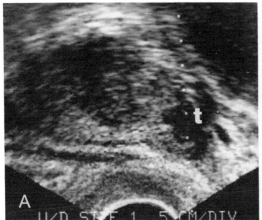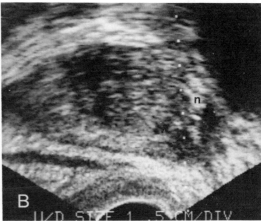

Figure 17.11. Use of end-firing sagittal probe for prostate biopsy. **A,** Lesion is shown at the prostatic apex (*t*). The end-fire probe allows the needle to run directly parallel to the direction of the probe. In this way, an apical lesion can be approached without traversing extraprostatic tissue, particularly the periprostatic venous plexus. **B,** The needle (*n*) has traversed the lesion. The use of this approach may be preferable in certain sites, also allowing for biplane visualization of the lesion.

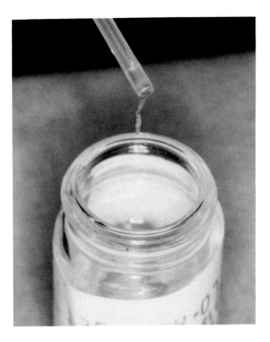

Figure 17.12. The biopsy specimen can be removed from the needle easily with a plastic straw or needle cover. The specimen is then fixed in formalin for histology.

Biopsy Results

Recent reports with ultrasound-guided biopsies yielded positive results in 30% to 67% of patients. The percentage of positives depends on clinical findings, age of the patients, and on whether patient selection was based on results of digital rectal examination or from a screening population (24, 26, 28). One study (22) suggests that ultrasound guidance is not necessary when an obviously palpable abnormality is detected. In our initial experience with ultrasound-guided biopsies, we performed transperineal biopsies in 44 patients. Fourteen were diagnosed as having carcinoma, giving a yield of 31%. This percentage is influenced by the patient selection criteria, which included a significant number of patients without obvious palpable disease, who only had abnormal sonograms.

Following the acquisition of appropriate equipment for transrectal biopsies, this approach became standard. In another recently reported series (25), 70 biopsies were performed in 68 patients. Thirty-six lesions were palpable by digital exam, and 34 were nonpalpable. The average size of all lesions was 9.8 mm. Biopsy results are listed in Table 17.1.

The data show that transrectal ultrasound is capable of diagnosing nonpalpable cancer, as was evidenced in six of 23 patients in this series. The average size of the benign and malignant lesions was not significantly different. Benign diagnoses were usually glandular hyperplasia, although a few cases of granulomatous prostatitis were biopsied (25).

When lesion size was analyzed, it was

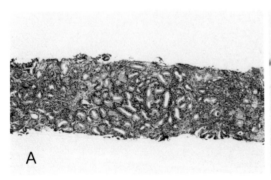

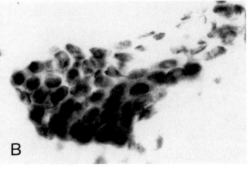

Figure 17.13. **A,** Histologic specimen from 18-gauge automatic Tru-cut needle demonstrating prostatic carcinoma. This extensive tissue core is typical of the cores obtained with this needle in almost every instance. **B,** Cytologic identification of prostatic carcinoma. Prostate specimens are usually quite cellular and prostatic carcinoma can be diagnosed with relative ease. There is some difficulty in grading the neoplasm cytologically.

Table 17.1
Transrectal Prostate Biopsy Results

	Palpable	Nonpalpable	Mean Diameter (mm)	Contralateral Positive
Benign (41) 59%	13	28	9	0
Malignant (29) 41%	23	6	11	5
TOTAL (70)	36	34		

The results of 70 transrectal prostate biopsies performed in 68 patients in whom a contralateral biopsy was performed.

found that 18 of 22 masses (82%) greater than 1.5 cm in maximum diameter were malignant. Five patients had cancer discovered on the contralateral side, two of these with small foci and the other three with diffuse carcinoma. This phenomenon is not surprising considering the propensity for prostate cancer to be present in scattered and multifocal areas throughout a single gland (31).

An additional small group of six patients who underwent biopsy during this time had a diagnosis of atypical hyperplasia (25). These biopsies were considered indeterminate since atypical hyperplasia is a premalignant condition (32). The results were therefore excluded from the data. Two patients were biopsied again with similar results. One patient was shown to have carcinoma on re-biopsy. Three others await further follow-up (Fig. 17.14).

Complications

Significant complications from prostate biopsy, regardless of the mode of guidance, needle size, or approach have been relatively low. Minor complications, including hematuria, hematospermia, and rectal blood are relatively common, with hematuria seen in at least 35% of transrectal biopsies and in a small number of transperineal procedures. Major complications include sepsis, large hematomas, and tumor seeding (27, 30, 33, 34). To date, with the ultrasound-guided transrectal technique, only a single septic complication has been reported. We have had one patient develop a rectal wall hematoma during a transrectal biopsy (Fig. 17.15). Careful attention to technique and use of antibiotics and enemas can help prevent these complications.

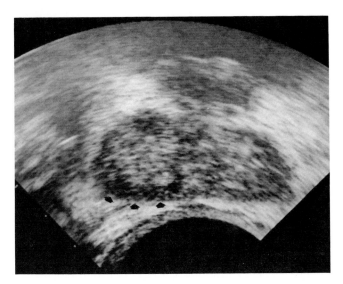

Figure 17.14. Atypical hyperplasia. Transverse image of patient with asymmetric prostate. The right lobe is enlarged and the peripheral zone is diffusely hypoechoic (arrowheads). Initial biopsy of this area revealed atypical hyperplasia on histology and cytology. Biopsy performed several months later revealed prostatic carcinoma.

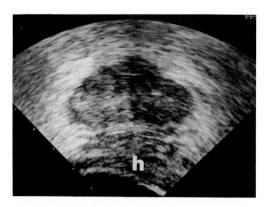

Figure 17.15. Rectal wall hematoma following prostatic biopsy. A biopsy was performed on a patient with normal coagulation studies. During the course of the biopsy, a large rectal wall hematoma (*h*) was noted. Patient continued to bleed from the rectum and required overnight hospitalization without further consequence.

OTHER ULTRASOUND-GUIDED PROCEDURES

Percutaneous Iodine-125 Seed Placement

Iodine-125 seed placement for radiotherapy, performed surgically, has had considerable criticism due to the difficulty in correctly spacing the seeds for uniform distribution. A percutaneous approach using a template and transrectal ultrasound guidance is popular (35, 36). This technique involves placing multiple needles into the gland with a transperineal approach and placing the seeds through the needles in a uniform distribution monitored with ultrasound. This procedure has a high response rate, although it is usually performed for more advanced stages of prostate cancer (36).

Percutaneous Cryotherapy of the Prostate

Hepatic cryosurgery with ultrasound guidance to monitor the probe position and extent of the freezing process has been in use clinically. Prostatic cryosurgery with open techniques has been sporadically performed in recent years, and results compare favorably with more conventional surgical

and radiation procedures. Recently, experimental work in animals has shown the ability of ultrasound to monitor a transperineal cryosurgical approach and determine when the freezing has extended into normal tissue (37). Clinical trials in humans are about to begin.

Prostate Abscess

Transrectal ultrasound can accurately diagnose inflammatory lesions of the prostate. When suspicion of abscess is raised, transrectal or transperineal puncture of the gland for culture and short-term drainage is possible (38; Fig. 17.16).

Nonprostatic Transrectal Biopsy and Aspiration

SEMINAL VESICLES

Except for agenesis of the seminal vesicles, the most common benign abnormality of this tissue is a cyst. These may be ejaculatory duct cysts or true cysts of the seminal vesicles related to Müllerian duct remnants. Small ejaculatory duct cysts are usually asymptomatic. Larger midline cysts may be symptomatic and are probably congenital. Symptoms such as perineal pain, ejac-

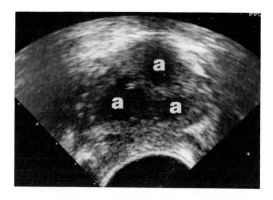

Figure 17.16. Prostate abscess. Multiple hypoechoic areas are noted within the central portion of the gland (*a*). Patient was febrile and tender and aspiration of one of the masses yielded purulent material. The patient was treated with antibiotic therapy with full recovery.

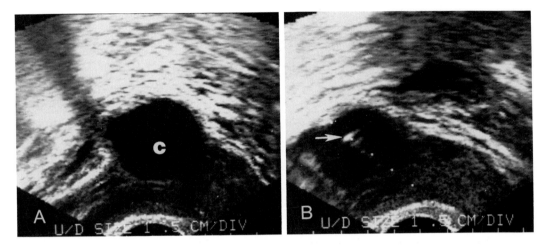

Figure 17.17. Seminal vesicle cyst. **A**, 20-year-old male complained of pelvic pressure and ejaculatory pain. Transrectal ultrasound revealed a large cyst (c) in region of the ejaculatory duct. **B**, A needle (*arrow*) was guided into the cyst with ultrasound guidance. The cyst was completely drained and the patient became asymptomatic. Repeat drainage could be performed if the cyst re-filled.

ulatory pain, or hemospermia may be associated. The cause of the pain and hemospermia has been related to calculi in the cysts. Ultrasonically guided aspiration of these cysts may be useful for symptomatic relief and analysis of the fluid (Fig. 17.17; 39). Hemospermia may also be related to seminal vesiculitis. When a swollen or tender seminal vesicle is identified, guided puncture for fluid analysis and instillation of steroids has been described with good clinical results (40).

Primary neoplasms of the seminal vesicles are rare and, when discovered, are usually so large that their origin is obscure. Extension of prostatic carcinoma into the seminal vesicle can be histologically proven with guided biopsy of the seminal vesicle. This can be important when accurate staging will affect the mode of therapy.

OTHER PELVIC MASSES

Transrectal and transperineal techniques have been described for biopsy of pelvic masses, particularly of recurrent neoplasms. The safety of this approach rivals that of prostate biopsy, and the technique is simpler and safer than transabdominal procedures with ultrasound or CT (Fig. 17.18; 41).

Transrectal sonography has been utilized for evaluation of rectal abnormalities, particularly in the staging of rectal neoplasms (42). Occasionally, based on results of digital palpation or symptoms, submucosal or perirectal abnormalities may be discovered that

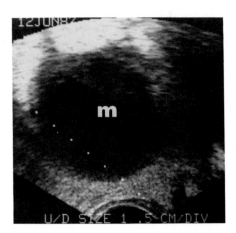

Figure 17.18. Recurrent bladder carcinoma. A patient with bladder carcinoma following a cystectomy was found under computed tomography to have a pelvic mass. Due to the mass's proximity to the rectum, a transrectal biopsy was performed. The mass (*m*) is illustrated in the sonogram and the direction of the needle shown with the guide marks. Cytologic biopsy of this area demonstrated recurrent bladder carcinoma.

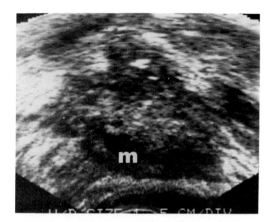

Figure 17.19. Rectal and perirectal inflammatory lesions. A patient with pelvic pain was examined with transrectal ultrasound and a perirectal mass (*m*) detected in the lateral side of the pelvis. Aspiration of this mass yielded inflammatory cells without neoplasm. A chronic diverticular abscess was proven at surgery.

can be further evaluated with transrectal ultrasound and guided aspiration. We have aspirated two rectal wall dermoids for diagnosis and therapy. Several perirectal abscesses have been aspirated utilizing a transrectal approach (Fig. 17.19). The ease and safety of a transrectal approach to a perirectal abscess has been established (43) and an aspiration or a catheter drainage can be performed.

REFERENCES

1. Dahnert WF: Ultrasonography of carcinoma of the prostate: A critical review. *Applied Radiology* 17: 39–44, 1988.
2. Lee F, Litrup PJ, Torp-Pederson ST, et al.: Prostate cancer: Comparison of transrectal US and digital rectal examination for screening. *Radiology* 168: 389–394, 1988.
3. McClennan BL: Transrectal US of the prostate: Is the technology leading the science? *Radiology* 571–575; 168: 1988.
4. Torp-Pederson ST, Littrup PJ, Lee F, Mettlin C: Early prostate cancer: Diagnostic costs of screening transrectal US and digital rectal examination. *Radiology* 351–354; 169: 1988.
5. Rifkin MD: Prostate ultrasound. *Seminars in US, CT and MR* 9: 352–369, 1988.
6. Rifkin MD: *Ultrasound of the Prostate.* New York, Raven Press, pp 51–91, 1988.
7. Rifkin MD: Endorectal sonography of the prostate: Clinical implications. *AJR* 1137–1142; 148: 1987.
8. Lee F, Gray JM, McLeary RD, et al.: Prostatic evaluation by transrectal sonography: Criteria for diagnosis of early carcinoma. *Radiology* 91–95; 158: 1986.
9. Rifkin MD, Friedland GW, Shortliffe L: Prostatic evaluation by transrectal endosonography: Detection of carcinoma. *Radiology* 158: 85–90, 1986.
10. Rifkin MD: *Ultrasound of the Prostate.* New York, Raven Press, pp 31–49, 1988.
11. Lee F, Torp-Pederson ST, Littrup PJ, et al.: Variable appearance of prostate cancer, clinical relevance of tumor size, digital rectal examination, and prostate specific antigen [abstract]. *Radiology* 169 (P): 237, 1988.
12. Kuligowska E, Delgado J, Curhan D, Babayan R: Comparative analysis of endosonography and prostate specific antigen in detecting prostatic carcinoma [abstract]. *Radiology* 169 (P): 23: 1988.
13. Stamey TA, Yang N, Hay AR, McNeal JE, Freiha FS, Redwine E: Prostate-specific antigen as a serum marker for adenocarcinoma of the prostate. *N Engl J Med* 317: 909–916, 1987.
14. Grayhack JT, Bockrath JM: Diagnosis of carcinoma of prostate. *Urology* 17 (Suppl): 54–60, 1981.
15. Graham JB, Ignatoff JM, Holland JM, Christ ML: Prostatic aspiration biopsy: An assessment of accuracy based on long-term observations. *J Urol* 139: 971–974; 1988.
16. Wajsman Z, Klimberg I: Needle aspiration and needle biopsy techniques. *Urol Clin N Am* 14: 103–113; 1987.
17. Layfield LJ, Mukamel E, Hilborne LH, et al.: Cytologic grading of prostatic aspiration biopsy: A comparison with the Gleason grading system. *J Urol* 138: 798–800, 1987.
18. Kaye KW, Horwitz CA: Transrectal fine needle biopsy of the prostate: Combined histological and cytological technique. *J Urol* 139: 1229–1231; 1988.
19. Holm HH, Gammelgaard J: Ultrasonically guided precise needle placement in the prostate and seminal vesicles. *J Urol* 125: 385–387; 1981.
20. Fornage BD, Didier HT, Deglaire M, Fardux MJ, Simatos A: Real-time ultrasound-guided prostatic biopsy using a new transrectal linear-array probe. *Radiology* 146: 547–548; 1983.
21. Lee F, Littrup PJ, McLeary RD, et al.: Needle aspiration and core biopsy of prostate cancer: Comparative evaluation with biplanar transrectal US guidance. *Radiology* 163: 515–520; 1987.
22. Resnick MI: Transrectal ultrasound guided versus digitally directed prostatic biopsy: A comparative study. *J Urol* 139: 754–757; 1988.
23. Rifkin MD, Kurtz AB, Goldberg BB: Sonographically guided transperineal prostatic biopsy: Preliminary experience with a longitudinal linear array transducer. *AJR* 140: 745–747; 1983.
24. Vallancien G, Leo JP, Brisset JM: Transperineal prostatic biopsy guided by transrectal ultrasonography. *Prog Clin Biol Res* 243B: 25–27; 1987.
25. Bree RL, Roberts JL, Jafri SZ: Transrectal US-guided biopsy of the prostate: Techniques and results [abstract]. *Radiology* 169 (P): 236–237, 1988.
26. Cooner WH, Mosley BR, Rutherford CL, et al.: Clinical application of transrectal ultrasonography and prostate specific antigen in the search for prostate cancer. *J Urol* 139: 758–761, 1988.
27. Rifkin MD: *Ultrasound of the Prostate.* New York, Raven Press, pp 113–139, 1988.

28. Torp-Pederson S, Lee F, Littrup PJ, et al.: Transrectal biopsy of the prostate guided with transrectal US: Longitudinal and multiplanar scanning. *Radiology* 170: 23–27; 1989.

29. Lindgren PG, Frödin L, Larsson E, Tufveson G, Wahlberg J: A new needle device from renal transplant biopsy. *Transp Proc* 18: 98–99; 1986.

30. Eaton AC: The safety of transrectal biopsy of the prostate as an outpatient examination. *Br J Urol* 53: 144–146; 1981.

31. McNeal JE, Price HM, Redwine EA, Freiha FS, Stamey TA: Stage A versus stage B adenocarcinoma of the prostate: Morphological comparison and biological significance. *J Urol* 139: 61–65; 1988.

32. McNeal JE: Normal anatomy of the prostate and changes in benign prostatic hypertrophy and carcinoma. *Seminars in US, CT and MR* 9: 329–334; 1988.

33. Choyke PL, Blei CL, Jaffe MH, Zeman RK, Lieberman M: Prevesical hematoma: a complication of prostatic biopsy. *Urol Radiol* 8: 32–34, 1986.

34. Haddad FS, Somsin AA: Seeding and perineal implantation of prostatic cancer in the track of the biopsy needle: Three case reports and a review of the literature. *J Surg Oncol* 35: 184–191; 1987.

35. Holm HH, Juul N, Pedersen JF, Hansen H, Stroyer I: Transperineal 125 iodine seed implantation in prostatic cancer guided by transrectal ultrasonography. *J Urol* 130: 283–286; 1983.

36. Rifkin MD: *Ultrasound of the Prostate.* New York, Raven Press, pp 185–190; 1988.

37. Onik G, Cobb C, Cohen J, Zabkar J, Perterfield B: US characteristics of frozen prostate. *Radiology* 168: 629–630; 1988.

38. Thornhill BA, Morehouse HT, Coleman P, Hoffman-Tretin JC: Prostatic abscess: CT and sonographic findings. *AJR* 148: 899–900; 1987.

39. Littrup PJ, Lee F, McLeary RD, Wu D, Lee A, Kumasaka GH: Transrectal US of the seminal vesicles and ejaculatory ducts: Clinical correlation. *Radiology* 168: 625–628; 1988.

40. Saitoh M, Watanabe H, Ohe H: Ultrasonically guided puncture for the prostate and seminal vesicles with transrectal real-time linear scanner. *J Kyoto Pref Univ Med* 90: 47–50; 1981.

41. Larsen T, Torp-Pederson S, Bostofte E, Rank F: Transperineal fine needle biopsy of gynecologic tumors guided by transrectal ultrasound: A new method. *Gynecol Oncol* 22: 281–287, 1985.

42. Rifkin MD, Marks GJ: Transrectal US as an adjunct in the diagnosis of rectal and extrarectal tumors. *Radiology* 157: 499–502, 1985.

43. Nosher JL, Needell GS, Amorosa JK, Krasha IH: Transrectal pelvic abscess drainage with sonographic guidance. *AJR* 147: 1047–1048, 1986.

18 Obstetrics

WITOLD M. ZALESKI
PHILIPPE JEANTY

Probably in no other clinical situation has ultrasound had more direct impact on patient management than in the imaging of pregnancy. As ultrasound uses no radiation and can provide visualization of the fetus in real time, it is ideally suited to examination of the pregnant uterus. In addition to determining menstrual age, placental location, fetal viability, and the presence of fetal anomalies, ultrasound has been used to guide a number of diagnostic and therapeutic obstetrical techniques. As needle or catheter insertion can be monitored with real-time ultrasound, it is well-suited to guide such procedures as amniocentesis, chorionic villous biopsy, and percutaneous umbilical blood sampling and transfusion. A number of interventional therapeutic procedures can also be guided with ultrasound. These will be reviewed in detail in this chapter.

Amniocentesis

HISTORICAL NOTES

The first reports of amniocentesis date from 1881 in Germany, where the procedure was used for the treatment of polyhydramnios (1). Subsequent applications included amniography in 1930 (2), spectrophotometric analysis of bilirubin in the 1950s, and X chromatin analysis for determination of fetal sex in 1956 (3). Chromosomal analysis of human amniotic fluid cells became possible in 1966 for the prenatal diagnosis of genetic disorders (4). In 1970, an enzyme deficiency in fetal amniotic fluid cells (galactosemia) was first detected (5).

INDICATIONS

The major indications for amniocentesis include prenatal genetic diagnosis, assessment of fetal lung maturity, and Rh isoimmunization.

Prenatal Genetic Diagnosis

Antenatal cytogenetic studies involve two major subgroups: chromosomal anomalies and single gene or polygenic disorders. Risk factors for chromosomal abnormalities include increasing maternal age, previous gestation with chromosomal anomaly, and parental translocation, inversion, or aneuploidy.

Advanced maternal age is associated with increased incidence of fetal chromosomal abnormalities. For instance, the frequency of trisomy 21, the most familiar chromosomal anomaly associated with advanced maternal age, increases exponentially above age 30. The incidence of other disorders, such as autosomal trisomies 13 and 18 as well as sex chromosomal trisomies 47,XXX and 47,XXY, also increases. (See Table 18.1).

These risk figures are calculated for liveborn infants. Importantly, at 16 to 18 weeks gestation, the prevelence of chromosomal abnormalities is approximately 30% higher than in liveborns (7) (and is even greater at 9 to 11 weeks gestation at the time of chorionic villus sampling). In most centers, genetic amniocentesis is offered to all

Table 18.1
Chromosomal Abnormalities in Liveborn
Infants at Various Maternal Ages (6)

Maternal age	Risk of trisomy 21 (average)	Risk of all chromosomal anomalies (excluding 47,XXX)
20	1/1667	1/526
25	1/1250	1/476
30	1/952	1/385
35	1/385	1/179
40	1/106	1/63
45	1/30	1/19

women who will be 35 years or older at the expected date of delivery.

Following the birth of a liveborn infant with a chromosomal abnormality, the risk of a subsequent gestation also having a chromosomal anomaly remains elevated even if parental chromosomal complements are normal. The relative increase in risk is greater for younger parents, whose initial risk prior to the birth of the first trisomic child was lower. The risk of recurrence with autosomal as well as sex chromosomal trisomies is generally considered to be 1% to 2% (8).

Balanced translocations occur in one of every 500 individuals who remain phenotypically normal but may produce offspring with aneuploidy (8). The risks vary with the type of translocation; for example, the likelihood of having a child with trisomy 21 is 2% or less if the father carries a 14/21 translocation, and about 10% if the mother is the carrier of the translocation (9).

Single gene and polygenic disorders may be divided into inborn errors of metabolism, neural tube defects (NTD), and sex-linked abnormalities. Most inborn errors of metabolism are autosomal recessive disorders, although some are inherited in an X-linked recessive or autosomal dominant fashion. Antenatal diagnosis is now possible for at least 80 of these disorders (1).

For example, hexosaminidase A levels can be assayed in amniotic fluid fibroblasts or chorionic villus cells for the diagnosis of Tay-Sachs disease (GM$_2$ gangliosidosis type

1). Screening programs can detect heterozygotes with diminished serum hexosaminidase A, which is needed for the metabolism of sphingolipids. A second example is cystic fibrosis, in which heterozygote detection is not yet reliably available. However, assays for decreased levels of various amniotic fluid intestinal microvillar enzymes, (10) as well as DNA analysis, show some promise in the prenatal diagnosis of this disorder.

Neural tube defects include anencephaly, spinal dysraphism (with associated meningocele or myelomeningocele), and other midline defects such as encephalocele. The likelihood that a first-degree relative will have either anencephaly or spina bifida is 2% in the United States and 5% in the United Kingdom, with approximately equal risk of having either malformation. The risk for second- and third-degree relatives is proportionately less but remains elevated above that for the general population even for first cousins (0.3%–1.0% versus a general incidence of 1.4 to 1.6 per 1000 live births in the U.S.) (11).

Ultrasound examination and amniotic fluid assay both contribute to the antenatal diagnosis of NTD. With assays of amniotic fluid alpha-fetoproteim (AFP), diagnosis of NTD is possible in all except the 5% to 10% of spina bifida cases in which skin covers the lesion. Ultrasound can readily exclude anencephaly, and the vertebral column can be examined for the presence of defects in the bony structures as well as the presence of a myelomeningocele sac.

The causes of elevated amniotic fluid AFP other than NTD include contamination by fetal blood, omphalocele, gastroschisis, cystic hygroma, congenital nephrosis, and fetal death. The presence of acetylcholinesterase in the amniotic fluid, an enzyme not detectable in maternal serum, serves as a check that elevated amniotic fluid AFP is due to an NTD or other fetal defect. If fetal hemoglobin is detected and acetylcholinesterase is absent, this suggests that the elevated AFP in the amniotic fluid results from contamination by fetal blood. Sometimes screening programs detect a persistently elevated maternal serum AFP, for which no obvious cause can be found. Amniocentesis may be required in these cases for assessment of amniotic fluid AFP, in conjunction with a careful ultrasound survey to exclude a visible neural tube defect.

Decreased maternal serum AFP (lower than 0.4 multiples of the median) has been associated with a three- to seven-fold increase in the risk of trisomy 21, compared to that expected on the basis of maternal age alone. Age-dependent cut-off levels of maternal serum AFP at 14 to 20 weeks gestation have been suggested as an indication for genetic amniocentesis ($\leq$0.5 at age 25–31, $\leq$0.6 at age 32–33, and $\leq$0.7 at age 34) (12).

Fetal sex determination is important in determining fetuses at risk for sex-linked abnormalities. Male fetuses only are affected in many x-linked or male-limited autosomal dominant disorders. For some of the most common of these disorders, such as Lesch-Nyhan syndrome, Fabry disease, G6PD deficiency, Hunter syndrome, fragile X syndrome, hemophilia, and Duchenne muscular dystrophy, a definitive diagnosis is now possible. (1) Using the technique of restriction fragment-length polymorphism (RFLP) for DNA analysis of the X chromosome, these disorders can now be identified, and the list of detectable X-linked traits should increase rapidly. For other X-linked disorders that are not at present diagnosable, pregnancies with male fetuses can be selectively terminated to avoid the delivery of an affected child. However, statistically, only half of these fetuses will have inherited the abnormal X chromosome, the remainder being genetically normal.

Analytical techniques in molecular genetics (gene probes, restriction enzymes, Southern blotting, and DNA hybridization) applied to DNA analysis are continually extending the range of disorders detectable in utero. Since these molecular genetic techniques can utilize any available fetal DNA, including amniotic fluid cells, indications for amniocentesis and chorionic villus sampling (see below) are almost certainly going to continue to expand. The following genetic disorders can now or soon will be diagnosed in utero: sickle cell anemia, beta-thalassemia, alpha-thalassemia, Duchenne muscular dystrophy, phenylketonuria, hemophilia A and B, Huntington chorea, and cystic fibrosis (majority of cases) (1).

Fetal Lung Maturity

Gluck and colleagues in 1971 noted an abrupt increase occurred in the amount of lecithin in the amniotic fluid at about 35 weeks gestation, with little or no change in the sphingomyelin. On the basis of 302 amniocenteses, they concluded that a sudden increase in the lecithin-sphingomyelin (L/S) ratio after 35 weeks "heralds the maturity of the pulmonary alveolar lining" (13). Other studies have confirmed that an L/S ratio greater than 2.0 predicts the absence of respiratory distress syndrome in the newborn. Gluck subsequently reported that the presence of phosphatidyl glycerol (PG) in the amniotic fluid improves the accuracy of an L/S ratio greater than 2.0 in predicting the absence of respiratory distress syndrome in the newborn infant (14).

Rh Isoimmunization

The management of the patient at risk for Rh sensitization begins with an initial antibody screen and titre to determine the presence and level of maternal antibodies. Amniocentesis is recommended if the maternal antibody titre is 1:16 or greater. The change in amniotic fluid optical density at 450 nm (ΔOD_{450}), measured by spectrophotometry, reflects the concentration of yellow bile pigments resulting from isoimmune fetal red cell hemolysis. The level of the ΔOD_{450} is compared to charts prepared by Liley (15).

Since the comparison of the measured ΔOD_{450} with Liley's charts is based on gestational age, a preliminary ultrasound examination early in pregnancy is essential for an accurate determination of fetal age using the crown-rump length. The timing of amniocentesis for Rh isoimmunization depends on the maternal antibody titre and the degree to which previous pregnancies were affected. If a previous infant was only mildly affected, the initial amniocentesis can be performed at 28 weeks gestation. If the degree of fetal compromise was moderate to severe in the previous pregnancy, amniocentesis should be performed at 21 to 22 weeks gestation, provided there is no evidence of fetal hydrops on prior ultrasound examinations. Finally, if there has been previous fetal loss due to Rh isoimmunization, amniocentesis should be performed 10 weeks prior to the time of the previous loss or before 21 weeks gestation.

Serial amniocentesis is repeated at 1- to 3-week intervals, depending on the severity of the disease. If the ΔOD_{450} reaches the upper 20% level in Liley zone II or an initial reading falls into Liley zone III after 34 weeks gestation, prompt induction and delivery should be carried out if the amniotic fluid L/S ratio indicates pulmonary maturity. A ΔOD_{450} level in Liley zone III prior to 34 weeks gestation is an indication for fetal blood transfusion on the basis of a single reading. In utero transfusion should also be considered if the ΔOD_{450} level rises into the upper 20% of Liley zone II prior to 30 weeks gestation or into zone III between 31 and 34 weeks gestation (16). If the ΔOD_{450} levels are in Liley zone II but decreasing at a rate >0.01 units/week, amniocentesis can be performed every 2 weeks and fetal transfusion deferred.

Ultrasound findings associated with immune hydrops include 1)polyhydramnios; 2) placental hypertrophy with loss of architecture, disappearance of the chorionic plate, loss of cotyledon definition, buckling of the fetal surface, and ground glass appearance; 3) fetal scalp and abdominal wall edema; 4) fetal ascites, pleural and pericardial effusions; 5) hepatosplenomegaly; and 6) rapid enlargement of the fetal abdominal circumference as a sign of impending hydrops (17).

TECHNIQUE

Although differences exist in the details of amniocentesis technique from center to center, the most commonly used variants will be described. A preliminary ultrasound survey is performed prior to the procedure in order to 1) detect the presence of multiple gestation, 2) confirm fetal viability, 3) assess fetal age by appropriate biometric measure-

ments, 4) detect gross fetal anomalies (18), 5) evaluate placental position as well as any maternal uterine/adnexal abnormalities, 6) determine fetal lie, and 7) select a site for needle insertion. Most recent reports recommend the use of real-time ultrasound guidance during needle insertion, as well as continuous monitoring of the needle tip position throughout the procedure (19–24). Three main variants of this technique have been described.

Ultrasound Guidance Techniques

Parallel freehand insertion. After sterile preparation of the patient's abdomen, the transducer is covered with a sterile glove or plastic bag and placed directly over the selected puncture site, with needle insertion alongside and parallel to the transducer (without angulation) (20, 23) (Fig. 18.1**B**). After approximately 2 cm penetration the needle enters the ultrasound beam, producing the characteristic flare of the bevelled tip. The needle is advanced into the selected amniotic fluid pocket, with adjustments being made should fetal position change during needle insertion.

Orthogonal free hand insertion. The patient's abdomen is prepared as above; however, the transducer is used without a sterile cover and is applied to the maternal abdomen at a site outside the sterile field that will still allow visualization of the needle entry site and proposed needle track aligned in the plane of the sector scan (Fig. 18.1**A**). The abdominal wall can be palpated gently to identify the position of the needle entry site on the margin of the image. The needle is then introduced and advanced slowly until the shaft and flare of the needle tip are visualized on the real-time image (19).

Care must be taken to maintain the entire needle in the scanning plane; otherwise, an oblique image of the needle shaft only may by obtained, without visualization of the needle tip. This may result in uncontrolled placement of the needle tip, with an increased risk of fetal puncture or needle misplacement in a posterior placenta or posterior uterine wall.

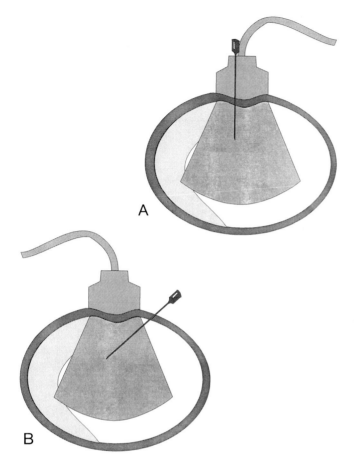

A

B

Figure 18.1. Using the freehand technique, the needle may be inserted perpendicularly to the plane of the ultrasound beam (orthogonal) (**A**) or parallel to the imaging plane (**B**).

Fixed-needle guidance. A third ultrasound technique has been described (24, 25) using a slightly angled approach via a Lucite needle guide attached to the sector scanning head (CIVCO Medical Instruments Co. Inc. Kalona, IA). Some authors (24) have soaked the Lucite in Cidex (activated dialdehyde) for 15 minutes between procedures, then rinsed with sterile saline, thus avoiding time consuming gas resterilization or the necessity of having several guides available for a series of consecutive amniocenteses.

The fixed-needle guidance method has some limitations for amniocentesis. First, the requirement for a needle guide restricts the choice of transducers available for amniocentesis. Losing the device may be cumbersome. In addition to these relatively minor drawbacks, the major hindrance of this technique is that needle and transducer are joined for the whole procedure. Thus,

checking the fetal heart or imaging a different area of the abdomen to search for a better fluid pocket should the fetus move, becomes cumbersome. This last restriction has made the procedure less attractive and it is not widely used. The choice between the techniques described above depends on personal preference: only one operator is needed to perform amniocentesis using the parallel insertion technique, whereas the orthogonal approach is slightly faster because a sterile covering for the transducer is not required.

There are a number of practical considerations when performing amniocentesis. The ideal pocket of amniotic fluid should be easily accessible with minimal risk to the fetus (Fig. 18.2). Thus, needle placement in proximity to the fetal head or face is contraindicated. We avoid uterine leiomyomas and contractions (26). For the patient's comfort

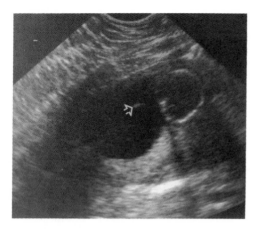

Figure 18.2. Using the parallel freehand technique, the needle is inserted in a spot free of placental tissue. Note the needle tip (*open arrow*) in the amniotic fluid.

we try to select a pocket near the fundus of the uterus, since skin entry is less painful with increasing distance from the pubis. It has also been suggested that fundal insertions have a lower risk of causing premature rupture of the membranes than suprapubic insertions.

When an appropriate spot has been localized, a small pressure mark is made on the patient's skin with a plastic straw to indicate the area of skin preparation. We do not use sterile drapes. It should be emphasized that one should not rely on the preliminary mark to insert the needle since in approximately 10% of cases the fetus will have changed position during the time it took to prepare the skin (19). Although the prescribed method of using a 10% povidine-iodine solution is to let it dry for maximal germicidal activity, we usually apply the solution with three separate swabs and then wipe off the excess in the area of needle insertion with a sterile 4 x 4 gauze.

Placental location

Although we make an effort to avoid the placenta, Crane and co-workers (22) as well as Hanson and colleagues (27) have shown that anterior or partly anterior placentas, which occur in 47% to 60% of patients, can be penetrated routinely during amniocentesis without increased complication. A site in the periphery of the placenta, at least a few

centimeters away from the cord insertion, should be chosen (Fig 18.3). We do not attempt to access the uterus via a lateral approach to avoid passing through an anterior placenta.

Needles commonly used range from 20-gauge to 23- and 25-gauge. At our institution, second trimester amniocentesis is performed with a 22-gauge spinal needle, and third trimester amniocentesis with a 20-gauge needle. Specially designed Teflon-coated needles as well as needles with a roughened external surface near the tip are theoretically more reflective and therefore easier to visualize on the ultrasound image (25). Another design modification is side holes that reduce the likelihood of clogging. These innovations are interesting; however, the increased cost of these needles seems to outweigh any advantage in their use. The addition of a sonically sensitive stylet has also been reported to enhance visualization of the needle tip, but leads to a more awkward technique requiring resterilization of the stylet (28).

The tip of the needle should be constantly monitored during insertion. It is usually not visible during the first few centimeters of penetration. In the parallel technique, this is due to the narrow near field (usually narrower than the physical width of the transducer); while in the orthogonal approach, it

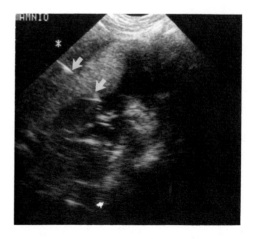

Figure 18.3. Again using the parallel freehand technique, the needle is inserted (*arrows*) transplacentally into the amniotic cavity.

is caused by limited skin contact of the end of the transducer closest to the needle. Nevertheless, even if the tip itself is not visible during the first few centimeters of penetration, tissue motion will be perceived in the region where the needle will appear. If the needle is inserted in an incorrect direction, it should be repositioned by withdrawal into the subcutaneous tissues and subsequent reinsertion, not by lateral movement.

Membrane tenting is another potential problem during amniocentesis (29). Localized separation of the membranes may occur at the site of needle puncture into the uterine wall with the tented membranes covering the advancing needle tip, resulting in a "dry" tap. When the needle reaches the chorion, it should be advanced with a clean thrust to perforate the membranes. Suspected tenting can be corrected by deeper penetration, reorientation, gentle thrusting or twisting so that the bevel can cut the amnion. We do not recommend advancing the needle into the posterior uterine wall (30), as this causes an unnecessary second perforation of the membranes with potential fluid accumulation (Fig. 18.4). "Pseudotenting," the appearance of a membrane-like structure covering the tip of the needle on the ultrasound image when fluid can easily be withdrawn, is usually caused by a side lobe

artifact arising from the tip of the needle (Fig. 18.5).

Whenever possible, the needle should be inserted as deeply as possible into the amniotic cavity, ideally, close to the posterior uterine wall. This reduces the risk of the fetus coming into contact with the sharp tip of the needle (Fig. 18.6). When the stylet is removed, fluid should spontaneously drip from the needle hub within 5 to 10 seconds. If no fluid is seen, aspirating with a syringe is usually not helpful and simply delays proper repositioning of the needle.

The use of plastic extension tubing (K50 or equivalent) to connect the needle hub to the aspirating syringe has two major advantages: 1) the needle is not "fixed" within the amniotic cavity, as it would be if it were attached directly to the syringe, and 2) motion of the obstetrician's hands is not translated into motion of the needle. If the needle is not fixed, fetal motion will simply displace it. In addition, the not uncommon tendency either to slowly advance or withdraw the needle during aspiration is avoided. Accessory tubing (Fig. 18.7) usually also allows the obstetrician to assume a more comfortable position during the procedure. We also use an Everest aspiration handle (Cook Urological, Spencer, IN) designed for a 20-cc syringe (Fig. 18.7). This device allows sin-

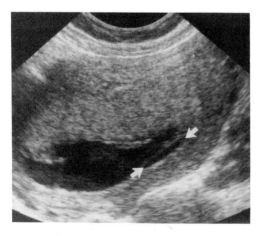

Figure 18.4. Fluid accumulated (*arrows*) outside the amniotic membranes after a through-and-through insertion into the posterior myometrium. Ultimately, this gestation miscarried.

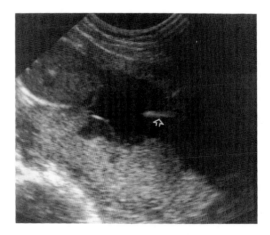

Figure 18.5. Using the parallel freehand technique, there is pseudotenting due to a side lobe artifact (*open arrows*) from the needle tip.

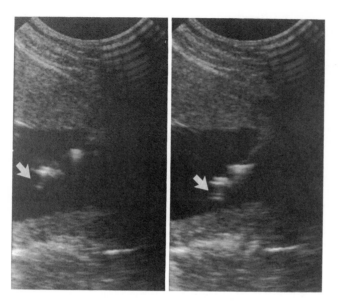

Figure 18.6. (*Left*) Initially the needle (*Arrow*) has been inserted into the midportion of the amniotic fluid, but (*Right*) deeper insertion prevents fetal injury from the tip of the needle (*Arrow*).

gle-handed aspiration, leaving the other hand free to manipulate the needle.

When satisfactory needle position is obtained, the stylet is removed from the needle and the first 1 or 2 ml of amniotic fluid are aspirated with a 3-cc syringe. This sample is discarded to avoid potential contamination of the aspirate by blood or tissue collected during the insertion. Fluid is aspirated into a 20-cc syringe using steady but gentle suction either directly or with plastic extension tubing connected to the needle hub. Increasing the suction does not significantly increase the flow of fluid through the needle, but may cause an adjacent loop of cord to be sucked onto the tip of the needle. If this occurs, the needle can be flushed with a very small amount of previously aspirated fluid, provided that the operator is confident that the needle tip still lies free within the amniotic cavity (Fig. 18.8).

Differentiation of amniotic fluid from maternal urine is rarely necessary. Should there be any doubt as to the origin of a particular sample, a drop of fluid can be aid dried in a few seconds on a glass slide. Amniotic fluid will form a characteristic crystalline arborization pattern that is not seen with maternal urine. Adequate sample size is usually 20 to 30 ml in total for genetic amniocentesis, 3 to 4 ml for fetal lung maturity assessment, and 5 to 10 ml for Rh isoimmunization studies.

Samples sent for evaluation of ΔOD_{450} must be protected from light to avoid oxidation of bilirubin to colorless compounds.

Difficulties in performing amniocentesis may occur in cases of maternal obesity, oligohydramnios, or multiple gestations. Amniocentesis in obese patients (greater than 4 cm of subcutaneous fat) may be a challenge. Needle localization will be more difficult and a longer needle may be necessary. Possible solutions involve a suprapubic approach, with the patient holding redundant

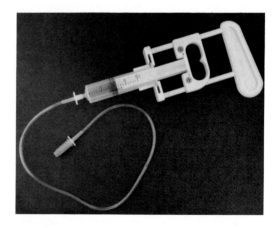

Figure 18.7. The connecting tubing and aspiration handle that may be used when performing amniocentesis.

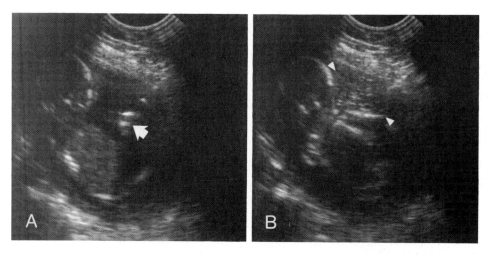

Figure 18.8. **A,** The needle was inserted into the amniotic cavity (*arrow*) but "dry tap" was obtained. **B,** The needle was flushed with 0.5 cc amniotic fluid, which resulted in numerous microbubbles (*arrowheads*) within the amniotic fluid. The needle is unclogged.

folds of the abdominal wall out of the way, or an insertion through the umbilicus.

Even in the presence of oligohydramnios, amniocentesis performed with ultrasound guidance should rarely result in a "dry" tap, except in some cases of premature rupture of membranes. Fluid can usually be found between the fetal abdomen and limbs. However, these pockets of fluid may also contain loops of cord, and very careful needle positioning is required. If Doppler color flow mapping is available, it may be helpful to outline the position of the cord. Instead of inserting the needle as far as possible into the amniotic cavity before removing the stylet, the latter may be removed and the tubing attached as soon as the membranes have been pierced. The needle is then advanced slowly, with gentle suction to the syringe until fluid is encountered. Fixed-needle guides have been advocated in these cases (25).

The overall frequency of twin gestations is approximately 1/90 pregnancies, occurring most frequently in blacks and least frequently in Orientals. Monozygosity occurs in 34% of white and 29% of black twin pregnancies in the United States. Twinning frequency increases overall with maternal age to approximately one in 65 between the ages of 35 and 39, the vast bulk of the increase being due to increased rates of dizygotic twinning. Although overall the risk of fetal anomaly in twins is double that of singleton pregnancies, because of an association with increased maternal age, dizygotic twins have six times increased risk that one or the other twin will be chromosomally abnormal (31).

Concerns about sampling both sacs of a twin gestation include 1) monozygosity, making genetic amniocentesis of the second sac redundant, 2) the possibility of alpha-fetoprotein diffusion from one sac to the other, and 3) coexistence of a normal and abnormal twin with subsequent therapeutic dilemma.

Multiple gestations are readily diagnosed by ultrasound. Amniocentesis may be performed via two separate punctures (31–33) or as recently reported from our institution, via a single puncture traversing the intervening membrane (34; Fig. 18.9). In the first method, a dye (2 to 3 ml of 0.8% indigo carmine diluted to 0.08% in bacteriostatic water) is injected into the first sac after withdrawal of the fluid sample. The second sac is then entered via a separate skin puncture, the absence of blue discoloration of the second sampling serving to confirm that the fluid indeed originates from the second gestational sac.

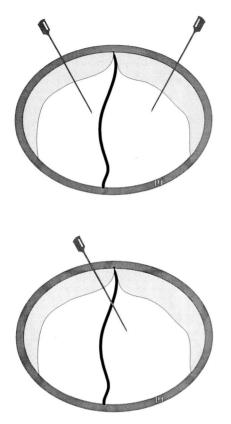

Figure 18.9. Twin gestational sac can be tapped by two separate needle punctures or conveniently through a single needle insertion, first tapping one sac and then piercing the membranes to tap the second sac.

Our experience with the instillation of indigo carmine suggests that the dye has a higher specific gravity than the amniotic fluid and settles at the bottom of the sac. Thus withdrawal of fluid immediately after instillation may not always demonstrate its presence. Some authors have recommended that the patient take a short walk or simply roll on the table between needle insertions to allow better mixing of the dye (31).

We have recently described a simpler technique using a single needle insertion. The needle puncture site that we select demonstrates both gestational sacs as well as the interamniotic membrane, through a region of myometrium that is free of placenta. The more proximal sac is tapped first and the syringe and plastic tubing are disconnected.

No dye is used. The stylet is replaced in the needle and the latter is advanced under ultrasound guidance through the interamniotic membrane. Initial tenting of the intervening membrane is seen, then perforation is accomplished by an easily visible "pop." When the needle tip has been positioned within the second sac, the first few ml of fluid are discarded, and a new syringe and plastic tubing are attached for the second tap.

Even is the membrane is not readily visualized by ultrasound, one should still assume the presence of a septum and attempt to sample both sacs. The two fetal bodies can be lined up in a single plane and the needle inserted on the side of the fetus furthest from the other twin, in order to increase the chances of penetrating the second sac (33).

COMPLICATIONS

After the procedure, the patient is instructed to report fluid loss per vagina, bleeding, uterine cramping or fever. Most authors also advise against strenuous exercise or coitus for 24 hours. Potential complications of amniocentesis can be divided into maternal risks and fetal risks.

Maternal Risks

Serious maternal complications are rare. These include amnionitis in approximately 1/1000 procedures according to one survey, usually without maternal sequelae (35). One maternal death in a combined survey of over 20,000 procedures has been reported, but details were not published (36). Minor problems include transient spotting or leakage of amniotic fluid per vagina in 1% to 3% of cases, and occasional uterine contractions. Persistent amniotic fluid leakage is a rare complication observed in only two of 5,200 procedures in a study by Crane and colleagues (37). These same authors reviewed the eight reported cases at the time and found preterm delivery (less than 32 weeks) occurred in three instances, with club foot deformity observed in two of the eight infants.

Fetal Risks

Although the routine administration of Rh-immunoglobulin (RHIG) has raised some concerns about possible risks to the fetus (38), the American College of Obstetricians and Gynecologists recommended in 1981 that a 300µ dose of RHIG be given to Rh-negative women following second trimester amniocentesis, to prevent Rh isoimmunization.

Potential fetal complications of amniocentesis include spontaneous abortion, premature rupture of membranes, premature labor, placental abruption, fetal transplacental hemorrhage, fetal trauma, and deformities that may be associated with withdrawal of amniotic fluid, such as arthrogryposis, or amniotic band syndrome. The United Kingdom collaborative study on the risks of amniocentesis suggested that there may be an association between genetic amniocentesis and an increased risk of talipes equino varus and congenital dislocation of the hip (39); however, this has not been found in other reports (40).

Direct fetal trauma is rare, but cases of ileocutaneous fistula, ileal atresia, gangrene of an arm, corneal perforation and blindness, porencephalic cysts, patellar disruption, peripheral nerve injury and umbilical hematoma have been associated with amniocentesis in case reports (1). Fetal cutaneous scarring is also rare.

Amniocentesis related abortion rates have varied from a low of 0.3% (41) to 2.9% (42, 43). The added risk of fetal loss attributable to amniocentesis is felt to be 0.5% or less (44).

Immediate and unexplained fetal death was found in 5 cases from a combined survey of 7,524 in four centres (45). A neurogenic mechanism is postulated since post mortem examination was not helpful.

THE ROLE OF ULTRASOUND

Ultrasound has been used as an adjunct to amniocentesis since the late 1960s and early 1970s. Initially, opinion in the literature was divided as to the usefulness of an ultrasound examination immediately prior to amniocentesis in reducing the incidence of certain complications such as bloody taps, failed amniocentesis, and fetal injury or loss. Several studies reported lower rates of bloody taps using ultrasonographic fetal, umbilical cord, and placental localization (44–48). On the other hand, studies also reported the converse, that the frequency of bloody taps was actually slightly higher using prior ultrasound localization. For example, in the British collaborative amniocentesis study (39) 14.6% of amniotic fluid samples were blood contaminated when ultrasound guidance was used, compared to 11.2% without the use of ultrasound.

Since the early 1980's the use of ultrasound guidance in amniocentesis has been modified to include real-time monitoring of needle placement during the procedure in addition to preliminary scanning for placental localization and exclusion of fetal anomalies.

In 1983, Benacerraf and Frigoletto (19) reported the use of continuous ultrasound monitoring in 232 of 235 consecutive amniocenteses (184 for prenatal genetic diagnosis, 51 for monitoring Rh incompatability or fetal lung maturity in older fetuses). Among these 232 procedures, the rate of unsuccessful dry taps was 2.6% and the initial bloody tap rate was 2.9%, "both substantially lower than those previously reported in the literature (19). In addition, in 10% of cases the initial site chosen had to be modified due to a change in fetal position during the time it took the operator to prepare the skin (approximately 30 to 60 seconds).

Romero and colleagues (23) compared 688 patients undergoing genetic amniocentesis after prior ultrasound localization to 612 undergoing amniocentesis with continuous real-time ultrasound guidance. In the group with continuous monitoring, there was a statistically significant decrease in the frequency of bloody or unsuccessful taps, as well as in the number of patients requiring multiple needle insertions. The greatest reduction in complication rates with continuous ultrasound monitoring was seen with relatively inexperienced operators whose rates of dry or bloody taps approached those of the most experienced obstetrician using this technique.

A reduction in the number of needle passes to obtain amniotic fluid as well as fewer bloody taps have been reported to be associated with a lower percentage of postamniocentesis complications, such as pregnancy loss, fetal injury, or fetal-maternal transfusion (49–51). In a study by Ron and co-workers (52), controls with clear fluid had a rate of fetal loss of 1.7%, but the fetal loss rate was 6.6% when amniotic fluid was contaminated by maternal blood, and 14.3% when contaminated by fetal blood. Fewer bloody taps may also avoid falsely elevated amniotic fluid AFP levels caused by contamination with fetal blood, as well as reduce the incidence of culture failure (19).

Chorionic Villus Sampling

Although successful genetic amniocentesis has been performed by some investigators as early as 11 to 15 weeks since the last menstrual period (53), others are of the opinion that amniocentesis cannot be safely performed prior to 15 to 16 weeks gestation (54). Proponents of early amniocentesis have found no difference in the mean time from amnicentesis to culture processing in early (less than 15 weeks) versus late (greater than 15 weeks) amniocentesis (53). Potential problems in early amniocentesis include a small total amniotic pool, estimated at around 75 ml at 12 weeks menstrual age, a lower concentration of amniotic fluid cells, and a higher culture failure rate. Since genetic amniocentesis involves a 2- to 3-week delay before the results of karyotyping are available, fetal diagnosis can be established consistently only around 18 weeks gestation.

Chorionic villus sampling (CVS) can advance the time of fetal diagnosis considerably, the optimal time for the procedure being 9 to 11 weeks from the onset of the last menstrual period (54–59). Some authors use slightly expanded gestational age criteria from 8 to 12–13 weeks (58–63). Cytogenic analysis is usually available within 24 to 48 hours using the direct method and between 5 and 7 days using the culture technique (54), allowing the parents to choose a

first trimester abortion. Thus the fivefold increased risk of maternal mortality associated with abortion between 16 and 24 weeks gestation may be avoided (64).

HISTORICAL NOTES

Transcervical biopsy of placental tissue was first reported in Sweden in 1973 by Kullander and Sandahl utilizing a 5-mm endoscope (65). In 1974 Hahnemann used a 2.5-mm hysteroscope introduced through a 4-mm cannula placed in the cervical canal to biopsy the "extraembryonic membranes" (66). A Chinese study of 100 patients at Tietung hospital in 1975 used a 3-mm metal cannula blindly introduced transcervically into the uterus to aspirate chorionic villi (67). Finally, in 1982, Kazy and co-workers in the Soviet Union compared the use of a 1.7-mm fetoscope (and direct-vision biopsy forceps) to the use of 2-mm flexible biopsy forceps placed in the placental tissue using real-time ultrasonographic guidance (68). In the same year Old and colleagues introduced a 1.5-mm plastic catheter with a malleable aluminum obturator placed transcervically into the placenta under simultaneous transabdominal ultrasound guidance (69).

After a number of single case reports and small series in 1983 describing CVS for cytogenic diagnosis in the first trimester, Simoni and colleagues published the first larger series of diagnostic CVS procedures in continuing pregnancies in 1984 (70).

INDICATIONS

Since cells derived from chorionic villi differentiate from the same blastocyst as does the fetus, chromosomal and DNA analysis of these cells reflects the status of the fetus in much the same way as do cultured amniotic cells. Although normal expression and range of activity have not been fully documented for many fetal enzymes in chorionic villus cells, CVS also has been applied to the diagnosis of some inborn errors of metabolism, such as gangliosidosis GM_1 and GM_2 (Tay-Sachs disease), Niemann-Pick disease and Hurler syndrome (70, 71).

The indications for CVS therefore are

similar to those for genetic amniocentesis, and include prenatal genetic diagnosis related to 1)advanced maternal age, 2) previous gestation with chromosomal anomaly, 3) parental translocation or aneuploidy, 4) single-gene and polygenic disorders, including some inborn errors of metabolism, and 5) fetal sex determination in X-linked disorders. The only major indication for genetic amniocentesis that cannot be assessed by CVS is the amniotic fluid alpha-fetoprotein level used for diagnosis of neural tube defects.

Generally accepted contraindications to CVS are 1) severe cervicitis, 2) active genital herpes, 3) undiagnosed cervical lesion, 4) active uterine bleeding, 5) large leiomyoma obstructing the projected pathway to the placenta, and 6) markedly angulated cervical canal (55). Multiple gestation is considered a contraindication by some, although limited reports of this technique in twin gestations have been published, particularly when the two placental sites can be easily distinguished on ultrasound (56, 70).

TECHNIQUE

CVS is ideally performed between 9 and 11 weeks from the onset of the last menstrual period. A preliminary ultrasound examination is used to 1) exclude multiple gestation, 2) document fetal viability, and 3) estimate gestational age from crown-rump length measurements. A rather high fre-

quency of missed abortion in patients seeking CVS has been demonstrated, with abnormal gestational sacs detected by initial ultrasound in up to 12.4% of cases (56, 58, 72). Patients are also screened in some centers by cervical culture for Neisseria gonorrhea prior to the procedure.

Different techniques of CVS have been described, but the most commonly used at present is the transcervical approach with ultrasonographic guidance (Fig. 18.10). Other methods that have been reported, mainly in Europe, consist of 1) transvaginal CVS using a needle guide attached to a transvaginal transducer (73), 2) transcervical CVS via a small endoscope (65, 66, 68, 74), and 3) transabdominal biopsy using a coaxial system of guide and aspiration needles (75–78). This latter technique has the theoretical advantage of a reduced risk of infectious complications and simplicity (77); however, it is not commonly used in North America.

Various CVS catheters are available, ranging from a 1.5-mm diameter polyethylene catheter with a malleable stylet (Portex Inc., Wilmington, MA: 56) to a round-ended nonmalleable 2-mm diameter 14-gauge hollow metal cannula with the distal 3 cm angulated 30° (79). Some investigators have attempted to increase the visibility of the sampling catheter on ultrasound by the addition of a highly echogenic strip in the catheter wall (60) or even by incorporating a

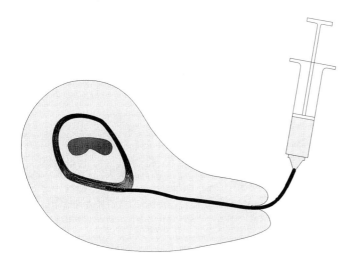

Figure 18.10. Schematic drawing demonstrating chorionic villous sampling catheter insertion.

small ultrasonic emitter into the end of the catheter (80). In our institution, we use the Angiomed catheter (Angiomed Aktiengesellschaft, Karlsruche, W. Germany) varying from 20 cm to 24 cm in length, depending primarily on the length of the vagina, as well as uterine/cervical configuration.

The procedure is performed with the patient in lithotomy position. The bladder should be full enough to allow good ultrasound visualization, but not to the point that the patient cannot comfortably endure the length of the procedure. After speculum insertion, the vaginal vault and cervix are prepared with a 10% povidine-iodine solution and wiped gently with gauze. An appropriate curve is formed in the malleable obturator. The CVS catheter and obturator assembly is then inserted into the external os and advanced into the chorion frondosum of the placenta under continuous ultrasound monitoring. A single-tooth tenaculum is used to grasp the anterior lip of the cervix only in cases where the external os cannot easily be visualized using the speculum alone.

Ultrasound guidance is provided from the suprapubic area. The catheter is seen as a bright line well identified by its motion (Fig. 18.11). As in any ultrasound-guided procedure, it is important to check the position of the distal end of the catheter, and not merely the portion visible at the level of he cervix. The ultrasonographer should look at the curve that the obstetrician has formed in the guide in order to appreciate how it should appear on the ultrasound image. A frequent problem for the ultrasonographer is that the catheter can be followed for some distance in the uterus, and then no apparent further progression is noted. This is often due to the fact that the obstetrician has turned or angled the catheter and therefore the portion of the catheter displayed on the screen is part of the distal shaft and not the tip (Fig. 18.12). If this is not appreciated quickly, the actual catheter tip may have penetrated much deeper. Communication between the obstetrician and ultrasonographer is critical. Even when the catheter tip is well located, small side-to-side move-

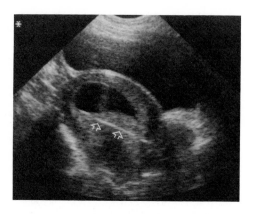

Figure 18.11. Longitudinal ultrasound demonstrating insertion of chorionic villous sampling catheter (*open arrows*).

ments of the transducer should be performed to ensure that the entirety of the catheter tip is visualized.

When the catheter with the appropriate shape formed in the malleable obturator reaches the gestational sac, it will usually dissect preferentially towards the trophoblast and not indent the membranes. Should the catheter push the membranes, a distinct tenting can be seen. The obstetrician should be immediately alerted, but without alarming the patient. When the trophoblast in on the lateral side of the uterine cavity, a sagittal scan may create the alarming appearance that the catheter is lying inside the gestational sac. This actually represents an artifact caused by volume averaging.

Catheter guidance is usually not a problem in an anteverted uterus, Occasionally, in a uterus with a steeper degree of anteversion, a high anterior trophoblast may be difficult to reach. Maneuvers that may help in this situation include pulling the cervix anteriorly and caudally or allowing increased bladder filling to displace the uterus posteriorly. Some of the most difficult cases involve a posterior placenta in a steeply retroverted uterus. Again, the only solution may be to apply gentle traction on the cervix or to form a more pronounced curve in the guide. Finally, the presence of a leiomyoma may make the procedure technically more difficult, but can be dealt with on an individual basis by varying the curve of the

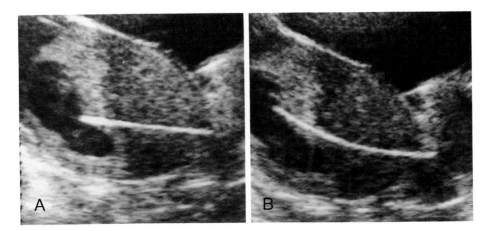

Figure 18.12. **A,** Longitudinal ultrasound of the uterus demonstrating partial visualization of the catheter with the tip angled out of the scanning plane. **B,** Scan angled slightly to the side to demonstrate the tip of the chorionic villous sampling catheter that has been inserted too deep.

catheter, the direction of traction on the cervix, and the degree of bladder distention, as well as by applying gentle suprapubic manual manipulation.

After removal of the stylet, a 20-ml syringe containing a 7-ml aliquot of F10 culture medium supplemented with heparin (10 IU/ml), penicillin (100 IU/ml) and streptomycin (100μ/ml) is attached to the catheter. Mild suction is applied by withdrawing the plunger to approximately the 5–10-ml mark on the syringe. A gentle to-and-fro movement is performed for a few seconds. This helps to dislodge the villi and increase the amount of material sampled. The suction is then released and the catheter withdrawn.

The sample is immediately examined on a Petri dish through a low-power dissecting microscope for the presence of chorionic villi. Good-quality specimens reveal the multiple buds, capillaries, and arborization pattern of villi. Sample size, as compared with photographically documented reference standards should be at least 3 to 5 mg, optimally 10 to 20 mg, particularly if enzyme assays are to be performed. Unsuccessful analysis will generally result from a sample containing edematous or degenerating villi.

Laboratory analysis, as for genetic amniocentesis, can be subdivided into two broad categories: cytogenetic studies including DNA analysis and biochemical studies.

Cytogenetic Studies

Two techniques of processing chorionic villi are available, a "direct" method and a culture method. The direct method allows cytogenetic analysis within 24 to 48 hours and consists of chromosomal preparations obtained from spontaneous mitoses freed from the cytotrophoblasts. The culture technique, on the other hand, requires 5 to 7 days, but provides a greater number of metaphases for analysis (54).

Initially, maternal cell contamination from aspirated decidua was thought to lead to the potential for erroneous diagnosis in patients whose results showed a 46,XX chromosomal complement, and follow-up genetic amniocentesis was offered to patients with this finding. However, at present, identification of villi has become reliable in experienced hands and reexamination by genetic amniocentesis is required infrequently.

Biochemical Studies

The same methods are used to prepare chorionic villus extracts as those used in the analysis of prepared fibroblasts or cultured amniotic fluid cell extracts after genetic amniocentesis. DNA analysis by molecular genetic techniques can be used in the diagnosis of hemoglobinopathies such as β-thalassemia and sickle cell anemia. Linkage analysis of DNA now allows the in utero detection of many X-linked recessive disorders, and provides prenatal diagnosis of cystic fibrosis in most cases in which one family member is affected.

A concern about the accuracy of CVS involves the possibility that trophoblastic cells may not necessarily accurately reflect fetal status. Up to one-third of abnormal chromosomal complements from villus biopsy demonstrate mosaicism (56, 61). Martin and colleagues (57) concluded that in these cases interpretation must be guarded and a confirmatory amniocentesis is warranted, particularly if mosaic 45,X or trisomy for lethal autosomes are detected.

COMPLICATIONS

Short-term complications include bleeding per vagina, infection, and spontaneous abortion. Spotting after CVS may be due to a small laceration on the anterior cervical lip if a tenaculum is used (55). Even without the use of a tenaculum, spotting is not uncommon, but should progressively decrease over the next few days. Significant uterine bleeding could theoretically arise from placental separation or perforation of the uterus, but neither to our knowledge has been reported to date.

A rare syndrome of fever and myalgias, progressing to generalized sepsis, has been described following CVS. Immediate evacuation of the uterus and broad spectrum antibiotic therapy were required (81, 82). In larger series, the rate of chorioamnionitis has been reported as 0.2% to 0.6% (56, 61).

Possible long-term complications have only recently begun to be evaluated in larger series. These include late complications involving the placenta (abruption, accretion), fetus (intrauterine growth retardation, prematurity, fetal malformations such as amniotic band syndrome), as well as maternal isoimmunization. In patients at risk for Rh isoimmunization, an indirect Coombs test is performed and 300 μg anti-D immune globulin are given if antibodies are not detected.

In order to reduce potential complications, many authors recommend that the number of catheter insertions be limited to a total of three (54, 55, 81). For every additional pass, a new sterile catheter should be used. Reporting a series of 940 cases, Green and colleagues (56) noted that over 80% of patients required only one catheter insertion for successful retrieval of tissue. Other studies (55, 58) report a somewhat lower frequency of success on the first catheter insertion, 45% to 55%, with adequate samples obtained after two aspirations in 25%, and after three in 14% to 30%.

A recent worldwide survey of centers performing CVS reported a 4.2% absolute pregnancy loss rate after the biopsy (83). The total spontaneous abortion rate after CVS in larger studies has varied from 2.4% (56) to 4.3% (60) with estimates of the real loss rate due to CVS ranging from 0.6% (56, 61) to 2.7% (84).

Assessments of the real spontaneous abortion rate due to CVS should be based on a comparison with spontaneous fetal losses in a matched sample of women who have had documentation of a sonographically normal pregnancy at about 8 weeks gestation and have not undergone CVS. Once pregnancy has been established clinically, it is accepted that between 12% and 15% undergo spontaneous abortion (84). On the other hand, the rate of spontaneous fetal loss after ultrasound-proven viability in early pregnancy has been reported in the range 2.0% to 5.2% (85–89). More specifically, Simpson and colleagues (84) reported a fetal loss rate of 3.2% in 220 controls from the Diabetes in Early Pregnancy Study, who had documented fetal vialibity by ultrasound at 8 weeks gestation.

This indicate that in a significant proportion of spontaneous abortions occurring after 8 weeks gestation, fetal demise is already present prior to 8 weeks and the dead fetus is retained in utero for several weeks until actual clinical fetal loss occurs. Significant risk factors for spontaneous abortion after first trimester sonographic detection of fetal cardiac activity include vaginal bleeding, advanced maternal age, and low socioeconomic status (89).

Percutaneous Umbilical Blood Sampling and Transfusion

HISTORICAL NOTES

Although fetal blood sampling was first reported in 1973 by Valenti and colleagues (90), available techniques were limited until recently to blind aspiration of the placenta under ultrasound guidance, fetal scalp sampling, and fetoscopy. Limitations of these procedures included a 76% rate of contamination of fetal blood samples by maternal blood with the blind aspiration technique (91), an associated pregnancy loss rate of 2% to 5% with fetoscopy (possible only after 24 weeks gestation) (92), and availability of fetal scalp sampling only after the patient is in labor, with cervical dilatation and ruptured membranes.

With introduction of direct percutaneous umbilical blood sampling (PUBS) by Daffos and co-workers (93), using an ultrasound-guided 20-gauge needle, many of these limitations have been obviated and PUBS has already in large part supplanted fetoscopy and blind placental aspiration. In utero blood transfusions directly into the fetal circulation have also replaced transfusions into the fetal peritoneal cavity in many centers.

INDICATIONS

Percutaneous umbilical blood sampling can be used for prenatal diagnosis or therapy from about 16 to 17 weeks since the last menstrual period to the 40th week of gestation. The list of major indications for PUBS continues to grow (94, 95). Applications to date can be considered under the following broad headings.

Rh isoimmunization. A direct Coombs titer, complete blood count, and blood smear (96) can be obtained from fetal blood samples in Rh hemolytic disease, with the potential for percutaneous umbilical blood transfusion (PUBT) during a single procedure. The pre- and posttransfusion fetal hematocrit (Hct) can be directly monitored.

Chromosomal analysis. A high-quality karyotype can be obtained from fetal lymphocytes, usually within 48 hours. This is an important application in cases where rapid karyotyping is necessary prior to the gestational limit for legal elective interruption of pregnancy.

Isoimmune or alloimmune thrombocytopenia. Fetal platelet levels can be obtained in cases of suspected thrombocytopenia at 38 weeks gestation, before the onset of labor, in order to help select the most appropriate mode of delivery. Prior to PUBS, fetal platelet counts could be estimated only from a fetal scalp sample after cervical dilatation and membrane rupture, which often precluded the possibility of an elective cesarean section (97, 98).

Coagulation deficiencies. Hemophilia A and B, as well as factor V deficiency have been detected in utero (99). The presence of normal factor VII and factor IX clotting activity in hemophilia A and B respectively, as well as adequate factor VIII coagulant antigen in hemophilia A, have helped identify normal fetuses in pregnancies at risk for these X-linked recessive coagulation disorders.

In utero infection. Toxoplasmosis, as well as rubella, CMV, and other viral infections have been diagnosed prenatally in pregnancies at risk, using fetal blood cultures and specific fetal IgM levels (100–102).

Hemoglobinopathies. The presence of sickle cell anemia as well as congenital hemoglobinopathies such as β-thalassemia can be assessed in the fetus, using DNA analysis techniques (90, 91).

Immune disorders. Diagnosis of agammaglobulinemia, chronic granulomatous disease, Chediak-Higashi syndrome, Wiscott-Aldrich syndrome, Bernard-Soulier syndrome, and severe combined immune deficiency have been reported (95, 103).

Promising developments based on fetal blood samples obtained by the PUBS technique include assessment of fetal renal function, treatment of cardiac arrhythmias as well as other in utero drug therapies, and analysis of fetal blood gases and acid-base balance in cases of fetal distress, hypoxia, or growth retardation (104, 105).

TECHNIQUE

As in the case of amniocentesis, a preliminary ultrasound survey is performed in order to 1) detect the presence of multiple gestation, 2) confirm fetal viability, 3) assess fetal age, 4) detect gross fetal anomalies or maternal adnexal/uterine abnormalities, 5) evaluate placental position, 6) determine fetal lie, and 7) select a site for needle insertion.

PUBS in most centers is performed in an operating suite under aseptic conditions, with the operator and assistants fully gowned and gloved. After preparation of the maternal abdomen with a 10% povidine-iodine solution, the transducer is placed in a sterile glove or sheath and the placenta, umbilical cord and fetus are relocalized using sterile gel as the coupling agent. Needle sizes vary from 20 gauge (106) to 25 gauge (98) in different centers, 22 gauge from 10 to 16 cm in length being the most commonly used. Some authors find the 25-gauge needle too pliable (107, 108).

Real-time ultrasonographic monitoring may take the form of either a parallel (98) or orthogonal (93, 94) free hand insertion under continuous guidance or insertion using a fixed-needle guide (109). Two percutaneous sampling techniques, intracardiac and intrafunicular, for obtaining fetal blood have been reported.

Intracardiac

Bang has reported the use of the fetal heart as a source of fetal blood samples (110). The tip os a 1.2-mm guide needle is placed in the fetal thorax, then a 0.6-mm needle is introduced through the guide and positioned in the left ventricle. The relatively large target presented by the heart is an advantage. Although this technique reportedly has no harmful effects on the fetal heart, its reported use has been limited to a single center.

Intrafunicular

The umbilical cord is punctured approximately 1 to 2 cm from its placental insertion, using either a transplacental approach with an anterior placenta or a transamniotic approach if the placenta is posterior (Fig 18.13). Either the umbilical vein or artery can be sampled, although some concerns have been raised about vascular spasm and fetal bradycardia after arterial puncture (109). The vein is larger, has thinner walls and a straighter course, and therefore is usually more easily sampled.

The midportion of the cord can be used in cases when the cord insertion is not accessible due to placental position and fetal lie, or in the presence of oligohydramnios. In the first instance, the cord can be pinned between the needle and the uterine wall or fetal trunk prior to definitive puncture with a gentle forward thrust. In the presence of oligohydramnios, cord fixation for puncture becomes less of a problem. Puncture of a free-floating cord loop is not recommended.

Correct placement of the needle tip in the selected vessel can be ascertained by demonstration of the needle tip "flare" within the vessel lumen imaged in cross-section approximately 1- to 2-cm from the placental insertion site of the cord. A small amount of Ringer's lactate can be injected after removal

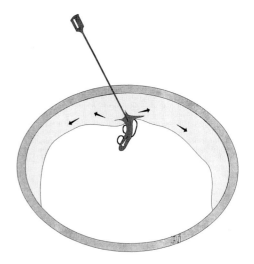

Figure 18.13. Schematic drawing of percutaneous umbilical blood sampling (PUBS). When saline is injected, the tiny bubbles either flow towards the fetus if injection is into the umbilical vein or towards the placenta if the injection is into the umbilical artery. If the saline does not move, this is a placental injection.

of the stylet, with typical intravascular turbulence visualized on the ultrasound image confirming correct needle positioning (Fig. 18.14). Some authors use duplex Doppler imaging with the Doppler sample volume placed in the vessel of interest, serving both as a target for needle placement and as a simultaneous monitor of fetal heart rate (94).

Once the needle is positioned, the stylet is removed and 0.5 ml of fetal blood is aspirated into a heparinized syringe. This initial sample is discarded to avoid maternal blood contamination. The subsequent diagnostic sample (0.5 ml to 3 ml) is drawn into a heparinized syringe and assayed by Kleihauer-Betke smear as well as by measurement of mean corpuscular volume (MCV) by Coulter counter, to exclude maternal blood or amniotic contamination (95, 109–112).

Under 20 to 25 weeks gestation, some authors replace the sample volume with an equivalent volume of lactated crystalloid solution (95, 109). However, this is rarely a problem, since small amounts of Ringer's lactate or normal saline are usually injected into the umbilical vessels to confirm needle position during the course of the procedure.

In certain cases, for example, to avoid needle dislodgement from a posterior placenta, the fetus can be paralyzed by an intramuscular injection of a neuromuscular blocking agent such as pancuronium (113). The cord can then sampled near its origin from the fetal abdomen if this is the only site available.

In a series of 96 procedures, Weiner and colleagues (109) reported the site of PUBS as placental umbilical cord insertion in 64%, free-floating loop of cord in 27%, and fetal umbilical cord origin in 9% of cases. Two attempts associated with anhydramnios failed. PUBS was successful in 63% of cases on the first attempt and 95% of cases after three or fewer attempts. Mean sample volume was 4.0 ml. Mean sampling time has been reported in a series of 100 cases as 5.5 minutes (111).

PUBS can be performed on an outpatient basis. After the procedure, if fetal heart monitoring is normal for 1 to 2 hours or a normal biophysical profile is obtained, the patient can be discharged home. In patients

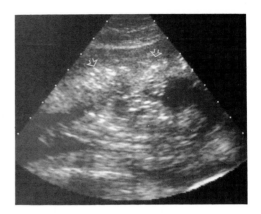

Figure 18.14. Air embolized into the placenta during a practice PUBS, appearing as multiple echogenicities within the placental substance (*open arrows*).

at risk for Rh isoimmunization, an indirect Coombs test is performed and 300 µg anti-D immune globulin are given if antibodies are not detected.

Many different parameters have been measured in fetal blood samples, and normal ranges for various blood and serum values have been published (114), including hematologic indices (111), blood gas values (104, 105, 109), blood group antigens (115), and coagulation factor assays (99).

COMPLICATIONS

The most frequent complications of percutaneous umbilical blood sampling are 1) blood leakage from the cord puncture site, 2) fetal bradycardia (usually transient), 3) chorioamnionitis, and 4) transient irregular uterine contractions. Transient bleeding from the cord puncture site has been reported to occur in 10% to 40% of cases (94, 106, 109), lasting less than 60 to 90 seconds in the great majority of reported instances. Fetal bradycardia has been observed in 3% (109) to 12% (94) of PUBS procedures. Weiner and colleagues noted that the frequency of transient fetal bradycardia was 20% if the umbilical artery was punctured and 1..5% if the umbilical vein was sampled, which they considered statistically significant (109). A case of chorioamnitis has been reported by Ludomirski and colleagues (111) who now prescribe a course of broad-spectrum antibiotics for 3 to 5 days after the procedure (94).

PERCUTANEOUS UMBILICAL BLOOD TRANSFUSION

Until recently, the bile pigment concentration in amniotic fluid, measured by spectrophotometry as the change in optical density at 450 nm and compared to Liley's charts, was the only method available as an indirect measure of the degree of fetal hemolysis secondary to Rh isoimmunization. This technique is known to be inaccurate in the second trimester, with a 68% false-negative rate between 18 and 25 weeks gestation (94, 107, 116).

PUBS provides determinations of fetal hematocrit (Hct), blood type and antibody level by direct Coombs test, allowing intravascular transfusion 4 to 5 weeks earlier than the older intraperitoneal method (94). The absorption of an intravascular transfusion is not affected by fetal ascites or lack of fetal breathing movements in hydropic fetuses, and the X-ray exposure previously required to confirm intraperitoneal placement of the transfusion catheter (after injection of radiopaque contrast) is eliminated. Moreover, some authors feel that intraperitoneal transfusion offers no hope for the moribund fetus when the biophysical profile score is 4 or less, and recommend the use of intravascular transfusion in these cases (117). More recently, ultrasound monitoring alone has been used for the guidance of fetal intraperitoneal transfusions by Watts and co-workers (118); however, five transfusion-related complications occurred in 77 transfusions including two fetal colon infusions, two fetal retroperitoneal infusions, and one fetal abdominal wall hematoma.

Percutaneous umbilical blood transfusion (PUBT) is usually undertaken if the fetal hematocrit is less than 20% to 25%. The fetus is paralyzed with pancuronium to avoid fetal movement during the procedure. Packed red blood cells (PRBC) compatible with maternal blood and previously irradiated to kill the leukocytes, are administered according to the formula (119, 120):

$$\begin{aligned} &\textit{volume of PRBC required} \\ &= (\textit{desired Hct} - \textit{actual Hct}) \\ &\quad \times \textit{estimated fetoplacental blood volume} \\ &\quad \times \textit{estimated fetal weight (kg)} \div \textit{donor Hct} \end{aligned}$$

Estimated fetoplacental blood volume is 150–160 ml/kg fetal weight, donor hematocrit varies between 75% and 85% for PRBC, and desired fetal hematocrit is approximately 40%. The transfusion is usually given at a rate of 1 to 3 ml/min (119). Some authors have recommended adjunctive maternal therapy with furosemide and digoxin, as well as prophylactic oral antibiotics during PUBT (121), while other reports conclude that this is unnecessary (108).

The transfusion is repeated at 1- to 3-week intervals, depending on maternal antibody titers, severity of fetal disease, measured posttransfusion hematocrit, and rate of decrease of the hematocrit as measured by serial PUBS (94).

FETAL INTRAPERITONEAL BLOOD TRANSFUSION

In spite of the rising popularity of percutaneous umbilical blood transfusion, fetal intraperitoneal transfusion remains a viable option (118). Intraperitoneal transfusion may provide an alternative route for therapy if the umbilical vessels prove to be poorly accessible due to a posterior placenta or unfavorable fetal lie.

Most fetal intraperitoneal blood transfusions are now guided by continuous real-time ultrasound. Preliminary ultrasound scanning is performed as in the PUBT technique and, after selection of a puncture site, a 17- to 19-gauge Tuohy needle is inserted into the amniotic cavity and directed against the fetal abdominal wall. A point is chosen superior and lateral to the bladder, away from the umbilical cord insertion, and the needle is advanced into the fetal peritoneal cavity. After removal of the stylet, the position of the needle tip is confirmed by injection of a small amount of saline to create a small amount of turbulence around the needle tip. As much ascitic fluid as possible is withdrawn prior to transfusion. To avoid needle displacement due to fetal motion, an 1.8-mm epidural catheter or infant feeding tube is inserted through the Tuohy needle. The tip is coiled in the fetal abdomen and a the needle is removed. Fresh O-negative packed red blood cells are then transfused, with the volume to be administered calculated by the formula (121):

$$vol = (gestation\ in\ weeks - 20) \times 10\ ml$$

Infusion rates vary from 1 to 2 ml/min to transfusion of the whole volume over 10-15 minutes (119). The fetal heart rate should be continuously monitored, and if bradycardia is detected, the infusion is stopped. In addition to the problem of diminished absorption of transfused intraperitoneal blood in hydropic fetuses, the intraperitoneal transfusion method is limited by unavailability of fetal pre- and posttransfusion hematocrit, other hematological indices, and serum bilirubin.

Fetal Interventional Techniques

Although in utero therapy aimed at reducing fetal morbidity and mortality has been a well established procedure for many years, the advent of high-resolution real-time ultrasound in the 1980s has resulted in many new attempts at treating conditions in the fetus that previously would have been allowed to run their natural course. Some of these interventions have raised not only concerns about potential benefit or risk to the fetus, but also ethical considerations related to possible conflicts between the physicians obligations to the mother versus his or her responsibility to promote the best interests of the fetus (122, 123).

After Liley's initial success with in utero intraperitoneal blood transfusions in fetuses with immune hydrops, indications for fetal interventional techniques have grown to include management of obstructive uropathy, decompression of fetal hydrocephalus, fetoscopy, fetal tissue biopsy, and fetal drug therapy. In general, any proposed therapy must be based on a consideration of the following factors: 1) the natural history of the disease or anomaly in question, including its ultimate prognosis, 2) the rate of progres-

sion of the disease process, 3) the gestational age and maturity of the affected fetus, and 4) the availability of suitable perinatal treatment modalities that will allow continuing therapy or corrective surgery postnatally (124).

MANAGEMENT OF OBSTRUCTIVE UROPATHY

Primary urethral obstruction, produced either by posterior urethral valves (almost exclusively in males) or, less commonly, urethral atresia (both sexes), is the only form of fetal obstructive uropathy for which in utero surgical intervention has been considered of proven value (124).

Fetal therapy is undertaken only if no other major anomalies are detected, if the disease process is severe and progressive, and if the fetus is too immature to survive as a neonate. Prior to intervention, stable or increasing fetal bladder distention must be demonstrated. Fetal renal function can be assessed by evaluation of the quantity of amniotic fluid, serial observation of fetal bladder volume, percutaneous fetal bladder puncture for drainage and urinalysis, or occasionally by prolonged fetal urinary system catheterization for analysis of urine production and fetal glomerular filtration rates (by measuring clearance of a placental soluble substance such as iodothionate or iothalamate). This last procedure has largely been abandoned due to the increased risk of perinatal infection (124).

Analysis of fetal urinary electrolytes and osmolarity has been proposed as a method of evaluating the functional status of an obstructed fetal urinary tract. Golbus and colleagues (125) reported that a poor prognosis was associated with urinary electrolytes above certain cut-off levels: Na > 100 mEq/ml, Cl > 100 mEq/ml, and osmolarity > 210 mOsm. However, other authors are of the opinion that fetal urinary electrolytes are not necessarily an accurate predictor of neonatal renal function (126).

Placement of a fetal vesicoamniotic shunt is undertaken in the operating suite. Manning and Harman (127) describe a technique using a 17-gauge Tuohy needle with 15°

angulation at the distal end inserted percutaneously into the fetal bladder under continuous ultrasound guidance. A 3 French single- or double-pigtail Teflon catheter with spiral holes is then threaded on a wire guide and is advanced down the needle. Prior to insertion, the catheter is cut so approximately 5 cm of proximal catheter will protrude from the fetal abdomen into the amniotic cavity. The wire guide is then partly withdrawn to allow the distal catheter to coil in the fetal bladder. The outer needle is then pulled back along with the guidewire, maintaining catheter position with a specially designed introducer. As the cut proximal catheter end drops into the amniotic cavity, the introducer and needle are withdrawn.

Potential complications immediately related to the procedure include injury to adjacent fetal structures and chorioamnionitis, as well as misplacement of the proximal catheter tip in the fetal peritoneal cavity, creating a vesicoperitoneal shunt and fetal urinary ascites. Shunt displacement or blockage also occur (128).

Proponents of early decompression of an obstructed fetal urinary system base their conclusions on a series of animal experiments that demonstrated that ligation of the ureters of fetal sheep late in pregnancy (22 weeks human equivalent) produced simple hydronephrosis, whereas obstruction earlier in pregnancy (13–19 weeks human equivalent) produced irreversible changes of renal dysplasia (124). Others regard these studies as inconclusive (129). On the other hand, the etiological relationship of pulmonary hypoplasia, by far the most common cause of perinatal death in obstructive uropathies, to the renal disease process has not been completely defined. Although chronic oligohydramnios is clearly associated with pulmonary hypoplasia, Manning has also observed pulmonary hypoplasia in obstructive uropathies with normal amniotic fluid volumes, suggesting that more than one etiological factor may be responsible for this lethal lung condition (124).

Results of 73 interventional procedures on obstructed fetal urinary tracts were included in the Report of the International Fetal Surgery Registry (130). Forty-one per cent of the fetuses survived, with a procedure-related death rate of 4.6%. Of the fetal deaths, approximately one-third occurred in utero and two-thirds postnatally, with pulmonary hypoplasia as the major cause of mortality. Of 28 fetuses with severe oligohydramnios, only six (21%) survived.

On the other hand, Sholder and colleagues (129) treated six fetuses suspected to have posterior urethral valves (five cases) or an obstructed megaureter (one case). They found that only two of these fetuses had posterior urethral valves postnatally, and concluded that "no fetus had any recognized benefit from the antenatal intervention."

DECOMPRESSION OF FETAL HYDROCEPHALUS

Neurosurgeons prefer that fetuses with hydrocephalus and macrocephaly be delivered by cesarean section to avoid birth trauma. On the other hand, obstetrical literature has advocated cephalocentesis to enable vaginal delivery and to avoid maternal birth trauma, particularly in cases with severe associated anomalies (122). According to the Report of the International Fetal Surgery Registry, the results of shunt procedures for obstructive hydrocephalus were even less encouraging than those for treatment of obstructive uropathy (130). Although 34 of 44 fetuses (83%) survived, the procedure-related death rate was 10.3%. Eighteen of the 34 survivors (53%) had serious neurological handicaps, four (12%) had less severe handicaps, and only twelve (35%) were developing normally at the time of publication of the report. All the neonates with normal development had aqueductal stenosis (125). At present, in utero CFS shunting into the amniotic cavity remains an experimental procedure (131), and is not generally considered a viable treatment option. Cephalocentesis in isolated fetal hydrocephalus with macrocephaly involves ethical dilemmas that have been discussed elsewhere (122).

FETOSCOPY

In 1973 Valenti and colleagues reported the use of a "surgical endoamnioscope" for fetal skin biopsy and umbilical cord blood sampling under direct vision in 11 patients scheduled for abortive hysterotomy during the second trimester (132). With the development of percutaneous umbilical blood sampling under continuous ultrasound monitoring in 1973, the need for blood sampling by fetoscopy has diminished considerably, although the procedure may still be used in some centers for fetal skin or liver biopsy (133), as well as fetal intravascular blood transfusions (134).

Fetoscopy generally requires hospitalization. It cannot be performed safely before 15 weeks gestation because of the inadequate size of the amniotic cavity, and is hindered after 20 weeks gestation by increasing cloudiness of amniotic fluid. Fetoscopy is difficult to perform with large fetuses in advancing pregnancy, and is generally unsuited for multiple sampling procedures (132, 133). The associated pregnancy loss rate has been 2% to 5% in the most experienced hands (135). Other complications include preterm labor (8% to 10%), amniotic fluid leakage (10%), and chorioamnionitis (0.5%) (133).

FETAL TISSUE SAMPLING

In utero sampling of fetal tissues other than blood has been reported using fetoscopy or percutaneous ultrasound-guided needle biopsy procedures. Tissues most commonly biopsied include skin, liver, and fetal tumors.

Fetal skin biopsy under ultrasound guidance has been performed in the gluteal region in 12 cases in one series, with no reported complications (136). In 10 cases (83%) there was enough tissue for analysis. The use of fetoscopy for skin biopsy allows precise identification of the area to be biopsied and even selection of the type of skin desired, for example, a hairy area for the diagnosis of oculocutaneous albinism (133). Other conditions that may be diagnosed prenatally include epidermolysis bullosa,

epidermolytic hyperkeratosis, Ehlers-Danlos syndrome, and Sjogren-Larsson syndrome (136).

Some inborn errors of metabolism such as rare enzyme deficiencies of the urea cycle, expressed only in the liver, for example, carbamyl phosphate synthetase and ornithine transcarbamylase deficiencies, can be diagnosed only by fetal liver biopsy. Again, the use of both an ultrasound-guided method and fetoscopy has been described (133, 137).

Fetal masses such as cystic hygroma, type 3 cystic adenomatoid malformation of the lung, and sacrococcygeal teratoma have all been punctured in utero both for diagnosis and to reduce tumor size. Fetal abdominal cyst aspiration has also been reported (136).

REFERENCES

Amniocentesis

1. Simpson JL, Elias S: Genetic amniocentesis. *In Diagnostic Ultrasound Applied to Obstetrics and Gynecology.* Sabbagha RE (ed): Philadelphia, Lippincott, pp. 64–82, 1987.
2. Menees TD, Miller JD, Holly LE: Amniography: Preliminary report. *Am J Roentgenol Radium Ther* 24: 363, 1930.
3. James F: Sexing foetuses by examination of amniotic fluid. *Lancet* 1:202, 1956.
4. Steele MW, Breg WR Jr: Chromosome analysis of human amniotic fluid cells. *Lancet* 1:383, 1966.
5. Nadler HL, Gerbie AB: Role of amniocentesis in the intrauterine detection of genetic disorders. *N Engl J Med* 282:596, 1970.
6. Hook EB: Rates of chromosome abnormalities at different maternal ages. *Obstet Gynecol* 58:282, 1981.
7. Hook EB, Cross PK, Schreinemachers DM: Chromosomal abnormality rates at amniocentesis and in liveborn infants. *JAMA* 249:2034, 1983.
8. Johnson M: Indications and techniques for genetic amniocentesis. *J Reprod Med* 27:557, 1982.
9. Boue A, Gallano P: A collaborative study of the segregation of inherited chromosome structural rearrangements in 13356 prenatal diagnoses. *Prenat Diagn* 4:45, 1984.
10. Brock CF: A comparative study of microvillar enzyme activities in the prenatal diagnosis of cystic fibrosis. *Prenat Diagn* 5:129, 1985.
11. Main DM, Mennuti MT: Neural tube defects: Issues in prenatal diagnosis and counselling. *Obstet Gynecol* 67:1, 1986.
12. Cuckle HS, Wald NJ: Maternal serum alpha-fetoprotein measurement: A screening test for Down syndrome. *Lancet* 2:926, 1984.
13. Gluck L, Kulovich M, Borer K et al.: Diagnosis of the respiratory distress syndrome by amniocentesis. *Am J Obstet Gynecol* 109:440, 1971.

14. Gluck L: Evaluation of fetal lung maturation by analysis of phospholipid indicators in the amniotic fluid. In *Lung Maturation and the Prevention of Hyaline Membrane Disease*. Proceedings of the 70th Ross Conference on Pediatric Research, Columbus, Ohio, Ross Laboratories, 1976.

15. Liley AW: Liquor amnii analysis in the management of the pregnancy complicated by rhesus sensitization. *Am J Obstet Gynecol* 82:1359, 1961.

16. Bowman JM: The management of Rh isoimmunization. *Obstet Gynecol* 52:1, 1978.

17. Harman CR, Manning FA, Bowman JM: Severe Rh disease: Poor outcome is not inevitable. *Am J Obstet Gynecol* 145:823, 1983.

18. Hegge FN, Prescott GH, Watson PT: Sonography at the time of genetic amniocentesis to screen for fetal malformations. *Obstet Gynecol* 71:522, 1988.

19. Benacerraf BR, Frigoletto FD: Amniocentesis under continuous ultrasound guidance: A series of 232 cases. *Obstet Gynecol* 62:760, 1983.

20. Jeanty P, Rodesch F, Romero R et al.: How to improve your amniocentesis technique. *Am J Obstet Gynecol* 146:593, 1983.

21. Defoort P, Thiery M: Amniocentesis with the use of continuous real-time echography: Experience with 200 consecutive cases. *Am J Obstet Gynecol* 147:973, 1983.

22. Crane JP, Kapta MM: Genetic amniocentesis: Impact of placental position upon the risk of pregnancy loss. *Am J Obstet Gynecol* 150:813, 1984.

23. Romero R, Jeanty P, Reese EA et al.: Sonographically monitored amniocentesis to decrease intraoperative complications. *Obstet Gynecol* 65:426, 1985.

24. Williamson RA, Varner MW, Grant SS: Reduction in amniocentesis risks using a real-time needle guide procedure. *Obstet Gynecol* 65:751, 1985.

25. McGahan JP, Tennant F, Hanson FW, Lindfos KK, Quilligan EJ: Ultrasound needle guidance for amniocentesis in pregnancies with low amniotic fluid. *J Reprod Med* 32(7): 513–516, 1987.

26. Finberg HJ, Frigoletto FD: Sonographic demonstration of uterine contraction during amniocentesis. *Am J Obstet Gynecol* 139:740, 1981.

27. Hanson FW, Tennant FR, Zorn EM et al.: Analysis of 2136 genetic amniocenteses: Experience of a single physician. *Am J Obstet Gynecol* 152:436, 1985.

28. McDicken WN, MacKenzie WE, Anderson T et al.: Ultrasonic identification of needle tips in amniocentesis. *Lancet* 2:198, 1984.

29. Platt LD, DeVore GR, Gimovsky ML: Failed amniocentesis: The role of membrane tenting. *Am J Obstet Gynecol* 144:479, 1982.

30. Bowerman RA, Barclay ML: A new technique to overcome failed second-trimester amniocentesis due to membrane tenting. *Obstet Gynecol* 70:806, 1987.

31. Elias S, Gerbie AB, Simpson JL: Genetic amniocentesis in twin gestations. *Am J Obstet Gynecol* 138:169, 1980.

32. Goldstein Al, Stills SM: Midtrimester amniocentesis in twin pregnancies. *Obstet Gynecol* 62:659, 1983.

33. Librach CL, Doran TA, Benzie RJ et al.: Genetic amniocentesis in seventy twin pregnancies. *Am J Obstet Gynecol* 148:585, 1984.

34. Jeanty P, Shah D, Roussis P: Single needle insertion in twin amniocentesis. (Submitted for publication).

35. Murken JA, Stengel-Rutkowski S, Schwinger E: Prenatal diagnosis. *Proceedings of the 3rd European Conference on Prenatal Diagnosis of Genetic Disorders*. Stuttgart, Ferdinand Enke, 1979.

36. Turnbull AC, MacKenzie IZ: Second-trimester amniocentesis and termination of pregnancy. *Br Med Bull* 39:315, 1983.

37. Crane JP, Rohland B: Clinical significance of persistent amniotic fluid leakage after genetic amniocentesis. *Prenat Diagn* 6:25, 1986.

38. Tabsh KMA, Lebherz TB, Crandall BF: Risks of prophylactic anti-D immunoglobulin after second trimester amniocentesis. *Am J Obstet Gynecol* 149:225, 1984.

39. Working Party on Amniocentesis: An assessment of hazards of amniocentesis. *Br J Obstet Gynecol* 85 Suppl 2: 1, 1978.

40. Wald NJ, Terzian E, Vickers PA et al.: Congenital taliopes and hip malformation in relation to amniocentesis: A case-control study. *Lancet* 2:246, 1983.

41. Philip J, Bang J: Outcome of pregnancy after amniocentesis for chromosomal analysis. *Br Med J* 2:1183, 1978.

42. NICHD National Registry for Amniocentesis Study Group: Mid-trimester amniocentesis for prenatal diagnosis. Safety and accuracy. *JAMA* 236:1471, 1976.

43. O'Brian WF: Mid trimester genetic amniocentesis: A review of the fetal risks. *J Reprod Med* 29:59, 1984.

44. Leschot NJ, Verjaal M, Treffers PE: Risks of mid-trimester amniocentesis: Assessment in 3000 pregnancies. *Br J Obstet Gynecol* 92:804, 1985.

45. Shapiro LR, Singer N, Mannor SM: Immediate and unexplained fetal death during mid-trimester amniocentesis. *Prenat Diagn* 3:151, 1983.

46. Crandall BF, Howard J, Lebhertz TB et al.: Follow up of 2000 second trimester amniocentesis. *Obstet Gynecol* 56:625, 1980.

47. Dacus JV, Wilroy RS, Summitt RL et al.: Genetic amniocentesis: A twelve year experience. *Am J Med Genet* 20:443, 1985.

48. Carpenter RJ, Hinkley CM, Carpenter AF: Mid-trimester genetic amniocentesis: Use of ultrasound direction versus blind needle insertion. *J Reprod Med* 28:35, 1983.

49. Varma TR: Amniocentesis in early pregnancy using free hand needle technique under ultrasonic control. *Int J Obstet Gynecol* 19:149, 1981.

50. Tabor A, Bang J, Norgaard-Pederson B: Feto-maternal haemorrhage associated with genetic amniocentesis: Results of a randomized trila. *Br J Obstet Gynecol* 94:528, 1987.

51. Kappel B, Nielsen J, Brogaard-Hansen K: Spontaneous abortion following mid trimester amniocentesis: Clinical significance of placental perforation and blood-stained amniotic fluid. *Br J Obstet Gynecol* 94:50, 1987.

52. Ron M, Cohen T, Yaffe H et al.: The clinical significance of blood contaminated mid-trimester amniocentesis. *Acta Obstet Gynecol Scand* 61:43, 1982.

Chorionic Villus Sampling

53. Hanson FW, Zorn EM, Tennant FR et al.: Amniocentesis before 15 weeks' gestation: Outcome, risks and technical problems. *Am J Obstet Gynecol* 156: 1524, 1987.

54. Elias S, Simpson JL, Martin AO et al.: Chorionic villus sampling for first-trimester prenatal diagnosis: Northwestern University program. *Am J Obstet Gynecol* 152:204, 1985.

55. Elias S, Simpson JL: Chorionic villus sampling. Diagnostic Ultrasound Applied to Obstetrics and Gynecology. Sabbagha RE (ed): Philadelphia, Lippincott, 1987.

56. Green JE, Dorfmann A, Jones SL: Chorionic villus sampling: Experience with an initial 940 cases. *Obstet Gynecol* 71:208, 1988.

57. Martin AO, Simpson JL, Rosinsky BJ et al.: Chorionic villus sampling in continuing pregnancies: Cytogenetic reliability. *Am J Obstet Gynecol* 154:1353, 1986.

58. Perry TB, Vekemans MJ, Lippman A et al.: Chorionic villi sampling: Clinical experience, immediate complications, and patient attitudes. *Am J Obstet Gynecol* 151:161, 1985.

59. Modell B: Chorionic villus sampling: Evaluating safety and efficiency. *Lancet* 1:737, 1985.

60. Holzgreve W, Miny P: Chorionic villi sampling with an echogenic catheter: Experiences of the first 500 cases. *J Perinat Med* 15:244, 1987.

61. Hogge WA, Schonberg SA, Golbus MS: Chorionic villus sampling: Experience of the first 1000 cases. *Am J Obstet Gynecol* 154:1249, 1986.

62. Maxwell D, Czepulkowski BH, Heaton DE et al.: A practical assessment of ultrasound-guided transcervical aspiration of chorionic villi and subsequent chromosomal analysis. *Br J Obstet Gynecol* 92:660, 1985.

63. Ward RHT, Modell B, Petrou M et al.: Method of sampling chorionic villi in first trimester of pregnancy under guidance of real-time ultrasound. *Br Med J* 286:1542, 1983.

64. Binkin NJ: Trends in induced legal abortion morbidity and mortality. *Clin Obstet Gynaecol* 13:83, 1986.

65. Kullander S, Sandahl B: Fetal chromosome analysis after transcervical placental biopsies in early pregnancy. *Acta Obstet Gynecol Scand* 52:355, 1973.

66. Hahnemann N: Early prenatal diagnosis: A study of biopsy technique and cell culturing from extraembryonic membranes. *Clin Genet* 6:294, 1974.

67. Department of Obstetrics and Gynecology, Tietung Hospital of Anshan Iron and Steel Company, Anshan: Fetal sex prediction by sex chromatin of chorionic villi cells during early pregnancy. *Clin Med J* 1:117, 1975.

68. Kazy Z, Rozovsky IS, Bakharev VA: Chorionic biopsy in early pregnancy: A method of early prenatal diagnosis for inherited disorders. *Prenat Diagn* 2: 39, 1982.

69. Old JM, Ward RHT, Karagozlu F et al.: First trimester fetal diagnosis for haemoglobinopathies: Three cases. *Lancet* 2:1413, 1982.

70. Simoni G, Brambati B, Danesino C et al.: Diagnostic application of first trimester trophoblast sampling in 100 pregnancies. *Hum Genet* 66:252, 1984.

71. Simoni G, Brambati B, Danesino C et al.: Efficient direct chromosome analysis and enzyme determination from chorionic villi samples in the first trimester of pregnancy. *Hum Genet* 63:349, 1983.

72. Gustavii B: Chorionic biopsy and miscarriage in first trimester, *Lancet* 1:562, 1984.

73. Ghirardini G, Popp WL, Camurri L et al.: Vaginosonographic guided chorionic villi needle biopsy (transvaginal chorionic villi sampling). *Eur J Obstet Gynecol Reprod Biol* 23:315, 1986.

74. Gustavii B: First trimester chromosomal analysis of chorionic villi obtained by direct vision technique. Letter to the Editor. *Lancet* 2:507, 1983.

75. Smidt-Jensen S, Hahnemann N, Hariri J et al.: Transabdominal chorionic villi sampling for first trimester fetal diagnosis: First 26 pregnancies followed to term. *Prenat Diagn* 6:125, 1986.

76. Maxwell D, Lilford R, Czepulkowski B et al.: Transabdominal chorionic villus sampling. *Lancet* 1:123, 1986.

77. Bovicelli L, Rizzo N, Mantacuti V et al.: Transabdominal versus transcervical routes for chorionic villus sampling. *Lancet* 1:290, 1986.

78. Hogdall CK, Doran TA, Shime J et al.: Transabdominal chorionic villus sampling in the second trimester. *Am J Obstet Gynecol* 158:345, 1988.

79. Liu DTY, Jeavons B, Preston C et al.: A purpose-designed cannula for transcervical chorion villus aspiration. *Br J Obstet Gynecol* 95:101, 1988.

80. Breyer B, Cikes I: Ultrasonically marked catheter: A method for positive echographic catheter position identification. *Med Biol Eng Comput* 22:268, 1984.

81. Blakemore K, Mahoney MJ, Hobbins JC: Infection and chorionic villus sampling. *Lancet* 2:339, 1985.

82. Brambati B, Varotto F: Infection and chorionic villus sampling. *Lancet* 2:609, 1985.

83. Jackson L: CVS Newsletter. Jefferson Medical College, Philadelphia. September 1985.

84. Simpson JL, Mills JL, Holmes LB et al.: Low fetal loss rates after ultrasound-proved viability in early pregnancy. *JAMA* 258:2555, 1987.

85. Cashner KA, Christopher CR, Dysert GA: Spontaneous fetal loss after demonstration of a live fetus in the first trimester. *Obstet Gynecol* 70:827, 1987.

86. Christiaens GC, Stoutenbeek ML: Spontaneous abortion in proven intact pregnancies. *Lancet* 2: 571, 1984.

87. Gilmore DH, McNay MB: Spontaneous fetal loss rate in early pregnancy. *Lancet* 1:107, 1985.

88. Wilson RD, Kendrick V, Wittman BK et al.: Spontaneous abortion and pregnancy outcome after normal first trimester ultrasound examination. *Obstet Gynecol* 67:352, 1986.

89. Siddiqi TA, Caligaris JT, Miodovnik M et al.: Rate of spontaneous abortion after first trimester sonographic demonstration of fetal cardiac activity. *Am J Perinatol* 5:1, 1988.

Percutaneous Umbilical Blood Sampling and Transfusion

90. Valenti C: Antenatal detection of hemoglobinopathies: A preliminary report. *Am J Obstet Gynecol* 115:851, 1973.

91. Cao A, Furbetta M, Angius A et al.: Haematological and obstetric aspects of antenatal diagnosis of beta-thalassemia: Experience with 200 cases. *J Med Genet* 19:81, 1982.

92. Special report: The status of fetoscopy and fetal tissue sampling. *Prenat Diagn* 4:79, 1984.

93. Daffos F, Capella-Pavlovsky M, Forestier F: A new procedure for fetal blood sampling in utero: Preliminary results of 53 cases. *Am J Obstet Gynecol* 146:985, 1983.

94. Ludomirski A, Weiner S: Percutaneous fetal umbilical blood sampling. *Clin Obstet Gynecol* 31:19, 1988.

95. Weiner CP: Percutaneous umbilical blood sampling. In Sabbagha RE (ed): *Diagnostic Ultrasound Applied to Obstetrics and Gynecology*. Philadelphia, Lippincott, pp. 414–422, 1987.

96. Pollock JM, Bowman JM, Manning FA: Fetal blood sampling in Rh hemolytic disease. *Vox Sang* 53:139, 1987.

97. Ludomirski A, Nemiroff R, Johnson A et al.: Percutaneous umbilical blood sampling: A new technique for prenatal diagnosis. *J Reprod Med* 32:276, 1987.

98. Hobbins JC, Grannum PA, Romero R et al.: Percutaneous umbilical blood sampling. *Am J Obstet Gynecol* 152:1, 1985.

99. Forestier F, Daffos F, Sole Y et al.: Prenatal diagnosis of hemophilia by fetal blood sampling under ultrasound guidance. *Haemostasis* 16:346, 1986.

100. Daffos F, Forestier F, Grangeot-Keros L et al.: Prenatal diagnosis of congenital rubella. *Lancet* 2:1, 1984.

101. Desmonts G, Daffos F, Forestier F et al.: Prenatal diagnosis of congenital toxoplasmosis: A prospective study of 278 pregnancies at risk. *Lancet* 1:500, 1985.

102. Hogge WA, Thiagarajh S, Brenbridge AN et al.: Fetal evaluation by percutaneous blood sampling. *Am J Obstet Gynecol* 158:132, 1988.

103. Durandy A, Griscelli C, Dumez Y et al.: Antenatal diagnosis of severe combined immune deficiency from fetal cord blood. *Lancet* 1:852, 1982.

104. Pardi G, Buscaglia M, Ferrazi E et al.: Cord sampling for the evaluation of oxygenation and acid-base balance in growth-retarded human fetuses. *Am J Obstet Gynecol* 157:1221, 1987.

105. Soothill PW, Nicolaides KH, Campbell S: Prenatal asphyxia, hyperlactemia, hypoglycemia, and erythroblastosis in growth retarded fetuses. *Br Med J* 294:1051, 1987.

106. Daffos F, Capella-Pavlovsky M, Forestier F: Fetal blood sampling during pregnancy with use of needle guided by ultrasound: A study of 606 consecutive cases. *Am J Obstet Gynecol* 153:655, 1985.

107. Benacerraf BR, Barss VA, Saltzman DH et al.: Fetal abnormalities: Diagnosis or treatment with percutaneous umbilical blood sampling under continuous ultrasound guidance. *Radiology* 166:105, 1988.

108. Socol ML, MacGregor SN, Pielet BW et al.: Percutaneous umbilical blood transfusion in severe rhesus isoimmunization: Resolution of fetal hydrops. *Am J Obstet Gynecol* 157:1369, 1987.

109. Weiner CP: Cordocentesis for diagnostic indications: Two years' experience. *Obstet Gynecol* 70:664, 1987.

110. Bang J: Ultrasound guided fetal blood sampling. Albertini A, Crosignani PG (eds): Progress in Peri-

natal Medicine. Amsterdam, *Excerpta Medica*, pp. 223–225, 1983.

111. Ludomirski A, Weiner S, Ashmead GG et al.: Percutaneous fetal umbilical blood sampling: Procedure safety and normal fetal hematologic indices. *Am J Perinat* 5:264, 1988.

112. Forestier F, Cox WL, Daffos F et al.: The assessment of fetal blood samples. *Am J Obstet Gynecol* 158:1184, 1988.

113. Moise KJ, Carpenter RJ, Deter Rl et al.: The use of fetal neuromuscular blockade during intrauterine procedures. *Am J Obstet Gynecl* 157:874, 1987.

114. Forestier F, Daffos F, Rainant M et al.: Blood chemistry of normal human fetuses at midtrimester of pregnancy. *Pediatr Res* 21:579, 1987.

115. Habibi B, Bretagne M, Bretagne Y et al.: Blood group antigens on fetal red cells obtained by umbilical vein puncture under ultrasound guidance: A rapid hemagglutination test to check for contamination with maternal blood. *Pediatr Res* 20:1082, 1986.

116. Nicolaides KH, Rodeck CH, Mibashan RS et al.: Have Liley charts outlived their usefulness? *Am J Obstet Gynecol* 155:909, 1986.

117. Harman CR, Manning FA, Bowman JM et al.: Use of intravascular transfusion to treat hydrops fetalis in a moribund fetus. *CMAJ* 138:827, 1988.

118. Watts DH, Luthy DA, Benedetti TJ et al.: Intraperitoneal fetal transfusion under direct ultrasound guidance. *Obstet Gynecol* 71:84, 1988.

119. Motew MN, Socol ML, Sabbagha RE: Intrauterine transfusion. Sabbagha RE (ed): *Diagnostic Ultrasound Applied to Obstetrics and Gynecology*. Philadelphia, Lippincott, pp. 423–430, 1987.

120. Grannum PA, Copel JA, Plaxe SC et al.: In utero exchange transfusion by direct intravascular injection in severe erythroblastosis fetalis. *New Engl J Med* 314:1431, 1986.

121. Harman CR, Manning FA, Bowman JM et al.: Severe Rh disease: Poor outcome is not inevitable. *Am J Obstet Gynecol* 145:823, 1983.

Fetal Interventional Techniques

122. Chervenak FA, McCullough LB: Ethical analysis of the intrapartum management of pregnancy complicated by fetal hydrocephalus with macrocephaly. *Obstet Gynecol* 68:720, 1986.

123. Arant BS: Prevention of hereditary nephropathies by antenatal interventions: Ethical considerations. *Pediatr Nephrol* 1:553, 1987.

124. Manning FA: Fetal surgery for obstructive uropathy: Rational considerations. *Am J Kid Dis* 10:259, 1987.

125. Golbus MS, Filly RA, Callen PW et al.: Fetal urinary tract obstruction: Management and selection for treatment. *Semin Perinatol* 19:91, 1985.

126. Wilkins IA, Chitkara U, Lynch L et al.: The nonpredictive value of fetal urinary electrolytes: Preliminary report of outcomes and correlations with pathological disease. *Am J Obstet Gynecol* 157:694, 1987.

127. Manning FA, Harman CR: In utero diversion shunts for urethral obstruction. In Sabbagha RE (ed): *Diagnostic Ultrasound Applied to Obstetrics and Gynecology*. Philadelphia, JB Lippincott, pp. 431–437, 1987.

128. Elder JS, Duckett JW, Snyder HM: Intervention for fetal obstructive uropathy: Has it been effective? *Lancet* 2:1007, 1987.
129. Sholder AJ, Maizels M, Depp R et al.: Caution in antenetal intervention. *J Urol* 139:1026, 1988.
130. Report of the International Fetal Surgery Registry: Catheter shunts for fetal hydronephrosis and hydrocephalus. *New Engl J Med* 315:336, 1986.
131. Depp R, Sabbagha RE, Brown JT et al.: Fetal surgery for hydrocephalus: Successful in utero ventriculo-amniotic shunt for Dandy-Walker syndrome. *Obstet Gynecol* 61:710, 1983.
132. Valenti C: Antenatal detection of hemoglobinopathies: A preliminary report. *Am J Obstet Gynecol* 115:851, 1973.
133. Soothill PW, Nicolaides KH, Rodeck CH: Invasive techniques for prenatal diagnosis and therapy. *J Prenat Med* 15:117, 1987.
134. Rodeck CW, Nicolaides KH, Warsof SL et al.: The management of severe rhesus isoimmunization by fetoscopic intravascular transfusion. *Am J Obstet Gynecol* 150:769, 1984.
135. Special report: The status of fetoscopy and fetal tissue sampling. *Prenat Diagn* 4:79, 1984.
136. Kurjak A, Alfirevic Z, Jurkovic D: Ultrasonically guided fetal tissue biopsy. *Acta Obstet Gynecol Scand* 66:523, 1987.
137. Holzgreve W, Golbus MS: Prenatal diagnosis of ornithine transcarbamylase deficiency utilizing fetal liver biopsy. *Am J Hum Genet* 36:320, 1984.

19 Ultrasound-guided Intervention in the Extremities

ROSS A. CHRISTENSEN
ERIC VANSONNENBERG

Ultrasound is indispensable for guiding interventional radiology procedures in the extremities. Pathologic processes that affect the soft tissues of the extremities typically are superficial; US is perfectly suited for evaluating these processes. Currently available linear-array and sector transducers enable accurate depiction of extremity soft tissue lesions and precise localization for diagnosis and biopsy. US can be effectively utilized for: 1) aspiration of musculoskeletal fluid collections, 2) therapeutic drainage of musculoskeletal abscesses, 3) needle biopsy of musculoskeletal lesions, and 4) sonographic identification of abnormal musculature to guide biopsy in muscle disorders (1).

Advantages of US as a Guidance Modality

US is advantageous compared to Computed Tomography (CT) and fluoroscopy for percutaneous intervention in the musculoskeletal system. The primary advantages are: 1) absence of radiation exposure, 2) constant real-time visualization of needle and/or catheter position, and 3) decreased cost compared to CT. US can detect subtle acoustic impedance differences between soft tissue pathology and surrounding normal structures. This results in characterization and precise localization of musculoskeletal masses and fluid collections.

Many patients referred to US-guided intervention have had successful attempts at fluid aspiration of palpable abnormalities by clinicians on the ward. This problem typically is due to the inability to identify a fluid component within a mass. By differentiating fluid texture from solid components with ultrasound imaging, the radiologist can achieve diagnosis and therapy.

Extremity Abscess and Fluid Drainage

Extremity abscesses are most commonly the sequelae of trauma, soft tissue hemorrhage, or osteomyelitis. Diseases that predispose to soft tissue hemorrhage, an altered immune status, or sources of sepsis are associated with these abscesses. These diseases include leukemia, bleeding dyscrasias, diabetes mellitus, lymphoma, autoimmune disease, occult bowel perforation, renal infection, and tuberculosis (2).

Joint hemorrhage or effusion may be loculated; in those cases, US guidance for aspiration may be essential. Primary or metastatic extremity neoplasms may necrose and become secondarily infected. Vascular grafts may become infected, and aspiration of surrounding fluid may be critical to the diagnosis of graft infection and viability of the graft.

THE THIGH

The thigh is the most common location for an extremity abscess. The typical US appearance is that of an anechoic or hypoechoic mass (Fig 19.1; 3). Debris or septation within the mass may be present. Most abscesses present as sonographically discrete masses, but some are poorly marginated or harbor ill-defined portions. Echogenic regions surrounding fluid components are frequent, and are thought to represent accompanying myositis or hematoma. Thigh abscesses typically are located anteriorly or anterolaterally. They can be situated superficial to, within, or deep to the quadriceps muscle. Abscesses abutting the femur are more characteristic of patients with underlying osteomyelitis (Fig. 19.2). US defines the cranial and caudal extent of an abscess, and may characterize the degree of loculation (2; Fig. 19.3).

In the evaluation of extremity masses and fluid collections a high index of suspicion must be maintained for false or true aneurysms masquerading as an abscess (1, 2). This is especially true for mycotic pseudo-aneurysms. Fluid collections located medially and posteriorly in the thigh, as well as those extending to the popliteal region of the groin, should be regarded as suspicious for a vascular origin. To assess for vascular pulsation, a real-time study should be con-

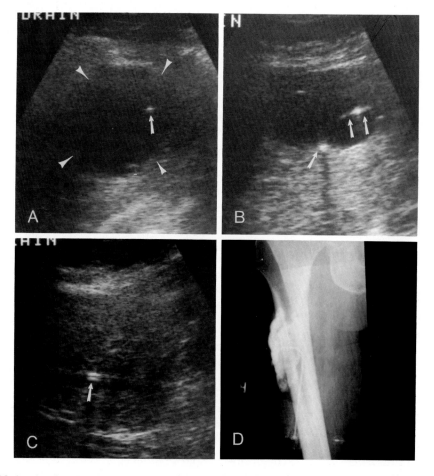

Figure 19.1. **A,** US-guided diagnostic aspiration of thigh abscess; echogenic 22-gauge needle (*arrow*) in hypoechoic abscess (*arrowheads*). **B,** Percutaneous catheter drainage of thigh abscess with 10F catheter (*arrows*) under US guidance. **C,** Postevacuation of 50 cc pus. Echogenic catheter (*arrows*) in minimal residual collection. **D,** Abscessogram demonstrates cavity size and extent.

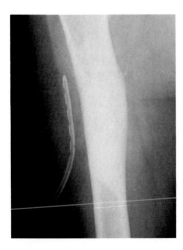

Figure 19.2. US-guided percutaneous drainage of thigh abscess. 12F sump catheter on plain x-ray parallels femur. Note sclerosis of associated chronic osteomyelitis of proximal femur.

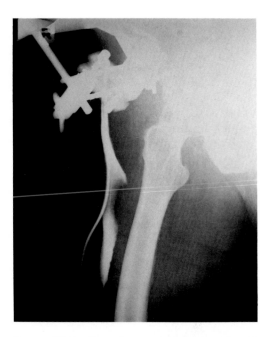

Figure 19.3. Percutaneous drainage of post-traumatic thigh abscess utilizing ultrasound. Abscess communicates to repaired fracture site in ileum. Orhthopedic hardware affixes fracture site.

ducted, and Doppler analysis should be performed on any suspicious mass (Fig. 19.4). Thrombus within a portion of an aneurysm may obscure the diagnosis, and all portions of mass should be scrutinized carefully.

Other pitfalls in diagnosis of thigh abscesses include inguinal hernia and a large synovial cyst of the hip (1, 2). Both usually are located more cephalad and near the groin. Bowel motion and bowel gas shadowing may be seen in a hernia. A synovial cyst is seen most typically in patients with rheumatoid arthritis. These cysts usually are fluid in nature, but internal debris and wall irregularity may be seen. A sterile or infected neoplasm can be confused with a thigh abscess. Needle aspiration or biopsy is necessary to differentiate tumor from infection (2; Fig. 19.5).

Technique

Percutaneous needle aspiration and drainage of extremity abscesses is technically straightforward compared to the more complex procedure in intraabdominal and intrathoracic abscesses. Coagulation studies are obtained routinely, and should be normalized if abnormal. Intravenous analgesia and sedation with midazolam and fentanyl are usual. Warnings for specific medications are presented in Chapter 1. A diagnostic ultrasound exam is performed immediately prior to skin preparation to confirm the presence of and to characterize the lesion and to plan the percutaneous approach. Transducers of 3.5, 5.0, and (rarely) 7.5 or 10 MHz are used. The selection of the transducer depends on which provides the best visualization of the lesion without an acoustic stand-off pad. Careful attention is paid to the identification of regional vascular structures. A thorough knowledge of the expected location of major nerves and their relation to the lesion is integrated into the selection of the access route.

The sterile field is prepared, and 1% lidicaine is used as local anesthetic. Nonsterile acoustic gel is placed within a commercially available sterile transducer sleeve or a sterile surgical glove. The transducer cord is wrapped with a sterile towel.

A 22-gauge needle is introduced into the fluid collection using a specially equipped

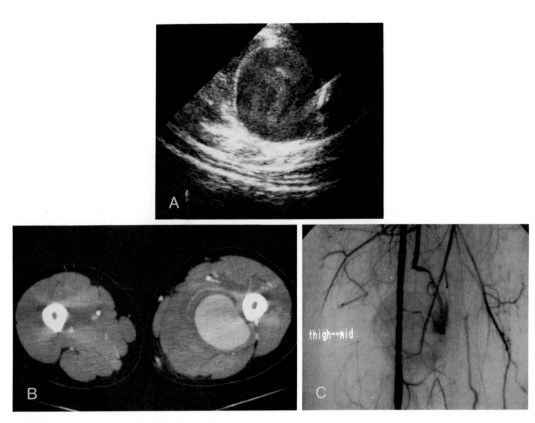

Figure 19.4. US showing large hypoechoic mass in posteromedial aspect of thigh in patient on Coumadin following aortic valve replacement. A swirling motion within the mass was detected at real-time examination. **B**, the mass was clinically suspected to be a hematoma. CT shows the mass to enhance homogeneously. **C**, Arteriography confirms a pseudoaneurysm of a branch of the profunda femoris artery. This was a mycotic pseudoaneurysm, a dangerous pitfall in the evaluation of extremity masses that can masquerade as an abscess. (Courtesy of Albert Nemcek, M.D., Chicago, IL.)

biopsy attachment to the transducer or by freehand technique with the needle introduced immediately adjacent to the transducer (Fig 19.1**A**). Once the needle is accurately localized within the fluid component of the mass, gentle suction is applied with a connecting tube. Less than 1 ml of fluid is removed for immediate Gram stain and culture. The amount of fluid aspirated should be minimal so the cavity is not decompressed. Overzealous aspiration of fluid may reduce target size, making catheter placement more difficult or impossible. A negative Gram stain for organisms and white cells should raise concern that the mass is neoplastic, and biopsy should be considered; necrotic fluid usually is bloody.

If initial aspiration is unsuccessful despite accurate needle placement, the needle should be repositioned by advancement, withdrawal, or angulation. A second needle may be placed into a different portion of the mass. Solid masses occasionally appear anechoic or hypoechoic. Large needles (20- and 18-gauge) may be necessary as fluid occasionally is quite viscous, particularly if hemmorhagic. If these maneuvers should fail to obtain fluid, the mass is assumed to be solid, and the lesion is biopsied.

If pus is obtained at aspiration, or the Gram stain indicates infection, a catheter is placed into the fluid collection (Fig. 19.1**B**). Even if a collection is judged to be sterile, a catheter may be placed to decompress the fluid component of a mass and to relieve pressure symptoms. A single- or double-lumen catheter with multiple side holes is chosen for drainage, based on the cavity size and viscosity of the fluid. Large and viscous collections require 12 or 14 French sump catheters. The catheter may be placed using the trocar technique in tandem with the localizing needle. Once a small amount of fluid is aspirated from the collection, a guidewire is placed coaxially through the trocar assembly to serve as a protective guidewire for catheter advancement (4). This prevents potentially erroneous placement of the catheter into surrounding normal or solid components of the mass and ensures smooth coiling of the catheter within the cavity. Smaller collections may require Seldinger technique for catheter placement. One risks decompressing the mass during the course of tract dilatation using Seldinger technique, which may prevent catheter insertion. Collections may be judged too small for catheter placement, and simple one-step needle aspiration is used in these cases.

Catheter position within the abscess is confirmed by ultrasound. Cavity contents then are evacuated. The cavity is reimaged to assess for undrained or loculated components (Fig 19.1C). Large or loculated fluid components may require placement of additional catheters. Once evacuated, the cavity is irrigated with sterile saline; small volumes of irrigant are used until the return of fluid is clear. We usually defer performance of an abscessogram for 24 to 48 hours because of the potential for bacteremia induced by the high pressures necessary for the performance of an abscessogram (Fig. 19.1D). By abscessogram, one is particularly looking for communication into the adjacent knee or hip joint (Fig. 19.3).

Follow-up Care

Follow-up consists of standard abscess-drainage care (2, 4). The catheter is connected to wall or bulb suction, and daily irrigation is performed. An abscessogram is performed at 24 or 48 hours to assess for joint space or enteric communication. Once

drainage has been decreased to fewer than 5 to 10 cc/day, and the cavity is nearly obliterated by sinography, the catheter is gradually withdrawn 1 to 2 cm daily and is removed.

Results and Complications

Ultrasound-guided percutaneous needle aspiration and drainage of thigh abscesses has been almost uniformly successful. Approximately 75% of our patients had undergone previous repeated and unsuccessful attempts at ward aspiration, and half had undergone surgery (2). Patients often will exhibit a dramatic clinical response following drainage; defervescence frequently occurs within 24 hours. Repeat US or CT should be performed on the patient who fails to improve clinically with 24-48 hours following drainage. Lack of improvement implies an undrained, loculated component, inappropriate antibiotic coverage, or an occult abscess elsewhere.

Potential complications include hemorrhage, sepsis, superinfection, and fistula formation. Extension of the abscess to the hip or knee joint may necessitate longer periods of catheter drainage, but should not alter a successful outcome. Arterial, venous, and major nerve damage are theoretic complications that should be avoided by proper access planning.

THE KNEE

Ultrasound-guided aspirations of knee effusions may be performed when nonguided clinical attempts fail. US provides precise guidance in localizing loculated fluid collections in and about the knee. This is especially helpful in patients with hemarthrosis where loculated components may exist. Sonographic guidance may be utilized for percutaneous aspiration and drainage of septic joints. Anterolateral approaches should be used to avoid transgression of the posteriorly located neurovascular bundle, and the laterally located ligamentous structures.

US may be used to guide aspiration and to diagnose suspected Baker's cysts in the popliteal fossa and posterior compartment of the calf (5–7). Aspiration is valuable when the cyst does not fill at arthrography due to

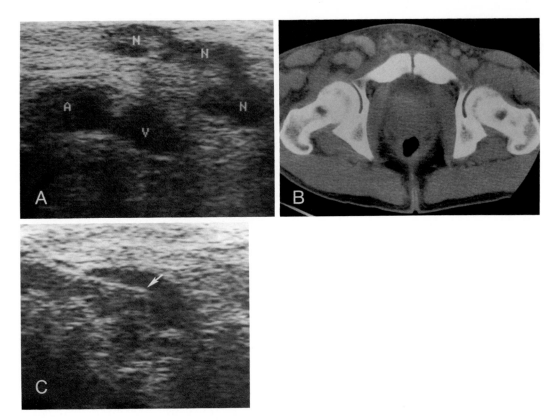

Figure 19.5. **A,** 70-year-old male with history of lymphoma. Transverse scan of right groin demonstrates several small nonpalpable lymph noeds (*N*). Femoral artery (*A*) and vein (*V*) are seen more posteriorly. **B,** CT through lower pelvis demonstrates bilateral inguinal adenopathy (right > left) and edema in soft tissue. **C,** US-guided biopsy. Transverse scan of 22-gauge Teflon-coated localizing needle in node (*arrow*). Biopsy was performed with a 16-gauge cutting needle.

obstructing debris or a one-way valve mechanism. Assessment for pulsation by real-time US and Doppler analysis as well as arteriorography or venography may be required to exclude a thrombosed pseudoaneurysm, a true aneurysm, or an arteriovenous malformation.

THE HIP

Ultrasound has been used to detect an effusion in the infant or pediatric hip (8–10). Arthrosonography is superior to plain radiography in diagnosing hip effusion. The normal capsular space is less than 3mm; the difference in measurement compared to the contralateral side should be less than 2mm.

Ten millimeters of fluid are required to increase the capsular distance by 2mm (11). Smaller amounts of fluid may go undetected by US. Fluid was obtained in 88% of 16 pediatric hips when effusion was suggested by ultrasound (8). The hypoechoic psoas muscle, as it crosses the hip joint, can mimic a joint effusion, and the sonographer needs to be aware of this pitfall.

US may be used to guide aspiration of a septic hip joint. An ancillary clue to septic arthritis is asymmetric thickening of the joint capsule (8). US allows accurate needle placement into the fluid component of a septic hip. The femoral vessels are identified and avoided.

THE UPPER EXTREMITY

US evaluation and guidance for percutaneous aspiration, drainage, and biopsy of upper extremity masses and fluid collections is similar to that in the lower extremities. A working knowledge or upper extremity vascular and nerve anatomy is essential prior to needle placement. As in the lower extremity, a high index of suspicion for mycotic pseudoaneurysm or aneurysm simulating a simple abscess should be maintained.

US has been utilized for identification, biopsy, and aspiration of infected and neoplastic nodes and masses within the axilla and arm (1). Axillary vessels can be quickly identified and avoided to prevent the complication of an axillary hemorrhage.

Renal dialysis shunts or arterial bypass grafts suspected of being infected can be evaluated by US (Fig. 19.6). If infected fluid about the graft is demonstrated, US is used to guide accurate needle placement for diagnostic aspiration. Diagnosis of infection is instrumental in salvaging a graft or dictating the need for removal.

Ultrasound-Guided Biopsy

Sonographically guided needle biopsy of soft tissue tumors in the extremities is performed with a high degree of accuracy. Zornoza and associates obtained representative material in 83% of 42 needle biopsies using US and CT guidance. A specific diagnosis was obtained in 76% of biopsies (12).

Twenty and 22-gauge needles are adequate for most biopsies. Needle localization within the lesion is confirmed by US. Five to ten milliliters of suction is exerted on a 15- or 20-cc syringe. A smooth, coring motion is applied when the needle is advanced to and fro within the lesion. Larger, 18-gauge needles are used when there is suspicion of lymphoma (Fig. 19.5). Eighteen-gauge Surecut needles with a beveled cutting edge are excellent for obtaining large cores of tissue (1).

The cytologist is present at the time of biopsy to perform immediate stains. Quick staining reduces the number of passes required for diagnosis (13). The cytologist can ascertain the adequacy of the tissue sample for diagnosis at the time of biopsy. Two or three needle passes typically are sufficient to make a diagnosis. Four or more passes are required in approximately 5% of cases (13). Material is submitted for histology in addition to cytology. Special stains, T- and B-cell markers, and material for electron microscopy all may be obtained by these methods.

Large lesions often contain necrotic portions. It is essential to obtain biopsy specimens from the solid peripheral portions of a necrotic mass to ensure a diagnosis. US affords precise localization of the needle within the solid portions, thereby reducing the incidence of false-negative results.

MUSCLE BIOPSY

Diseases that affect the muscles, particularly childhood neuromuscular disorders, have not been easily amenable in percutaneous needle biopsy in the past. Neuromuscular diseases may affect only selected muscles within a muscle group. Nonimage guided, "blind" biopsy may miss these focal areas of involvement. US is capable of identifying subtle differences in acoustic impedance in these focal muscle diseases. US has been used to identify isolated muscle involvement in limp girdle dystrophy and to guide needle biopsy. Abnormally increased

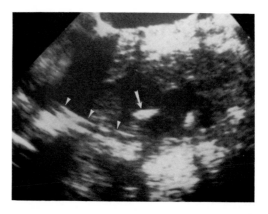

Figure 19.6. US-directed percutaneous drainage of perigraft hematoma surrounding forearm dialysis shunt. Note echogenic catheter (*arrows*) coiled in collection and echogenic graft located posteriorly (*arrowheads*).

echogenicity of selected muscles with sparing of adjacent muscles within the same muscle group can be demonstrated by US. Successful US-guided needle biopsy of these abnormal muscles has been performed (1, 14).

REFERENCES

1. Christensen RA, vanSonnenberg E, Casola G, Wittich GR: Interventional ultrasound in the musculo-skeletal system. *Radiol Clin Am* 26(1): 145–156, 1988.
2. VanSonnenberg E, Wittich GR, Cabrera OA et al.: Sonography of thigh abscesses: Detection, diagnosis, and drainage. *AJR* 149:769, 1987.
3. Beckman CRB, Thomason JL, Sampson EE et al.: Ultrasonographic confirmation of a thigh abscess. *Ill Med J* 167:126–127, 1985.
4. Mueller PR, vanSonnenberg E, Ferrucci JT: Percutaneous drainage of 250 abdominal abscesses and fluid collections: II. Current procedural concepts. *Radiology* 151:343–347, 1984.
5. Hermann G, Yeh HC, Lehr-Janus C et al.: Diagnosis of popliteal cyst: Double-contrast arthrography and sonography. *AJR* 137:369–372, 1981.
6. Lukes PJ, Herberts P, Zachrisson BE: Ultrasound in the diagnosis of popliteal cysts. *Acta Radiol Diagn* 21:663–665, 1979.
7. Cooperberg BL, Tsang I, Truelove L, et al.: Gray scale ultrasound in the evaluation of rheumatoid arthritis of the knee. *Radiology* 126:759–763, 1978.
8. Adam R, Hendry MA, Moss J et al.: Arthrosonography of the irritable hip in childhood: A review of 1 year's experience. *Br J Radiol* 59:205–208, 1986.
9. Boal DKB, Schwenkter EP: The infant hip: Assessment with real-time US. *Radiology* 157:667–672, 1985.
10. Clark NMF, Harcke HT, McHugh P et al.: Real-time ultrasound in the diagnosis of congenital dislocation and dysplasia of the hip. *J Bone Joint Surg* 67: 406–412, 1985.
11. Selzer S, Finberg HJ, Weissman BN: Arthrosonography: technique, sonographic anatomy, and pathology. *Invest Radiol* 15:19–26, 1979.
12. Zornoza J, Bernardino ME, Ordonez NG et al.: Percutaneous needle biopsy of soft tissue tumors guided by ultrasound and computed tomography. *Skeletal Radiol* 9:33–36, 1982.
13. Rowley VA, Cooperberg PL: Ultrasound guided biopsy in interventional ultrasound. *Clin Diagn Ultrasound* 21:59–76, 1987.
14. Heckmatt JZ, Dubowitz V: Diagnostic advantage of needle muscle biopsy and ultrasound imaging in the detection of focal pathology in a girl with limp girdle dystrophy. *Muscle Nerve* 8:705–709, 1985.

Index

Page numbers in *italics* denote figures; those followed by "t" denote tables.

Abdominal abscesses, 129–143
   choice of imaging modality for, 132–133
   clinical features of, 129–130
   diagnosis of, 129–133
      accuracy of, 133
      by CT, *130–131*, 130–132
      by ultrasound, 130, *130–133*
   etiology of, 129
   intraoperative ultrasonography of, 125–126
   percutaneous drainage of, 133–143
      bacteremia/septicemia after, 142
      catheter irrigation after, 141–142
      catheter management and patient follow-up
         after, 141–143
      catheters for, 138–139, *140*
      contraindications to, 134
      CT guidance for, *134*, 134–137, *138*, *140*
      patient preparation for, 135
      patient response to, 142
      patient selection for, 133–135
      in patients with fistulas, 142–143
      sinographic follow-up after, 139–141
      sonographic guidance for, 135, *136–137*, 137–
         138, *139*
      study of, 139
      techniques for, 135–138
   vs. phlegmons, 130
Abdominal ultrasonography, 31–32, 115–197. *See
      also* specific applications
   of abscesses, 129–143
   of gallbladder, 159–167
   of hepatobiliary tract, 145–156
   intraoperative, 115–127
      of abscesses, 125–126
      appearance of gastrointestinal wall on, 126, *126*
      benefits of, 126–127
      of biliary tract, 121–123, *122*
      contact vs. probe-standoff techniques for, 115–
         116, *116*
      of extrahepatic bile duct, 116, *116*
      instrumentation for, 115
      of liver, 117–121, *118–121*
      of malignancies, 126, *126*
      for needle placement, 117
      of pancreas, 116–117, *117*, 123–125, *124–125*
      probe preparation for, 115
      timing of, 117
   of pancreas, 171–189
   for percutaneous gastrostomy, 193–197

Abscess sinography, 139–141
Abscesses
   abdominal. *See* Abdominal abscesses
   breast, 74
   extremity, 267–273
      factors predisposing to, 267
      of thigh, *268–270*, 268–271. *See also* Thigh ab-
         scesses
      ultrasound guidance for, 267
   hepatic, *131*, 153, *153*
   intracerebral, 50–51
   lung, 88
   pancreatic, 179
   pelvic, 215, 218, *220*
   perinephric, *207*, 207–208
   perirectal, 236, *236*
   prostatic, 234, *234*
   renal, *131*
   spinal, 54
   testicular, 209, *209*
   tubo-ovarian, 219
Abscessogram, 271
Adenocarcinomas, pancreatic, 175
Adenoma
   hepatic, 146
   pancreatic, 176
   parathyroid, 65
      ablation of, 66–67, *68*
   vs. carcinoma, 22
Adrenal lesions, 32, 203–204, *204*
Agammaglobulinemia, 255
Alpha-fetoprotein
   elevated amniotic fluid levels of, 240–241
   maternal serum levels of, 240–241
Amniocentesis, 239–250
   early vs. late, 250
   fetal risks of, 249
   guidelines for
      amniotic fluid vs. maternal urine, 246
      aspiration, 246, *247*
      avoiding membrane tenting, 245, *245*
      depth of needle insertion, 245, *246*
      monitoring needle tip, 244–245
      needle placement, 243–244
      needles, 244
      placental location, 244
      sample size, 246
      use of plastic extension tubing, 245–246, *246*
   history of, 239

indications for, 239–242
    determination of fetal lung maturity, 241
    prenatal genetic diagnosis, 239–241, 240t
        alpha-fetoprotein levels, 240–241
        of chromosomal anomalies, 239–240, 240t
        of inborn errors of metabolism, 240
        molecular genetic techniques, 241
        of neural tube defects, 240
        of sex-linked anomalies, 241
        Rh isoimmunization, 241–242
    maternal risks of, 248
    in multiple gestations, 247–248, 248
    in obese patients, 246–247
    in oligohydramnios, 247
    role of ultrasound in, 249–250
    time delay to results of, 250
    ultrasound-guided techniques for, 242–243
        fixed-needle guidance method, 243
        orthogonal freehand insertion, 242, 243
        parallel freehand insertion, 242, 243–245
    ultrasound survey prior to, 242
Anatomy
    brain, 45–46, 46
    parathyroid, 64–65
    pericardial, 101
    prostate, 221–222, 223
    spinal, 51–52, 52–53
    thyroid, 61, 61–62
Anencephaly, 240
Anesthesia, 3
Aneuploidy, 22–23, 240
Aneurysms
    of renal artery, 199, 200
    vs. knee cysts, 272
    vs. thigh abscesses, 268–269
Angioplasty, echocardiographic guidance for, 111
Antilirium. See Physostigmine
Antiplatelet medications, 3
Aortocoronary grafting, intraoperative echocardiog-
        raphy for, 111–112
Arnold-Chiari syndrome, 49
Arteriovenous malformations, renal, 199, 200
Astrocytoma, closed-brain biopsy of, 48
Atrial septostomy, echocardiographic guidance of,
        109–110

Bernard-Soulier syndrome, 255
Biliary ultrasonography, intraoperative, 121–123
    to assess biliary tumors, 123
    to detect gallstones, 121
    indications for, 121
    to localize extrahepatic bile duct, 123
    vs. cholangiography to screen for common bile
        duct stones, 121–123, 122, 122t
Biopsy needles
    guidance systems for, 7–9, 8–10
        attachable needle guides, 7–8, 9–10
        dedicated biopsy transducers, 7, 8
        for use with endoluminal scanners, 8–9, 11
    manufacturers of, 20
    needle stops, 16, 17
    needle tips, 14–16
    selection of, 13–15, 14–15
    suction devices, 16, 18

visualization of, 10–13
    acoustic impedance and, 10
    air or water injection and, 11
    beam scattering, 11
    guidance systems and, 10–11
    methods for improving, 11, 13t
    needle design and, 11, 12
    needle size and, 11
Biopty gun, 16–18
Bladder carcinoma, 235
Bleeding time, preoperative measurement of, 3
Brain, 45–51
    abscess of, 50–51
    biopsy of, 46–48, 47–49
    intraoperative sonographic applications in, 49–50
    normal anatomy of, 45–46, 46
    shunt catheter placement in, 48, 49, 51
    sonographic appearance of masses of, 50–51
Breast masses, aspiration biopsy of, 30–31, 71–81
    abscess, 74
    carcinoma, 24, 75–76, 78–81
    cystosarcoma phyllodes, 74
    cysts, 73, 75–76, 76–77
    false-negative results of, 31
    false-positive results of, 31
    fat necrosis, 74, 75
    fibroadenoma, 73–74, 74, 82
    instrumentation for, 71–72
    nonpalpable masses
        intraoperative localization and in vitro scanning
            of, 81, 82
        preoperative localization of, 80–81, 81
    pneumocystography and, 75–76
    postprocedural hematoma, 74–75, 75
    postsurgical lymphocele, 75
    preparation of smears from, 73
    proliferative fibrocystic disease, 76
    technique for, 72–73, 72–73
    ultrasound guidance for
        accuracy of, 77–79, 79t
        vs. mammography, 71, 79–80
        vs. palpation, 71
Bronchiopleural fistula, 92

Carbuncle, renal, 201, 202
Carcinoma
    bladder, 235
    breast, 24, 75–76, 78–81
    cholangiocarcinoma, 147
    gallbladder, 155, 159, 160
    hepatocellular, 25, 32, 117–118, 118, 147
    pancreatic, 123–124, 124, 171, 173, 175, 187
    prostatic, 222–223, 223–225, 232
    renal cell, 203
    thyroid, 24, 62, 63–65
    vs. adenoma, 22
Cardazo, Paul Lopes, 25
Cardiac function analysis, intraoperative echocar-
        diography for, 112–113
Cardiac tamponade, 103–105
    echocardiographic features of, 104
    imaging technique for, 104
    physiology of, 103–104
Catheter drainage techniques, 18

Catheters
  for chorionic villus sampling, 251–252
  for drainage of abdominal abscesses, 138–139, *140*
  manufacturers of, 20
  for pleural space drainage, 90–92, *92*
  visualization of, 13, *13*
Cell blocks
  preparation of, 29
  staining and fixation of, 29
Cephalocentesis, for fetal hydrocephalus, 260
Chediak-Higashi syndrome, 255
Chiba needles, 11, *12*, 13, *15*, *16*
Cholangiocarcinoma, 147
Cholangiography
  percutaneous transhepatic, 154–155, *154–155*
  vs. intraoperative ultrasonography, 121–123, *122*,
    122t
Cholecystitis
  cholecystectomy for, 163
  diagnosis of, 162
Cholecystography, diagnostic, 159–162, *161–162*
Cholecystostomy, 163–165
  percutaneous, 164–165, *165–169*
    advantages of, 164
    catheters for, 164–165, *165*, *166*
    complications of, 165
    guidewire exchange method of, 165, *168–169*
    trocar method of, 165, *167*
  surgical, 164
  vs. cholecystectomy, 163–164
Cholelithiasis
  percutaneous treatment of, 165–167
    contact dissolution, 166–167
    mechanical stone removal, 166
  prevalence of, 159
Chorionic villus sampling, 250–254
  catheters for, 251–252
  complications of, 254
  contraindications to, 251
  history of, 250
  indications for, 250–251
  patient positioning for, 252
  sample analysis, 253–254
    biochemical studies, 253–254
    cytogenetic studies, 253
  techniques of, *251*, 251–253
  timing of, 250
  ultrasound guidance for, 252, *252–253*
  ultrasound survey prior to, 251
Chromosomal anomalies
  detection of
    amniocentesis for, 239–240
    percutaneous umbilical blood sampling for, 255
  maternal age and, 239–240, 240t
  recurrence risk of, 240
  risk factors for, 239
Chronic granulomatous disease, 255
Coagulation deficiencies, percutaneous umbilical
    blood sampling for, 255
Coagulation studies, preprocedural, 2–3
Coaxial needle technique, 6, *7*
Computed tomography
  of abdominal abscesses
    for diagnosis, *130–131*, 130–132

  to guide percutaneous drainage, *134*, 134–137,
    138, *140*
  to guide liver biopsy, 150–151
  to guide pancreatic biopsy, 172
Congenital heart disease treatments, echocardi-
    ographic guidance of, 109–110, *111*
Cope needle assembly, for pleural biopsy, 93–94, *94*
Coumadin, preoperative, 3
Cystadenocarcinoma, pancreatic, 176
Cystosarcoma phyllodes, 74
Cysts
  Baker's, 271
  breast, 73, 75–76, *76–77*
  hepatic, 119, 153–154
  intracranial, 50
  renal, 199–201
  seminal vesicle, 234–235, *235*
  spinal, 53, *54*
Cytology, 21–22
  adenoma vs. carcinoma, 22
  criteria for malignancy, 23–24, *23–26*
  DNA quantitation and morphometry, 22–23
  of fine-needle aspirate smears, 23–25
  preparation of cell blocks for, 29
  preparation of smears for, 28–29
  staining and fixation for, 29–30

Demerol. *See* Meperidine
DGBS needle, to obtain lung tissue cores, 96
Diazepam, preprocedural, 4
Dionosyl. *See* Propyliodone oil suspension
Disk herniations, 55
DNA quantitation, 22–23
  euploid, aneuploid, hyperploid lesions, 22–23
  methods of, 22–23
Duchenne muscular dystrophy, 241
Ductal epithelial hyperplasia, of breast, 76

Echocardiographic applications, 101–113
  angioplasty and thrombolysis therapy, 111
  electrophysiologic studies, 110
  expansion of, 113
  intraoperative, 111–113
    aortocoronary grafting, 111–112
    cardiac function analysis, 112–113
    structural revision and palliative procedures,
      112
    valve surgery, 112
  myocardial ablation procedures, 110–111
  myocardial biopsy, 109, *110*
  pericardiocentesis, 101–109. *See also* Pericardiocen-
    tesis
  treatments for congenital heart defects, 109–110,
    111
  valvuloplasty, 111, *112*
Embryo transfer. *See also* Follicular aspiration
  cystic aspiration before, 217, *218*
  transvaginal sonographic guidance for, 220
Empyema
  anechoic, 89
  drainage of, *91–92*, 91–93
Encephalocele, 240
Endoscopic retrograde cholangiopancreatography,

vs. percutaneous pancreatography, 188t, 188–189
Euploidy, 22
Extrahepatic bile duct, intraoperative sonography of
  for localization, 123
  technique of, 116, *116*
Extremity procedures, 267–273
  abscesses and fluid collections, 267–273. *See also*
    Abscesses
    of hip, 272
    of knee, 271–272
    of thigh, *268–270,* 268–271
    of upper extremity, 272–273, *273*
  biopsy
    of muscle, 273
    of soft tissue tumors, 273
  ultrasound guidance for, 267
    advantages of, 267
    applications of, 267

Fabry disease, 241
Fan needle technique, 6, *6*
Fentanyl, preprocedural, 3–4
Fetus. *See also* Obstetrics
  amniocentesis risks to, 249
  chorionic villus sampling risks to, 254
  determining lung maturity of, 241
  fetoscopy in, 261
  hydrocephalus in, 260
  hydronephrosis in, 206
  interventional techniques for, 259–261
  intraperitoneal blood transfusion in, 258–259
  management of obstructive uropathy in, 259–260
  percutaneous umbilical blood transfusion in, 258
  prenatal genetic diagnosis in, 239–241, 240t
  tissue sampling in, 261
Fibroadenoma, of breast, 73–74, *74, 82*
Fine-needle aspiration biopsy. *See also* Cytology;
    specific sites
  of abdominal masses, 31–32
  of benign cystic lesions, 30
  of brain, 46–48, *47–48*
  of breast masses, 30–31, 71–81
  causes of false negative aspiration, 30
  causes of sampling difficulty, 22
  of cervical lymph nodes, 64, *64–65*
  definition of, 25–26
  equipment for, 26, *28*
    preparation of, 39, *40*
    selection of, 36–38, *36–38,* 37t
  guidance systems for, 5–9
    freehand puncture, 6, *8, 47*
    indirect ultrasound guidance, 5–6, *5–7*
    needle guidance systems, 7–9, *8–10*
  guidelines for obtaining representative sample,
    21–22
  of head and neck lesions, 30, 59–61
  history of, 24–25
  of liver, 31–32, 145–146
  of masses under image guidance, 27–28
  of muscle, 273
  needles for. *See* Biopsy needles
  of palpable or superficial masses, 26–27
  of pancreatic masses, 171–179

of parathyroid
  sonographically guided, 66, *67*
  technique of, 61
portable techniques for, 26, *27*
of renal cyst, 199–201
of renal solid masses, 201–204
of retroperitoneal lesions, 32
sensitivity of, 30
of soft tissue tumors of extremities, 273
sonographer's role in, 35–41. *See also* Sonographer
technique for, 15–16, *16–18*
of thoracic masses, 31, 90–97
of thyroid
  by direct palpation, 62–63
  sonographically guided, 63–64, *63–65*
  technique of, 59–61, *60*
Fistulas
  abdominal abscesses and, 141–143
  bronchiopleural, 92
Flow cytometry, 22
Fluid collections. *See also* Abscesses; Cysts
  abdominal, 129–143. *See also* Abdominal abscesses
  hip, 272
  knee, 271–272
  perinephric, *207,* 207–208
  pleural, 85–95. *See also* Pleural space
  renal, 199–201
  upper extremity, 272–273
Fluoroscopic guidance
  for lung biopsy, 95–96
  for pancreatic biopsy, 172
  for percutaneous gastrostomy, 193–194, 196
Follicular aspiration, 213–216, *214–217*
  complications of, 215
  methods of, 213
  results of, 216t
  transvaginal technique for, 213–216
Fractures, spinal, 55, *55*
Fragile X syndrome, 241
Franseen needle, 14, *14–16*
Franzen, Sixten, 25
Freehand puncture technique, 6, *8*
  needle visualization with, 10–11

Gallbladder carcinoma, *155, 159, 160*
Gallbladder procedures, 159–167
  biopsy, 159, *160*
  diagnostic aspiration, 162–163, *163–164*
  diagnostic cholecystography, 159–162, *161–162*
  percutaneous cholecystostomy, 163–165, *165–169*
  percutaneous cholilithiasis treatments, 165–167
    mechanical stone extraction, 166
    methyltertiary-butyl ether stone dissolution,
    166–167
Gamete intrafallopian transfer, *217,* 219
Gastric cancer, *126*
Gastrinoma, intraoperative ultrasonography of, 124–
  125, *125*
Gastrostomy, percutaneous, 193–197
  alimentation after, 196
  anesthesia for, 193
  complications of, 193, 196–197
  disadvantages of, 193
  indications for, 193

role of ultrasonography in, 195–196
  guidance for needle puncture, 196
  preprocedure localization of parenchymal or-
    gans, 195–196, *197*
technique of, 193–195
  balloon distension, 194, *194*
  coiling of guidewires, 195, *196*
  instrumentation, 195, *195*
  skin puncture site, 194–195
  use of glucagon, 194
  vs. surgical gastrostomy, 193
Gliomas
  of brain, *48, 50*
  of spine, 52
Glucose 6-phosphate deficiency, 241
Greene needles, 13, *15, 16*

Hawkins catheter, 164–165, *165*
Heimlich valve, 95, *95, 96*
Hemangioma, hepatic, 146–147
Hematomas
  after breast biopsy, 74–75, *75*
  after follicular aspiration, 215
  after prostatic biopsy, 233, *234*
  after renal biopsy, 203, *203*
Hemoglobinopathies, percutaneous umbilical blood
  sampling for, 255
Hemophilia, 241, 255
Hemoptysis, due to mediastinal biopsy, 97
Hemospermia, 235
Hepatic procedures
  core biopsy, 152
  fine-needle aspiration biopsy, 31–32, 145–152
    of benign lesions, 146–147
      hemangiomas, 146–147
    complications of, 151–152
    contraindications to, 152
    CT guidance for, 150–151
    of cysts and abscesses, 145, *153*, 153–154
    of malignancies, 147
    MRI guidance for, 151
    sensitivity and specificity of, 151
    of solid lesions, 146
    ultrasound guidance for, 147–150, *148–150*
      checking adequacy of samples, 150
      indirect scanning technique for, 147
      with linear-array transducer, 149
      with needle guides, 149, *149–150*
      needles and syringes for, 150
      number of passes required for, 150
      patient preparation for, 147
      real-time scanning technique for, 147–149
  intraoperative ultrasonography, 117–121, *118–121*
    to detect cysts, 119
    to detect hepatocellular carcinoma, 117–118, *118*
    to detect intrahepatic stones, 119
    to detect metastases from colorectal cancers,
      118–119, *119*, 119t
    to differentiate benign from malignant lesions,
      120
    future applications of, 155
    to guide needle placement, 120, *120*
    role in hepatic resection, 120–121, *121*
Hepatocellular carcinoma, 25, 32, 147

daughter tumor of, 118, *118*
  intraoperative ultrasonography of, 117–118, *118*
Hepatoma, *150*
Herniated disk, 55
Hip, effusions of, 272
Hodgkin's disease, *23*
Hunter syndrome, 241
Hydrocephalus, fetal, 260
Hydronephrosis, fetal, 206
Hyperparathyroidism, 65–66
  causes of, 65
  incidence of, 65
  indications for sonographic localization in, 66
  with multiple gland involvement, 66
Hyperploidy, 22–23
Hypertensive crisis, due to biopsy of pheochromo-
  cytoma, 203–204

Image analysis, 22–23
Immune disorders, prenatal diagnosis of, 255
In utero infections, percutaneous umbilical blood
  sampling for, 255
In vitro fertilization
  cystic aspiration before, 217, *218*
  transvaginal sonographic guidance for, 219–220
Inborn errors of metabolism, 240
Indirect ultrasound guidance, 5–6, *5–7*
Interventional ultrasound
  advantages of, 1–2, 2t
  development of, 1
  disadvantages of, 2, 2t
  patient preparation for, 2–5
    anesthesia, 3
    coagulation data, 2–3
    informed consent, 2
    intravenous catheter placement, 3
    narcotic premedication, 3–4
    respiratory monitoring, 4
    tranquilizers, 4–5
  techniques for
    aspiration biopsy, 15–16, *16–18*. See also Fine-
      needle aspiration biopsy
    Biopty gun, 16–18
    catheter drainage, 18
    transducer sterilization for, 9
Islet cell tumors, 175–176, *177*
  differential diagnosis of, 176
  intraoperative ultrasonography of, 124–125, *125*
  percutaneous biopsy of, 175

Knee, effusions of, 271–272

Lee-Ray needle, 14, *14*
Lesch-Nyhan syndrome, 241
Lipoma, intradural, 53
Lobular hyperplasia, of breast, 76
Lung
  abscess of, 88
  biopsy of
    complications of, 96
    technique for, 96
  consolidation of, 87–88, *89*
  sonographic signs of diseased lung vs. pleural
    fluid, thickening, or masses, 87

sonographic vs. fluoroscopic or CT guidance in,
    95–96
squamous cell cancer of, *25*
Lymphoceles
    due to axillary node dissection, 75
    management of, 207
    perinephric, 207
Lymphoma, testicular, *208*

Madayag needles, 13, *16*
Mammography, 30
Manufacturers, 20
McGahan drainage catheter, 92, *92*, 165, *166*
Mediastinal masses
    biopsy of
        complications of, 97
        technique for, 97
    ultrasound diagnosis of, 97
Menghini needles, 13, *16*
Meningioma
    of brain, 50
    of spine, 52
Meningocele, 240
Meperidine, preprocedural, 3–4
Metastases, spinal, 53, *54*
Metastatic lesions
    of brain, 50
    of spine, 52
Methyltertiary-butyl ether, for gallstone dissolution,
    166–167
Microspectrophotometry, 22
Midazolam, preprocedural, 4
Morphine, preprocedural, 3–4
Morphometry, 22–23
Mueller empyema drainage catheter, 92, *92*
Multiple gestations, 247–248, *248*
Muscle biopsy, 273
Myelomeningocele, 240
Myocardial ablation, echocardiographic guidance
    for, 110–111
Myocardial biopsy, 109, *110*
    complications of, 109
    echocardiographic guidance of, 109
    technique of, 109

Naloxone, 4
Narcotic analgesics, preprocedural, 3–4
Neck. *See also* Parathyroid; Thyroid
    fine-needle aspiration biopsy in, 59–61, *60*
    parathyroid, 64–67
    sonographic evaluation of, 59
    thyroid, 61–64
Needles. *See* Biopsy needles
Nephroblastoma, *26*
Nephrostomy, percutaneous, 204–206, *205*
    techniques for, 205–206
    ultrasound guidance for, 204–206
Neural tube defects, 240
Neurinoma, 52
Neurosurgical sonography, intraoperative. *See also*
        Brain; Spine
    advantages of, 43–44
    applications of, 43
    of brain, 45–51

of spine, 51–56
technical considerations in, 44–45, *45–46*
    artifacts, 45
    coupling agents, 45
    craniotomy/laminectomy, 44–45
    instrument adjustments, 45
    sterile technique, 44
    transducers, 44

Obstetrics, 239–261. *See also* Embryo transfer; Follic-
        ular aspiration; specific procedures
    amniocentesis, 239–250
    chorionic villus sampling, 250–254
    fetal interventional techniques, 259–261
        decompression of fetal hydrocephalus, 260
        fetal tissue sampling, 261
        fetoscopy, 261
        management of obstructive uropathy, 259–260
    fetal intraperitoneal blood transfusion, 258–259
    percutaneous umbilical blood sampling, 255–258
    percutaneous umbilical blood transfusion, 258
Obstructive uropathy, fetal, 259–260
    assessment of renal function in, 259
    indications for therapy of, 259
    vesicoamniotic shunt placement for, 259–260
        complications of, 260
        results of, 260
Oligohydramnios, fetal, 206
Orbital lesions, 30

Pancreatic carcinoma, *173, 175, 187*
    diagnosis of, 171–172
    differentiation from pancreatitis, 171
    focal vs. diffuse, 171
    prevalence of, 171
Pancreatic procedures, 171–189
    intraoperative ultrasonography
        for cancer diagnosis and staging, 123–124, *124*
        for detection of metastases, 124
        for detection of pancreatitis complications, 123
        indications for, 123
        for islet cell tumor detection and localization,
            124–125, *125*
        for lesion localization, 123, *124*
        technique of, 116–117, *117*
        value of, 125, 125t
    percutaneous biopsy, 32, 171–179
        access route for, 172–173
        accuracy of, 171, 177
        complications of, 171, 178–179
        cytology results of, 174–176
            acinar cells, 174–175
            adenosquamous carcinoma, 175
            benign and malignant cystic tumors, 176
            ductal adenocarcinoma, 175
            ductal hyperplasia, 175
            ductal structures, 174–175
            epidermoid carcinoma, 175
            islet-cell tumors, 175–176, *177*
            mucinous adenocarcinoma, 175
            pleomorphic giant cell carcinoma, 175
            solid and papillary neoplasm, 175, *176*
        to differentiate carcinoma vs. pancreatitis, 171
        efficacy of, 177–178

failure of, 177
guidance modalities for, 172, *172–173*
  CT, 172
  fluoroscopy, 172
  ultrasound, 172, *172–173*
needles for, 174
results of, 177–178, 178t
vs. intraoperative biopsy, 171–172
wet vs. dry aspiration methods, 174
percutaneous drainage of fluid collections, 179–
  185
abscesses, 179
infected fluid collections, 184–185
in pancreatitis, 179
phlegmons, 179
pseudocysts, 179–184. *See also* Pancreatic pseudocyst
percutaneous pancreatic duct drainage, 189
percutaneous pancreatography, 171, 186–189
guidance modalities for, 186
indications for pancreatic duct opacification,
  188
requirements for, 186
results of, 187–188
technique of, 186–187, *187*
vs. endoscopic cannulation, 188t, 188–189
Pancreatic pseudocyst, 123
infected, *132*
  treatment of, 184–185
internal drainage of, 179
percutaneous treatment of, 179–184
  CT vs. ultrasound guidance for, 179, 180
  cystogastrostomy, 184
  endoscopy, 184
  external drainage, 180–181, *181–182*
  needle aspiration procedure, 180, *180*
  surgical treatments and, 185
  transgastric drainage, 181–184, *183*, 184t
recurrence of, 171
treatment of, 171
vs. acute fluid collection, 179
workup of, 179–180
Pancreatitis
due to percutaneous biopsy, 178
fluid collections in, 179
vs. carcinoma, 171
Papanicolaou, George, 21, 24
Papillomatosis, of breast, 76
Parathyroid
anatomy of, 64–65
fine-needle aspiration biopsy of
  sonographically guided, 66, *67*
  technique of, 61
primary hyperparathyroidism, 65–66
sonographic localization of, 66
therapeutic ablation of, 66–67, *68*
Partial thromboplastin time, 2–3
Pelvic procedures
obstetrics, 239–261
transrectally guided, 221–236
transvaginally guided, 211–220
PercuCut needle, 14, 15
to obtain lung tissue cores, 96
Pericardiocentesis, 101–109

complications of, 109
for detection of cardiac tamponade, 103–105
  criteria for evaluation, 104–105
  echocardiographic features, 104
  physiology, 103–104
for detection of pericardial effusion and clot, 101–
  103
  one- vs. two-dimensional imaging techniques,
    101
  pericardial anatomy, 101
  pericardial vs. pleural effusion, 103, *104*
  ultrasound imaging techniques, *102*, 102–103
guided by echocardiography, 105–109
  equipment for, 105
  information needed prior to procedure, 105
  needles and catheters for, 105–106, *107*
  postprocedural evaluation, 108–109
  technique of, 105–107, *106–108*
Perinephric fluid collections, *207*, 207–208
Pheochromocytoma
diagnosis of, 203, *204*
inadvertent biopsy of, 203
hypertensive crisis due to, 203–204
Phlegmon, vs. abscess, 130, 179
Physostigmine, 4
Platelets, preprocedural measurement of, 3
Pleural space, 85–95
anechoic empyema, 89
biopsy technique, 93–94, *93–94*
catheter drainage of empyema, *91–92*, 91–93
  catheters for, 91–92, *92*
  patient care after, 92–93
  portable ultrasound procedure for, 91, *91*
  technique of, 91–92
  vs. thoracostomy tube drainage, 91
complications of interventions in, 94–95
  pneumothorax, 95
  use of Heimlich valve, 95, *95*
diagnostic thoracentesis, 90
normal sonographic appearance of, 85–87, *86–87*
  dirty air shadow, 85
  linear array vs. sector scanner, 85, *86*
  liver mirror image artifact, 87, *87*
pleural thickening, 88–89, *90*
sclerotherapy to prevent recurrent effusions, 93
septations across, 88, *89*
sonographic signs of lung consolidation, 87–88,
  89
sonographic signs of pleural fluid, 87, *88*
therapeutic drainage of effusions, 90–91
viscous pleural fluid, 89
Pneumoconiosis, 31
Pneumocystography, of breast masses, 75–76
Pneumothorax
due to lung biopsy, 96
due to mediastinal biopsy, 97
due to percutaneous thoracic procedures, 95
Heimlich valve system for, 95, *95*, 96
Pregnancy. *See also* Obstetrics
biopsy of breast masses in, 71, 80, *80*
ruptured ectopic, 218–219
Prenatal diagnosis
amniocentesis for, 239–241, 240t
chorionic villus sampling for, 250–254

percutaneous umbilical blood sampling for, 255–258

Propyliodone oil suspension, to detect bronchio-pleural fistula, 92

Prostate
abscess of, 234, *234*
carcinoma of
atypical hyperplasia preceding, 233, *233*
cytological and Gleason grading of, 225
predictive value of ultrasound for, 223–224
screening for, 223
sonographic appearance of, 222–223, *223–225*
complications of biopsy of, 233, 234
conventional techniques for biopsy of, 224–225
normal anatomy of, 221–222, *223*
percutaneous cryotherapy of, 234
percutaneous iodine–125 seed placement in, 234
transrectal sonography of, 221, *222*
ultrasound-guided biopsy of, 225–233
equipment for, 225–226, *226–228*
patient preparation for, 226–227
results of, 232–233, 233t
specimen for, 231, *232*
transperineal technique for, 228–229, *229*
transrectal technique for, 229–231, *230–231*
Prostate specific antigen, 223–224
Prothrombin time, 2
Pulmonary lesions, aspiration biopsy of, 31

Rectal masses, 235–236, *236*
Reed-Sternberg cells, *23*
Renal artery aneurysm, 199, *200*
Renal cell carcinoma, *203*
Renal procedures, 32, 199–206
core biopsy, 204, *204*
complications of, 204
necessity for, 204
technique of, 204
cystic masses, 199–201
aspiration of
contraindications to, 199
indications for, 199
purpose of, 199
technique for, *200*, 200–201
drainage of, 201, *202*
sclerotherapy for, 201
sonographic criteria for cyst, 199
fetal hydronephrosis, 206
percutaneous nephrostomy, 204–206, *205*
techniques for, 205–206
ultrasound guidance for, 204–206
solid masses, 201–204
purposes of aspiration biopsy of, 201
technique of aspiration biopsy of, 201–204, *202–204*
vs. pseudotumors, 201
Restriction fragment-length polymorphism technique, 241
Retroperitoneal fluid collections, 207–208
Rh isoimmunization, 241–242
amniocentesis for, 241–242
fetal blood transfusion for, 242
intraperitoneal, 258–259
percutaneous umbilical, 258

percutaneous umbilical blood sampling for, 255
ultrasound features associated with, 242
Rotex needle, 11, *12*, 14, *15*
for lung biopsy, 96

Sacks drainage catheter, 91–92, *92*
Sclerosing adenosis, of breast, 76
Sclerotherapy
for perinephric lymphoceles, 207
pleural, 93
for renal cysts, 201
Scrotal masses, 209, *209*
Seminal vesicles, 234–235
cyst of, 234–235, *235*
primary neoplasms of, 235
Shunt placement, 48, *49*, *51*
Sickle cell anemia, percutaneous umbilical blood sampling for, 255
Sinography, abscess, 139–141
Smears
preparation of, 28–29
staining and fixation of, 29–30
Soderstrom, Nils, 25
Solid and papillary neoplasm of pancreas, 175, *176*
Sonographer, 35–41
intraprocedural role of, 41
patient preparation by, 39–41
explanations, 39–40
positioning, 40
postprocedural role of, 41
cleaning room and equipment, 41
record keeping, 41
procedural planning by, 35–39
checking equipment, 41
collecting patient data, 38
communicating with team members, 35, 38
determining location, 38
preparing equipment, 39, *40*
selecting equipment, 36–38, *36–38*, 37t
understanding procedure, 35
training of, 35
Spinal needle, *16*
Spine, 51–56
advantages of sonography for masses of, 52–53
decompression of, 52
dysraphism of, 56, 240
extradural lesions of, 54
extramedullary lesions of, 53–54
fractures of, 55, *55*
herniated disks of, 55
intramedullary lesions of, 53, *54*
normal anatomy of, 51–52, *52–53*
sonographic applications in, 55–56
tethered cord syndrome, 56
Surecut needle, 15, *16*
to obtain lung tissue cores, 96

Tandem needle technique, 6, *6*
Testicular masses, 209, *209*
abscess, 209, *209*
identification of, 209
lymphoma, *208*
Tethered cord syndrome, 56
Thigh abscesses, *268–270*, 268–271

aspiration and drainage of, 269–271
  complications of, 271
  follow-up care after, 271
  results of, 271
  location of, 268
  sonographic appearance of, 268
  vs. aneurysms, 268–269
  vs. inguinal hernia, 269
  vs. synovial cyst, 269
Thoracentesis, diagnostic, 90
Thoracic procedures, 31, 85–97
  in lung parenchyma, 95–96
    biopsy complications, 96
    biopsy technique, 96
    sonographic vs. fluoroscopic or CT guidance,
      95–96
  in mediastinum, 97
    biopsy complications, 97
    biopsy technique, 97
    ultrasound diagnosis, 97
  in pleural space, 85–95
    anechoic empyema, 89
    catheter drainage of empyema, 91–92, 91–93
    complications, 94–95
    diagnostic thoracentesis, 90
    normal sonographic appearance, 85–87, 86–87
    pleural biopsy, 93–94, 93–94
    pleural fluid and lung consolidation, 87–88, 88–
      89
    pleural sclerotherapy, 93
    pleural space septations, 88, 89
    pleural thickening, 88–89, 90
    therapeutic drainage of effusions, 90–91
    viscous pleural fluid, 89
Thrombocytopenia, percutaneous umbilical blood
      sampling for, 255
Thrombolysis therapy, echocardiographic guidance
      for, 111
Thyroid
  anatomy of, 61, 61–62
  aspiration biopsy of
    by direct palpation, 62–63
    sonographically guided, 63–64, 63–65
    technique of, 59–61, 60
  carcinoma of, 24, 62, 63–65
  nodules of, 62, 63
Tranquilizers, preoperative, 4–5
Transhepatic cholangiography, percutaneous, 154–
      155, 154–155
Transrectally guided procedures, 221–236. See also
      Prostate
  aspiration and biopsy of seminal vesicle masses,
      234–235
  evaluation of rectal masses, 235–236
  other prostate procedures, 234
  prostate biopsy, 224–233
  prostate imaging, 221–224
Transvaginally guided procedures, 211–220
  aspiration of fluid in ruptured ectopic pregnancy,
      218–219
  aspiration of pelvic cystic masses, 217, 218–219
  catheter placement for gamete intrafallopian
      transfer, 217, 219
  catheter placement for tubo-ovarian abscess, 219

cystic aspiration in embryo transfer patients, 217,
      218
  embryo transfer, 220
  follicular aspiration, 213–216, 214–217
    complications of, 215
    methods of, 213
    results of, 216t
    transvaginal approach for, 213–216
  instrumentation for, 211, 212
  suspected pelvic abscesses, 218, 220
  technique of, 211–213, 212
  theoretic complications of, 217–218
Trisomy 21, 239–240
Tru-Cut needle, 14
  to obtain lung tissue cores, 96
  for prostate biopsy, 225, 226, 228
Turner needles, 13, 16

Umbilical blood sampling, percutaneous, 255–258
  complications of, 257–258
  history of, 255
  indications for, 255
    chromosomal analysis, 255
    coagulation deficiencies, 255
    hemoglobinopathies, 255
    immune disorders, 255
    iso- or autoimmune thrombocytopenia, 255
    Rh isoimmunization, 255
    in utero infection, 255
  outpatient, 257
  sampling time for, 257
  site for, 257
  technique of, 256–257
    intracardiac, 256
    intrafunicular, 256–257, 256–257
    sample, 256–257, 256–257
  ultrasound survey prior to, 256
Umbilical blood transfusion, percutaneous, 258
Urinary tract procedures. See also Renal procedures
  aspiration of renal cystic masses, 199–201
  aspiration of renal solid masses, 201–204
  drainage of perinephric fluid collections, 207–208
  localization and treatment of scrotal masses, 209
  percutaneous nephrostomy, 204–206
  renal core biopsy, 204
  treatment of fetal hydronephrosis, 206
Urinoma, perirenal, 207

Valium. See Diazepam
Valve surgery, echocardiographic guidance for, 111,
      112, 112
Versed. See Midazolam

Wescott needle, 14
Wilms' tumor, 26
Wiscott-Aldrich syndrome, 255

X-linked anomalies, 241

Zajicek, Josef, 25